T0362300

# Observation Medicine

*Editors*

CHRISTOPHER W. BAUGH
R. GENTRY WILKERSON

# EMERGENCY MEDICINE CLINICS OF NORTH AMERICA

www.emed.theclinics.com

*Consulting Editor*
AMAL MATTU

August 2017 • Volume 35 • Number 3

**ELSEVIER**

1600 John F. Kennedy Boulevard • Suite 1800 • Philadelphia, Pennsylvania, 19103-2899

http://www.theclinics.com

**EMERGENCY MEDICINE CLINICS OF NORTH AMERICA Volume 35, Number 3**
**August 2017 ISSN 0733-8627, ISBN-13: 978-0-323-53227-3**

Editor: Katie Pfaff

Developmental Editor: Casey Potter

*Emergency Medicine Clinics of North America* (ISSN 0733-8627) is published quarterly by Elsevier Inc., 360 Park Avenue South, New York, NY, 10010-1710. Months of issue are February, May, August, and November. Business and Editorial Offices: 1600 John F. Kennedy Boulevard, Suite 1800, Philadelphia, PA 19103-2899. Customer Service Office: 6277 Sea Harbor Drive, Orlando, FL 32887-4800. Periodicals postage paid at New York, NY, and additional mailing offices. Subscription prices are $100.00 per year (US students), $323.00 per year (US individuals), $608.00 per year (US institutions), $220.00 per year (international students), $455.00 per year (international individuals), $747.00 per year (international institutions), $220.00 per year (Canadian students), $389.00 per year (Canadian individuals), and $747.00 per year (Canadian institutions). International air speed delivery is included in all *Clinics'* subscription prices. All prices are subject to change without notice. **POSTMASTER:** Send address changes to *Emergency Medicine Clinics of North America*, Elsevier Periodicals Customer Service, 11830 Westline Industrial Drive, St. Louis, MO 63146. Customer Service (orders, claims, online, change of address): Elsevier Periodicals **Customer Service, 11830 Westline Industrial Drive, St. Louis, MO 63146. Tel: 1-800-654-2452 (U.S. and Canada); 314-453-7041 (outside U.S. and Canada). Fax: 314-453-5170. E-mail: journalscustomerservice-usa@elsevier.com (for print support); journalsonlinesupport-usa@elsevier.com (for online support)**.

*Reprints.* For copies of 100 or more of articles in this publication, please contact the Commercial Reprints Department, Elsevier Inc., 360 Park Avenue South, New York, NY 10010-1710. Tel.: 212-633-3874; Fax: 212-633-3820; E-mail: reprints@elsevier.com.

*Emergency Medicine Clinics of North America* is covered in *MEDLINE/PubMed (Index Medicus), Current Contents/Clinical Medicine, EMBASE/Excerpta Medica, BIOSIS, SciSearch, CINAHL, ISI/BIOMED,* and *Research Alert.*

# Contributors

## CONSULTING EDITOR

**AMAL MATTU, MD, FAAEM, FACEP**
Professor and Vice Chair of Education, Department of Emergency Medicine, University of Maryland School of Medicine, Baltimore, Maryland

## EDITORS

**CHRISTOPHER W. BAUGH, MD, MBA, FACEP**
Assistant Professor, Department of Emergency Medicine, Brigham and Women's Hospital, Harvard Medical School, Boston, Massachusetts

**R. GENTRY WILKERSON, MD, FACEP**
Assistant Professor, Department of Emergency Medicine, University of Maryland School of Medicine, Baltimore, Maryland

## AUTHORS

**TARUNA K. AURORA, MD**
Director, Clinical Decision Unit, Department of Emergency Medicine, Virginia Commonwealth University Health System, Richmond, Virginia

**CHRISTOPHER W. BAUGH, MD, MBA, FACEP**
Assistant Professor, Department of Emergency Medicine, Brigham and Women's Hospital, Harvard Medical School, Boston, Massachusetts

**J. STEPHEN BOHAN, MD, MS**
Department of Emergency Medicine, Brigham and Women's Hospital, Harvard Medical School, Boston, Massachusetts

**JOSEPH B. BORAWSKI, MD, MPH**
Division of Emergency Medicine, Duke University Medical Center, Durham, North Carolina

**CHRISTOPHER G. CASPERS, MD**
Chief, Observation Medicine, New York University Langone Health System, Assistant Professor, New York University School of Medicine, New York, New York

**JARED CONLEY, MD, PhD, MPH**
Department of Emergency Medicine, Massachusetts General Hospital, Harvard Medical School, Department of Emergency Medicine, Brigham and Women's Hospital, Harvard Medical School, Boston, Massachusetts

**KATHLEEN T.P. DAVENPORT, MD**
Department of Emergency Medicine, Brigham and Women's Hospital, Harvard Medical School, Boston, Massachusetts

**JEREMIAH D. GADDY, MD**
Department of Emergency Medicine, Wake Forest School of Medicine, Winston-Salem, North Carolina

**LOUIS G. GRAFF, MD**
Department of Emergency Medicine, The Hospital of Central Connecticut, New Britain, Connecticut

**MICHAEL GRANOVSKY, MD, CPC, FACEP**
Adjunct Professor, Department of Emergency Medicine, George Washington University, President, LogixHealth, Bedford, Massachusetts

**JASON J. HAM, MD**
Assistant Professor, Departments of Emergency Medicine and Internal Medicine, University of Michigan Medical School, Ann Arbor, Michigan

**MICHAEL N. HELMREICH, MD**
Department of Emergency Medicine, St. John Hospital and Medical Center, Detroit, Michigan

**BRIAN C. HIESTAND, MD, MPH**
Department of Emergency Medicine, Wake Forest School of Medicine, Winston-Salem, North Carolina

**VIVIANE M. KAZAN, MD**
Department of Emergency Medicine, St. John Hospital and Medical Center, Department of Emergency Medicine, Wayne State University School of Medicine, Detroit, Michigan

**ALEXANDER T. LIMKAKENG, MD, MHS**
Division of Emergency Medicine, Duke University Medical Center, Durham, North Carolina

**SHARON E. MACE, MD, FACEP, FAAP**
Professor of Medicine, Emergency Services Institute, Cleveland Clinic, Department of Emergency Medicine, Cleveland Clinic Lerner College of Medicine, Case Western Reserve University, Cleveland, Ohio

**EDGAR ORDONEZ, MD, MPH, FAAEM, FACEP, FACP**
Director, Clinical Decision Unit, Ben Taub Emergency Center, Assistant Professor, Department of Emergency Medicine, Baylor College of Medicine, Houston, Texas

**ANWAR DAYAN OSBORNE, MD, MPM, FACEP**
Assistant Professor, Department of Emergency Medicine/Internal Medicine, Emory University School of Medicine, Emory University Hospital, Atlanta, Georgia

**MARGARITA E. PENA, MD**
Department of Emergency Medicine, St. John Hospital and Medical Center, Associate Professor, Department of Emergency Medicine, Wayne State University School of Medicine, Detroit, Michigan

**MICHAEL A. ROSS, MD, FACEP, FACC**
Chief of Service, Observation Medicine, Professor, Department of Emergency Medicine, Emory University School of Medicine, Emory University Hospital, Atlanta, Georgia

**PAWAN SURI, MD**
Chief, Division of Observation Medicine, Department of Emergency Medicine, Virginia Commonwealth University Health System, Richmond, Virginia

**MATTHEW A. WHEATLEY, MD, FACEP**
Assistant Professor, Department of Emergency Medicine, Emory University School of Medicine, Emory University Hospital, Atlanta, Georgia

**R. GENTRY WILKERSON, MD, FACEP**
Assistant Professor, Department of Emergency Medicine, University of Maryland School of Medicine, Baltimore, Maryland

# Contents

The history of observation medicine has paralleled the rise of emergency medicine over the past 50 years to meet the needs of patients, emergency departments, hospitals, and the US health care system. Just as emergency departments are the safety net of the health system, observation units are the safety net of emergency departments. The growth of observation medicine has been driven by innovations in health care, an ongoing shift of patients from inpatient to outpatient settings, and changes in health policy. These units have been shown to provide better outcomes than traditional care for selected patients.

The current health care landscape and evidence support the establishment of observation units (OUs) for safe and efficient care for observation patients. Careful attention is required in the design of OU process, location, and layout to enable optimal care and finances. Developing and maintaining protocols to guide patient selection and clinical care are critical. OU management requires a strong, collaborative leadership model, appropriate staffing, and a robust monitoring system for quality, safety, and finances. With a better understanding of these principles of OU establishment and management, hospital leaders can generate and sustain service excellence.

Care of the patient presenting to an emergency department (ED) with chest pain remains a common yet challenging aspect of emergency medicine. Acute coronary syndrome presents in nonspecific fashion. The development and evolution of the ED-based observation unit has helped to safely assess and diagnose those most at risk for an adverse cardiac event. Furthermore, there are several provocative testing modalities to help assess for coronary artery disease. This article serves to describe and discuss the modern ED-based observation unit approach to patients with chest pain and/or angina equivalents presenting to an ED.

The first emergency department observation units (EDOUs) focused on chest pain and potential acute coronary syndromes. However, most EDOUs now cover multiple other conditions that lend themselves to protocolized, aggressive diagnostic and therapeutic regimens. In this article, the authors discuss the management of 4 cardiovascular conditions that have been successfully deployed in EDOUs around the country.

The Emergency Department Observation Unit (EDOU) provides a viable alternative to inpatient admission for the management of many acute gastrointestinal conditions with additional opportunities of reducing resource utilization and reducing radiation exposure. Using available evidence-based criteria to determine appropriate patient selection, evaluation, and treatment provides higher-quality medical care and improved patient satisfaction. Discussions of factors involved in creating an EDOU capable of caring for acute gastrointestinal conditions and clinical protocol examples of acute appendicitis, gastrointestinal hemorrhage, and acute pancreatitis provide a framework from which a successful EDOU can be built.

Accelerated therapeutic protocols targeting metabolic conditions are ideal for observation unit care. Because many conditions, such as hypokalemia and hyperglycemia, have little to no diagnostic uncertainty, the care in the unit is often straightforward. Additionally, some components of care for the endocrine condition may exhaust services, such as phlebotomy. Hence, this discussion focuses resource utilization and management considerations for the purposes of matching the level of care to the severity of the conditions. When carefully selected candidates are cared for in the observation unit, hospital resources can enable a safe, efficient hospital stay.

As a group, neurologic conditions represent a substantial portion of emergency department (ED) visits. Cerebrovascular disease, headache, vertigo and seizures are all common reasons for patients to seek care in the ED. Patients being treated for each of these conditions are amenable to care in an ED observation unit (EDOU) if they require further diagnostic or therapeutic interventions beyond their ED stay. EDOUs are the ideal setting for patients who require advanced imaging such as MRIs, frequent neuro checks or specialist consultation in order to determine if they require admission or can be discharged home.

In adults, respiratory disorders are the second most frequent diagnoses treated in emergency department observation units (EDOUs) and account for the most frequent indication for placement of pediatric patients into an EDOU. With appropriate patient selection, chronic obstructive pulmonary disease exacerbations, and community-acquired pneumonia can be managed in the EDOU. EDOU management results in equivalent or better outcomes than inpatient care with decreased length of stay, increased patient satisfaction, lower cost and in some studies decreased mortality. Evidence-based protocols are important to ensure appropriate patients are placed in the EDOU, standardize best practice interventions, and guide disposition decisions.

Infectious conditions such as skin and soft tissue infections (SSTIs), Urogenital infections and peritonsillar abscesses frequently require care beyond emergency stabilization and are well-suited for short term care in an observation unit. SSTIs are a growing problem, partly due to emergence of strains of methicillin-resistant S. aureus (MRSA). Antibiotic choice is guided by the presence of purulence and site of infection. Purulent cellulitis is much more likely to be associated with MRSA. Radiographic imaging should be considered to aid in management in patients who are immunosuppressed, have persistent symptoms despite antibiotic therapy, recurrent infections, sepsis or diabetes.

Patients presenting to the emergency department with certain traumatic conditions can be managed in observation units. The evidence base supporting the use of observation units to manage injured patients is smaller than the evidence base supporting the management of medical conditions in observation units. The conditions that are eligible for management in an observation unit are not limited to those described in this article, and investigators should continue to identify types of conditions that may benefit from this type of health care delivery.

Infants and children and the elderly comprise a large and growing (especially the elderly) segment of the US population. The benefits of observation medicine have been documented in these two age groups: Based on the success of observation medicine, and recognizing the growth of these special populations, it is likely that observation medicine will be expanding in the future, especially within the pediatric and geriatric populations. Future studies should be able to provide further evidence regarding the value of observation medicine in these two diverse population age groups.

Matthew A. Wheatley

ED observation units (EDOUs) are designed for patients who require diagnostics or therapeutics beyond the initial ED visit to determine the need for hospital admission. Best evidence is that this care be delivered via order-sets or protocols. Occasionally, patients present with conditions that are amenable to EDOU care but fall outside the commonly used protocols. This article details a few of these conditions: abnormal uterine bleeding, allergic reaction, alcohol intoxication, acetaminophen overdose and sickle cell vaso-occlusive crisis. It is not meant to be exhaustive as patient care needs can vary hospital to hospital.

# EMERGENCY MEDICINE
# CLINICS OF NORTH AMERICA

---

**RELATED INTEREST**

*Critical Care Nursing Clinics of North America,* June 2017 (Vol. 29, Issue 2)
**Pediatric Critical Care**
Jerithea Tidwell and Brennan Lewis, *Editors*

---

**THE CLINICS ARE NOW AVAILABLE ONLINE!**
Access your subscription at:
**www.theclinics.com**

## PROGRAM OBJECTIVE

The goal of *Emergency Medicine Clinics of North America* is to keep practicing emergency medicine physicians and emergency medicine residents up to date with current clinical practice in emergency medicine by providing timely articles reviewing the state of the art in patient care.

## LEARNING OBJECTIVES

Upon completion of this activity, participants will be able to:
1. Review the history and development of observational medicine.
2. Recognize principles of care for acute conditions in the observation unit.
3. Discuss care of special populations in the observation room.

## ACCREDITATION

The Elsevier Office of Continuing Medical Education (EOCME) is accredited by the Accreditation Council for Continuing Medical Education (ACCME) to provide continuing medical education for physicians.

The EOCME designates this enduring material for a maximum of 15 *AMA PRA Category 1 Credit*(s)™. Physicians should claim only the credit commensurate with the extent of their participation in the activity.

All other healthcare professionals requesting continuing education credit for this enduring material will be issued a certificate of participation.

## DISCLOSURE OF CONFLICTS OF INTEREST

The EOCME assesses conflict of interest with its instructors, faculty, planners, and other individuals who are in a position to control the content of CME activities. All relevant conflicts of interest that are identified are thoroughly vetted by EOCME for fair balance, scientific objectivity, and patient care recommendations. EOCME is committed to providing its learners with CME activities that promote improvements or quality in healthcare and not a specific proprietary business or a commercial interest.

**The planning committee, staff, authors and editors listed below have identified no financial relationships or relationships to products or devices they or their spouse/life partner have with commercial interest related to the content of this CME activity:**

Taruna Auroa, MD; Christopher W. Baugh, MD, MBA, FACEP; J. Stephen Bohan, MD, MS; Joseph Borawski, MD, MPH; Christopher G. Caspers, MD; Jared Conley, MD, PhD, MPH; Kathleen T.P. Davenport, MD; Anjali Fortna; Jeremiah D. Gaddy, MD; Louis G. Graff, MD; Michael Granovsky, MD, CPC, FACEP; Jason J. Ham, MD; Michael N. Helmreich, MD; Viviane M. Kazan, MD; Alexander T. Limkakeng, MD, MHS; Amal Mattu, MD, FAAEM, FACEP; Edgar Ordonez, MD, MPH, FAAEM, FACEP, FACP; Anwar Dayan Osborne, MD, MPM, FACEP; Margarita E. Pena, MD; Katie Pfaff; Michael A. Ross, MD, FACEP, FACC; Pawan Suri, MD; Vignesh Viswanathan; Matthew A. Wheatley, MD, FACEP; Katie Widmeier; R. Gentry Wilkerson, MD, FACEP.

**The planning committee, staff, authors and editors listed below have identified financial relationships or relationships to products or devices they or their spouse/life partner have with commercial interest related to the content of this CME activity:**
**Brian C. Hiestand, MD, MPH** is a consultant/advisor Novartis AG and AstraZeneca.
**Sharon E. Mace, MD, FACEP, FAAP** has research support from Janssen Global Services, LLC; F. Hoffmann-La Roche Ltd; and Hospital Quality Foundation, has an employment affiliation with Cleveland Clinic, and receives royalties/patents from McGraw-Hill Education and Cambridge University Press.

## UNAPPROVED/OFF-LABEL USE DISCLOSURE

The EOCME requires CME faculty to disclose to the participants:
1. When products or procedures being discussed are off-label, unlabelled, experimental, and/or investigational (not US Food and Drug Administration [FDA] approved); and
2. Any limitations on the information presented, such as data that are preliminary or that represent ongoing research, interim analyses, and/or unsupported opinions. Faculty may discuss information about pharmaceutical agents that is outside of FDA-approved labelling. This information is intended solely for CME and is not intended to promote off-label use of these medications. If you have any questions, contact the medical affairs department of the manufacturer for the most recent prescribing information.

## TO ENROLL

To enroll in the *Emergency Medicine Clinics* Continuing Medical Education program, call customer service at 1-800-654-2452 or sign up online at http://www.theclinics.com/home/cme. The CME program is available to subscribers for an additional annual fee of $235 USD.

## METHOD OF PARTICIPATION

In order to claim credit, participants must complete the following:

1. Complete enrolment as indicated above.
2. Read the activity.
3. Complete the CME Test and Evaluation. Participants must achieve a score of 70% on the test. All CME Tests and Evaluations must be completed online.

## CME INQUIRIES/SPECIAL NEEDS

For all CME inquiries or special needs, please contact elsevierCME@elsevier.com.

# Foreword

# Observation Medicine

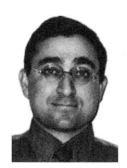

Amal Mattu, MD, FAAEM, FACEP
*Consulting Editor*

In the immortal words of Bob Dylan, "The times they are a-changin'." I recall a time earlier in my career when we were encouraged by hospital administrators and in-patient services to increase admissions, "when appropriate" of course. There were subtle financial incentives to inpatient services for admission, and patients seemed to expect that when they were sick they would be admitted to the hospital for others to care for them.

In recent years, however, there has been a change in emphasis to increase discharges from the Emergency Department (ED) whenever possible. Financial incentives have pushed more toward outpatient evaluations for initial visits, and monetary penalties are imposed for readmissions of certain conditions within a short time from their recent discharge. It seems that there has also been a cultural shift among patients, who more frequently want to avoid admission as well.

Unfortunately, many acute medical conditions are not quite so amenable to making simple choices of admit versus discharge. Many dispositions fall into the gray area whereby we as clinicians do not feel strongly about a prolonged admission, but we may not feel comfortable with immediate discharge from the ED either. To address this issue, Observation Medicine has emerged as a new area of medicine to address these difficult dispositions. Observation Medicine focuses on caring for the patient during the first 12 to 24 hours prior to discharge. Experts in this field have also developed innovative protocols to initiate care for patients that have traditionally been admitted, but now allow for discharge. For example, patients with low-risk chest pain, new onset atrial fibrillation, or transient ischemic attack can now get expedited workups and care over the course of a short observation stay, and then they can be discharged for further outpatient care. Not only is this care more efficient, but it is also associated with lower health care costs and increased patient satisfaction.

Emerg Med Clin N Am 35 (2017) xv–xvi
http://dx.doi.org/10.1016/j.emc.2017.05.002
0733-8627/17/© 2017 Published by Elsevier Inc.

emed.theclinics.com

In this issue of *Emergency Medicine Clinics of North America*, Guest Editors Drs Christopher Baugh and Gentry Wilkerson have assembled a group of experienced and expert physicians in Observation Medicine to discuss this growing and exciting field. Initial articles focus on the history and principles of Observation Medicine as well as how to set up an Observation Unit. Specific medical conditions are then addressed, including cardiovascular, neurologic, infectious, and other areas. An article addresses how to use Observation Medicine to help in caring for extremes of age, and a final article discusses additional conditions amendable to Observation Medicine.

The Guest Editors and authors are to be commended for their innovative and hard work. This issue of *Emergency Medicine Clinics of North America* represents an invaluable addition to the emergency medicine literature and can serve as a definitive resource to all those that are looking to find more cost-effective and safe ways of managing a potpourri of medical conditions in the ED. I anticipate that within our own ED we will be directly adopting many of the protocols from this text. I hope that all of our readers will take this opportunity to present the ideas contained within to their own administrators and medical directors and work toward creating observation protocols in their EDs. This issue will help in laying the groundwork for future care in the ED.

Amal Mattu, MD, FAAEM, FACEP
Department of Emergency Medicine
University of Maryland School of Medicine
110 South Paca Street
6th Floor, Suite 200
Baltimore, MD 21201, USA

*E-mail address:*
amalmattu@comcast.net

# Preface

# Observation Medicine: Providing Safe and Cost-Effective Care Beyond the Emergency Department

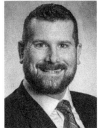
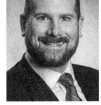

Christopher W. Baugh, MD, MBA, FACEP   R. Gentry Wilkerson, MD, FACEP
*Editors*

Observation units fill a ubiquitous need by providing a setting of care for patients not clearly requiring an inpatient admission to receive additional diagnostic workup or therapeutic intervention beyond the scope of a typical Emergency Department visit. Care for the patient with chest pain in whom the initial evaluation did not reveal a diagnosis and sufficient concern remained for myocardial infarction or ischemia was one of the earliest examples of observation care and remains the most common complaint encountered there today. More than three decades ago, chest pain units emerged to provide the right setting to continue care for these patients, reducing both avoidable admissions and inappropriate discharges. Since that time, the conditions routinely managed during an observation stay have multiplied, and continue to evolve as progressive clinicians search for novel conditions amenable to care in the observation setting. Patients with conditions previously cared for routinely in an inpatient setting now rarely need this level of care. Inpatient admission for hyperemesis gravidarum, migraine, asthma, transient ischemic attack, syncope, and many other similar conditions is becoming increasingly rare. Providers working with access to an observation unit can hardly imagine practicing without one.

This shift in care to observation units resulted from many trends, including payer policy changes, advances in diagnostics and treatments, improved understanding of pathophysiology, Emergency Department and inpatient crowding, and the pioneering work of early adopters, thought leaders, and mentors who have created and disseminated best practices for safe and efficient observation care. We are grateful for these individuals, many of whom have contributed to this special issue of *Emergency*

**emed.theclinics.com**

*Medicine Clinics of North America*. They have led the way to demonstrate that an observation stay can reduce hospital length of stay and thus cost, while also improving patient satisfaction and protocol compliance without compromising quality and safety.

Observation care is more relevant today than ever before. Looking forward, we expect the use of observation care to continue to expand. In order to create value, this care needs to be delivered by providers who embrace the best practices of a dedicated unit and condition-specific protocols to guide patient care. Many questions remain about how to optimize care, and as our tools and understanding change over time, new opportunities will emerge for further investigation into how to provide optimal care. For example, the introduction of highly sensitive troponin assays in the United States will fundamentally change the Emergency Department evaluation of patients presenting with chest pain and the role that observation care plays in this population.

In addition, as new conditions are explored for observation care, they need to be studied to establish criteria for patient selection, evidence-based interventions, and specific criteria for safe discharge. Such deliberate plans will enable further shifts of eligible patients out of inpatient beds, avoiding unnecessary admissions while still providing patient-centered care. Payer policy will surely continue to evolve, incentivizing lower costs while still demanding high-quality outcomes. In such an environment, a well-run observation unit shines as a valuable asset for hospitals with sufficient Emergency Department visit volume to operate one.

We hope you find this compilation a comprehensive representation of the most current and enlightened thinking on the topic of observation medicine. We have organized this issue to give a general understanding of observation medicine and observation units followed by a series of articles that focus on specific diagnoses and organ systems. We want to inspire readers to establish or improve observation units in their own hospitals and intend this issue to serve as a valuable resource for that purpose.

Christopher W. Baugh, MD, MBA, FACEP
Department of Emergency Medicine
Brigham & Women's Hospital
75 Francis Street
Neville House 2nd Floor
Boston, MA 02115, USA

R. Gentry Wilkerson, MD, FACEP
Department of Emergency Medicine
University of Maryland School of Medicine
110 South Paca Street
6th Floor, Suite 200
Baltimore, MD 21201, USA

*E-mail addresses:*
cbaugh@bwh.harvard.edu (C.W. Baugh)
gwilkerson@em.umaryland.edu (R.G. Wilkerson)

# History, Principles, and Policies of Observation Medicine

Michael A. Ross, MD[a],*, Michael Granovsky, MD, CPC[b,c]

## KEYWORDS

- Emergency medicine • Observation medicine • Observation units • Health policy

## KEY POINTS

- The history of observation medicine parallels the rise of emergency medicine over the past 50 years to meet the needs of patients, emergency departments (EDs), hospitals, and the US health care system.
- Type 1 protocol-driven observation units are best managed using 7 basic principles. These units have consistently been shown to provide better outcomes than traditional care for selected patients.
- The growth of observation medicine has been driven by innovations in health care, ongoing shift of patients from inpatient to outpatient settings, and changes in health policy.
- To fully understand observation medicine, it is important to understand observation services payment policy, history, and ramifications.

---

*Leave nothing to chance, overlook nothing: combine contradictory observations and allow enough time…A great part, I believe, of the art is to be able to observe.*
—*Hippocrates 410 BC*

## A BRIEF CLINICAL HISTORY OF OBSERVATION MEDICINE

The act of observing patients is not unique to the present. Observation has been fundamental to the care of patients since the time of Hippocrates, when he argued that understanding the nature of the humans and disease processes was best achieved through the active observation of their condition. This new approach,

---

Disclosure Statement: Dr M.A. Ross has no disclosure of any relationship with a commercial company that has a direct financial interest in subject matter or materials discussed in article or with a company making a competing product. Dr M. Granovsky is president of a company that does coding and billing for emergency physicians but has no other disclosures.

[a] Observation Medicine, Department of Emergency Medicine, Emory University School of Medicine, 531 Asbury Circle - Annex, Suite N340, Atlanta, GA 30322, USA; [b] LogixHealth, 8 Oak Park Drive, Bedford, MA 01730, USA; [c] Department of Emergency Medicine, George Washington University, Washington, DC, USA
* Corresponding author.
*E-mail address:* maross@emory.edu

Emerg Med Clin N Am 35 (2017) 503–518
http://dx.doi.org/10.1016/j.emc.2017.03.001          emed.theclinics.com

recorded in the Hippocratic Corpus, became the foundation of medicine as it is known today.

Jumping forward more than 2 millennia to the 1960s, the creation of EDs addresses a public health need. It was recognized that patients were dying of time-sensitive conditions, such as trauma and cardiac arrest, because they could not reach lifesaving experts and equipment soon enough — such as trauma surgeons, emergency physicians, operating rooms, and defibrillators. This led to the creation of emergency medicine, a new specialty whose defining feature was time rather than an organ system, age, or technology. EDs and emergency physicians specialized in the management of time-sensitive conditions. Between 1955 and 1971, ED visits increased by 367%.[1]

As EDs grew and became more differentiated, the first descriptions of observation beds appeared. In a 1965 edition of the journal, *Hospital Forum*, Lynn Boose, an administrative resident with the Bellflower California Kaiser Foundation Hospital, described "the use of observation beds in emergency service units" where it was recommended that an observation patient's stay "should not exceed 24 hours" based on his review of 1094 cases.[2]

Observation medicine research over the ensuing decades evolved along with innovations in health care.[3] In the 1970s, studies focused broadly on the use of short-stay units in EDs.[4] This focus continued in the 1980s with an increasing focus on specific conditions, in particular chest pain.[5,6] Studies explored other clinical areas, such as pediatrics, geriatrics, trauma, asthma, and abdominal pain.[7–9] The prevalence and scope of ED observation units (EDOUs) were described.[10,11] The 1990s saw high-quality observation medicine research flourish with federally funded prospective randomized clinical trials.[12–14] Chest pain research refined patient selection and diagnostic testing using the term, *accelerated diagnostic protocols* (*ADPs*).[14] Chest pain protocols in dedicated units were reported to have better outcomes than inpatient admission in terms of shorter length of stays, lower costs, less diagnostic uncertainty, and improved patient satisfaction.[13,14] Similar findings were reported in accelerated treatment protocols for asthma with shorter stays.[15] In the new millennium, EDOU research addressed new conditions, including syncope, transient ischemic attack, and atrial fibrillation.[16–18] Studies described the role of observation for pediatric conditions, the elderly, and hospital operations.[19–22] In the second decade of the millennium, clinical research continued as health services research focused on the impact of observation medicine on hospitals, health systems, and health policy.[23–25] Studies further defined which chest pain patients may not need observation or advanced cardiac imaging.[26]

In parallel with these advances, clinical practice also evolved. The American College of Emergency Physicians formed an Observation Medicine Section and adopted policies for the management of observation units, stating, "(o)bservation of appropriate ED patients in a dedicated ED observation area, instead of a general inpatient bed or an acute care ED bed, is a 'best practice' that requires a commitment of staff and hospital resources."[27] In the early 1990s, chest pain centers, which usually included chest pain ADPs and dedicated beds, became more common.[28,29] To represent this group, the Society of Chest Pain Centers was formed and has accredited more than 1000 hospitals nationally.[30]

## PRINCIPLES OF OBSERVATION MEDICINE

Observation care, like emergency care, is defined by time. Most ED visits occur in less than 6 hours, whereas the national average inpatient length of stay is approximately 4.5 days.[31,32] Hospitals are often penalized for patients whose inpatient length of stay is less than 24 hours.[33] These parameters defines a group of patients whose health care needs exceed what can realistically be achieved in less than 6 hours in the ED but if managed actively requires less than 24 hours of hospitalization. Left with an admit or discharge only model, they become orphans of the system and are either admitted unnecessarily or discharged inappropriately. These 6-hour to 24-hour patients have care that falls between the ED and inpatient settings and is best provided in a dedicated observation unit, otherwise known as a type 1 setting (**Table 1**). The principles of observation medicine describe how to best manage these 6-hour to 24-hour patients based on clinical research and national policies[27,34,35] (**Box 1**).

| Table 1 |||
| Observation care settings |||
| **Observation Settings** | **Description** | **Comments** |
| --- | --- | --- |
| Type 1 | Protocol driven Observation unit | Highest level of evidence for favorable outcomes Care typically directed by ED |
| Type 2 | Discretionary care Observation unit | Care directed by a variety of specialists Unit typically based in ED |
| Type 3 | Protocol driven Hospital bed anywhere | Often called a virtual observation unit |
| Type 4 | Discretionary care Hospital bed anywhere | Most common practice Unstructured care Poor alignment of resources with patients' needs |

**Box 1**
**Principles of observation medicine**

1. Focused patient care goals — a well-defined condition-specific patient care goal defined at the time of initiating observation services. Condition-specific guidelines specify patient selection for the observation unit, interventions, and criteria for discharge or admission from the EDOU.

2. Limited duration and intensity of service — the average length of stay of observation patients is 15 hours to 18 hours. Patients requiring a higher intensity of service are generally admitted.

3. Appropriate hospital setting — optimal clinical, operational, and economic outcomes occur in a type 1 setting, as proximate to the ED as possible.

4. Appropriate staffing — appropriate staffing levels of nurses, ancillary, associate providers, and physicians is essential, as is administrative oversight.

5. Providing ongoing care in an outpatient setting — clinical guidelines, care pathways, and protocols fall under 2 broad categories: ADPs (eg, chest pain) and accelerated treatment protocols (eg, asthma).

6. Intensive review — critical metrics must be collected to assure that benchmark targets are being achieved, for example, discharge rates (70%–90%), length of stay (15–18 hours), and financial metrics. These targets are tracked for the whole EDOU and for specific clinical conditions.

7. Economical service — to be successful, an EDOU must be cost-effective and equitable for all involved. Equitability should include the hospital, the physician, and those paying for these services.

## MEDICARE OBSERVATION SERVICES — HOSPITAL PAYMENT POLICY HISTORY

To understand observation services, it is important to understand past and present Medicare observation policy. To put this in context, in 2014 the United States spent approximately $3 trillion on health care, with the largest portion (32%) spent on hospital care. The largest individual payer of health care was the Centers for Medicare & Medicaid Services (CMS), which covered 36% of health insurance payments.[36] Control of escalating hospital costs has been a central issue for Medicare for decades. Medicare policy is developed at CMS headquarters in Baltimore, Maryland, and then administered via 10 regional offices located throughout the United States.[37] Medicare has 4 parts, which were developed in chronologic order to meet societal needs: Medicare Part A covers inpatient admissions and skilled nursing facility (SNF) care after admission; Part B covers outpatient visits, such as clinic, ED, or observation visits as well as physician services; Part C covers Medicare Managed Care (or Advantage) plans; and Part D covers prescription drug plans.[38,39] Observation services fall under Medicare Part B.[34]

To control rising hospitalization costs, in 1983 Medicare launched an inpatient prospective payment system, which adopted a payment methodology called diagnosis-related groups (DRGs).[40] Under this model, inpatient hospitalization is only paid for specific conditions with corresponding DRG codes and payment rates. Shortly thereafter, it was realized that this created a population of patients who were "too sick to go home, but not sick enough to be admitted" as inpatients. A policy correction was needed. To address this issue, Medicare introduced observation services, where a patient could be managed as an outpatient in a bed anywhere in a hospital for up to 24 hours to determine the need for inpatient admission. This definition, with minor modifications, remains:

> Observation care is a well-defined set of specific, clinically appropriate services, which include ongoing short-term treatment, assessment, and reassessment that are furnished while a decision is made regarding whether patients require further treatment as hospital inpatients or if they are able to be discharged from the hospital. Observation services are commonly ordered for patients who present to the ED and who then require a significant period of treatment or monitoring to make a decision concerning their admission or discharge. Observation services are covered only when provided by the order of a physician or another individual authorized by state licensure law and hospital staff bylaws to admit patients to the hospital or to order outpatient services.

> Observation services must also be reasonable and necessary to be covered by Medicare. In only rare and exceptional cases do reasonable and necessary outpatient observation services span more than 48 hours. In a majority of cases, the decision whether to discharge a patient from the hospital after resolution of the reason for observation care or to admit the patient as an inpatient can be made in less than 48 hours, usually in less than 24 hours.[34]

Initial ambiguity with the definition of observation led to misuse of observation services. The 2 most common examples were misuse of observation for scheduled elective outpatient procedures and prolonged observation stays.[41,42] For outpatient procedures, standard recovery periods after those procedures were allowed. In rare and unusual cases, a patient might require a few additional hours for recovery due to unforeseen complications. Initially, Medicare allowed hospitals to bill these rare and unanticipated additional hours of recovery using the observation codes. For various reasons Medicare was frequently double-billed for both the procedure and observation time, often from the time patients first arrived in the hospital.[43] In other cases, patients were held in inpatient beds as observation outpatients for several days to weeks. Both examples increased costs to Medicare, with prolonged stays increasing patient out-of-pocket costs.[41] Neither of these examples was relevant to EDOUs, but they drove policies that influenced observation unit funding.

To address these issues, in 2000 when Medicare launched its outpatient version of the DRG program, called ambulatory payment classifications (APCs), it stopped paying separately for observation services.[41,42] Observation payments were added to the associated ED or clinic visits payments, leading to a slight increase in payment for those visits but no identifiable separate payment for observation. This created a powerful incentive for hospitals to admit most, if not all, observation patients as short-stay inpatients. This policy change likely contributed to a significant rise in short-stay inpatient admissions, which later became a target of the recovery audit contractors (RACs). Based on provider input, in 2002 Medicare began paying again for observation services but with several stipulations for 3 specific conditions: chest pain, asthma, and heart failure.[44] In 2005, most stipulations were lifted; then in 2008, Medicare began paying for all conditions.[44]

In parallel with these events, in 2006 a Medicare demonstration project, called the RAC, collected more than $900 million in overpayments made by Medicare to hospitals. The largest collection category was for short inpatient admissions that should have been billed as outpatient. In 2010 this program was expanded to the entire country. In a 2014 report to Congress, the RAC program reported that it had collected $2.3 billion in Medicare overpayments to hospitals for inpatient services.[33] One of its largest over-payment collection categories was for patients admitted as inpatients whose medical records indicated that they "could have safely and effectively been treated as an outpatient." This finding encouraged hospitals to admit patients only if they were certain that they would meet inpatient criteria, which was becoming increasingly vague.

Not surprisingly, between 2007 and 2009 there was a 34% increase in the ratio of observation visits relative to inpatient admissions for Medicare patients.[45] Observation stays increased from 26 hours to 28 hours, with 40% of stays lasting more than 24 hours and 10% more than 48 hours. This increase in observation relative to inpatient was due to both an increase in observation stays and a decrease in inpatient admissions. The increase in observation volumes was likely due to several factors: a return to baseline when Medicare resumed payment for observation services in 2008, hospital fears of being targeted by RAC auditors for inappropriate inpatient admission, a lack of clarity regarding the definition of an inpatient, and medical innovations shifting care from inpatient to outpatient settings.

## THREE MEDICARE OBSERVATION POLICY ISSUES
### Observation Visits and Hospital Readmissions

In recent years, there has been a decline in hospital readmission rates, driven in part by Medicare inpatient readmission penalties.[46] This decline raised concerns that hospitals were keeping inpatient readmission rates down by keeping patients in outpatient observation status to avoid these penalties. Zuckerman and colleagues[46] found that between 2007 and 2015, for Medicare patients with acute myocardial infarction, heart failure, and pneumonia, inpatient readmission decreased more (21.5% to 17.8%) than the increases in observation visit (2.6% to 4.7%). More importantly, they found no patient-level association between inpatient readmissions and observation stays. Venkatesh and colleagues[47] found that for these targeted conditions, observation bed days represented less than 2.5% of visits.

## Patient Out-of-Pocket Costs for Observation Care

Concerns have been raised that observation care leads to higher patient out-of-pocket costs than inpatient admission, prompting some patients to demand that they be admitted rather than observed. The best way to avoid higher out-of-pocket costs is to manage them in a type 1 setting. Hockenberry and colleagues[48] reported that observation stays of less than 24 hours were associated with costs that were lower than the Medicare Part A deductible. Patients treated in a protocol-driven observation unit had fewer visits with a length of stay beyond 24 hours (10.4%) compared with local state (44%) and national (29%) data.[23] Unfortunately, between 66% and 80% of US hospitals do not have an observation unit.[24,49] Not surprisingly, Wright and colleagues[50] found that hospital, patient, and health system characteristics were associated with the duration of observation services.

Medicare patients are likely to pay less out of pocket as observation patients than as inpatients. Patient out-of-pocket costs are different for inpatient (Medicare Part A) and outpatient (Medicare Part B) services. In 2016, Medicare patients admitted as inpatients paid a $1288 deductible for that admission, which covers all hospital and SNF costs and associated readmissions within 60 days of discharge. Patients managed as outpatients (clinic, ED visits, and observation visits) paid a 20% copayment of Medicare-negotiated charges. Additionally, self-administered medications are not covered, and outpatient time does not qualify toward the inpatient 3-day minimum to establish an SNF benefit. An analysis of all 2012 Medicare claims found that 94% of patient out-of-pocket costs were lower with observation care than with inpatient care. Average out-of-pocket costs for inpatient care were almost twice those of observation: $725 versus $401. When the costs of self-administered medications ($127) were added, out-of-pocket costs for observation care were still less than those for inpatient[51] 2016 observation policy adjustments (discussed later) have made observation savings even less likely to exceed the inpatient deductible.[52] 1.6% of Medicare observation patients have more than 1 observation visits within 60 days, with the potential for higher costs.[53] A majority of Medicare patients, however, have supplemental insurance to cover these deductibles, making the likelihood of higher out-of-pocket costs even less.[54]

## Risk of Losing Medicare Skilled Nursing Facility Benefits due to Observation Services

Medicare allows inpatients requiring a prolonged inpatient convalescence after the acute phase of their inpatient illness to be moved to a SNF. Under this provision, the SNF stay is covered by the inpatient DRG payment. To qualify, patients must have spent at least 3 midnights as inpatients, with the inpatient clock starting when the inpatient order is written. Time in the ED or observation does not qualify.[55,56] An analysis of 2009 Medicare data by Feng and colleagues[57] found that only 0.75% of Medicare observation patients were at risk of losing SNF payment due to time spent in observation. A subsequent government analysis of all 2012 Medicare claims data found that 0.6% of Medicare observation patients were at risk of losing their SNF coverage.[51] Based on an analysis of Medicare Advantage claims, where the 3-day rule is not used, Grebla and colleagues[58] proposed that CMS consider waiving the 3-day rule because it seems to increase hospital length of stays. For these plans, the absence of the 3-day rule was associated with average hospitals stays that were 0.7 days shorter with no increase in the use of SNFs. By decreasing observation length of stays, observation units can minimize patient risks of losing their SNF benefits due to time spent in observation.[23]

## MEDICARE POLICY CHANGES TO DISCOURAGE PROLONGED OBSERVATION CARE

Beyond Medicare policy, which specifies that observation should rarely extend beyond 24 to 48 hours, Medicare has introduced 3 policy changes that discourage prolonged observation services.

### Two-Midnight Rule

To decrease RAC pressures and prolonged observation stays and provide greater clarity regarding the definition of an inpatient, CMS launched the two-midnight rule in October 1, 2013.[59] This is relevant to observation services since the objective of observation is to determine the need for inpatient admission. The hospital setting where patients are most likely to comply with this policy is an EDOU.[23] The two-midnight rule states that

- Inpatient admissions generally are payable under Part A if the admitting practitioner expects a patient to require a hospital stay that crosses 2 midnights and the medical record supports that reasonable expectation.
- Medicare Part A payment is generally not appropriate for hospital stays not expected to span at least 2 midnights.
- All treatment decisions for beneficiaries are based on the medical judgment of physicians and other qualified practitioners.

### The Notice of Observation Treatment and Implication for Care Eligibility Act

Responding to pressures from patient advocacy groups, Congress passed a bill called the Notice of Observation Treatment and Implication for Care Eligibility (NOTICE) Act (HR 876).[60] Hospitals are required to notify Medicare patients whose observation stay has exceeded 24 hours, both verbally and in writing, why they are still under observation status and what the financial consequences of this will be. The standardized notice letter is called the Medicare Outpatient Observation Notice.[61] Requirements of the NOTICE Act are for hospitals:

*To give each individual who receives observation services as an outpatient for more than 24 hours an adequate oral and written notification within 36 hours after beginning to receive them, which*
- *Explains an individual's status as an outpatient and not as an inpatient and the reasons why*
- *Explains the implications of that status on services furnished (including those furnished as an inpatient), the implications for cost-sharing requirements, and subsequent coverage eligibility for services furnished by an SNF*
- *Includes appropriate additional information*
- *Is written and formatted using plain language and made available in appropriate languages and is signed by the individual or a person acting on the individual's behalf (representative) to acknowledge receipt of the notification; or, if the individual or representative refuses to sign, the written notification is signed by the hospital staff who presented it*

### The Comprehensive Observation Services Ambulatory Payment Classification 8011

In 2016 Medicare packaged a majority of costs associated with an observation visit into a single payment called a comprehensive APC (C-APC 8011).[34] This includes payment for all services associated with an observation visit, such as the ED visit, diagnostic tests (such as stress tests), imaging, laboratory tests, treatments, and intravenous medications — making it unlikely that observation outpatient out-of-pocket costs exceed the inpatient deductible.[52] This APC, however, does not include self-administered medications and does not count time in observation toward the 3-day SNF rule. To qualify for this APC, there cannot be an associated major or T status procedure. Examples of T status procedures include a cardiac catheterization, endoscopy, or an appendectomy. This prevents double-billing observation time with procedures, discussed previously. The 2017 payment for C-APC 8011 is $2222 (**Box 2**).

Over the past 3 and a half decades, multiple Medicare policy revisions have shifted incentives toward, then away, and then toward observation services. Currently, observation services cost Medicare approximately 3 times less than inpatient admission.[51] It is unlikely that CMS will abandon observation services. Medicare policy changes have addressed several prior issues by incentivizing hospitals to avoid prolonged observation stays, decrease patient out-of-pocket costs, minimize loss of SNF benefits, and address confusion over outpatient status. These outcomes are most likely to occur in a well-run type 1 observation unit.

## PHYSICIAN OBSERVATION SERVICES — CODING AND REIMBURSEMENT
### Centers for Medicare & Medicaid Services Observation Regulations Shape Physician Documentation Requirements

CMS defines observation care to include short-term treatment, assessment, and reassessment and periodic monitoring and to be covered only when provided by order of a physician.[62] Based on these CMS directives, the following are typically accepted general documentation requirements for physician observation services:[62]

- An initial note with a plan demonstrating the medical necessity for the observation stay
- A clearly dated and timed order to place a patient in observation
- Progress note(s) demonstrating periodic assessments as appropriate
- A short discharge summary reviewing a patient's course in the unit and plans (if any) for additional postobservation treatment and follow-up

---

**Box 2**
**Synopsis of Centers for Medicare & Medicaid Services payment policy requirements for comprehensive observation services ambulatory payment classification 8011[a]**

1. A physician order and documentation supporting the need for observation

2. A preceding (packaged) hospital visit—any of the following:
   a. Type A ED visit — level 1 to level 5 (HCPCS codes 99281–99285)
   b. Type B ED visit — level 1 to level 5 (G0380–G0384)
   c. Outpatient clinic visit (HCPCS code G0463)
   d. Critical care (*CPT* code 99291)
   e. Direct referral to observation (G0463)

3. A minimum of 8 hours of observation: Observation services of substantial duration (HCPCS code G0378 × 8 or more hours)

4. No procedure with an associated T status on the claim for the same or preceding day of service.

5. Status indicator J2 for C-APC — a unique indicator for this C-APC category

[a] Effective 2016.

*Abbreviation:* HCPCS, Healthcare Common Procedure Coding System.

### Current Procedural Terminology Coding for Observation Services

*Current Procedural Terminology* (*CPT*) instructs that when observation status is "initiated in the course of an encounter in another site of service," such as an ED, all "Evaluation and Management" (E/M) services provided by the same physician (defined as a physician of the same specialty, from the same group) in conjunction with initiating observation status are bundled into the initial observation care when performed on the same date. This means that when the same group provides both emergency and observation services, the observation *CPT* E/M codes replace the emergency E/M codes for the initial E/M services provided in the ED. Reimbursement for these codes is similar. The observation codes provide payment for the work of discharging the patient, however, which the emergency codes do not.

*CPT* observation codes are divided into 2 categories. The first category involves care all delivered on the same calendar date. The second category involves care that spans past the midnight hour, involving care delivered during 2 or more calendar dates (**Table 2**).

### Care all on the same date (Current Procedural Terminology codes 99234, 99235, and 99236)

In this situation, all care takes place on a single calendar day. For example, a patient is placed in observation at 9:00 AM and discharged home at 9:00 PM the same day. The observation code set for same day services 99234 to 99236 was officially recognized in 1998. The Relative Value Update Committee (RUC) developed formal vignettes that were submitted to CMS as a component of the relative value unit (RVU) valuation of the services[63] (**Box 3**). The initial valuations were put forth in 1998 and have not changed much since that time. The CMS has a requirement of 8 hours of care on the same date of service by the provider reporting observation codes 99234 to 99236. When emergency and observation services are combined for a single group model, the clock starts at the beginning of the ED visit because this service is bundled.

### Care spans 2 calendar days (Current Procedural Terminology codes 99218, 99219, and 99220)

In this situation, a patient is observed for a period of time on the first day and the care continues past midnight ending on the second calendar day. For example, a patient is placed in observation status at 4:00 PM and discharged home the following day at 10:00 AM (see **Table 2**). Observation provided on calendar date #1 is reported with the code set 99218 to 99220, which was first officially recognized in 1993. The original valuations were put forth in 1993 and have increased since their initial publication.

**Table 2**
**Examples of evaluation and management services across different timeframes**

| Complexity | Emergency Care Without Observation[a] | Observation and Discharge Care on the Same Day | Observation and Discharge Care Covers 2 D | Observation, Subsequent, and Discharge Care Covers 3 (Plus) D[a] |
|---|---|---|---|---|
| Low | 99283 | 99234 | 99218 + 99217 | 99218 + 99224 + 99217 |
| Moderate | 99284 | 99235 | 99219 + 99217 | 99219 + 99225 + 99217 |
| High | 99285 | 99236 | 99220 + 99217 | 99220 + 99226 + 99217 |

[a] For the emergency codes and the subsequent care codes, these are common examples but not an automatic cross-walk between services.

> **Box 3**
> *Current Procedural Terminology* Relative Value Update Committee vignettes
>
> - RUC vignette: 99234 — a 19-year-old pregnant patient (9 weeks' gestation) presents to the ED complaining of persistent vomiting for 1 day.
> - RUC vignette: 99235 — a 48-year-old patient presents to the ED with a history of asthma in moderate respiratory distress. The patient is placed in the observation unit and discharged later the same day.
> - RUC vignette: 99236 — a 52-year-old patient comes to the ED because of chest pain. The patient is managed in the observation unit and discharged later on the same day.
> - RUC vignette: 99218 —an intoxicated 52-year-old man presents after a fall. He has a blood alcohol concentration of 0.325% and has vomited several times. The patient is kept for observation.
> - RUC vignette: 99219 — a 57-year-old woman presents with an allergic reaction after a bee sting, complaining that "her throat is constricting" and she is having "difficulty breathing." The patient is managed in observation.
> - RUC vignette: 99220 — a 78-year-old man with a history of congestive heart failure presents complaining of shortness of breath and lower extremity edema. He admits to not taking his "heart pills" and admits to drinking beer and eating hotdogs recently at a baseball game. He is dyspneic and able to complete 3-word to 5-word sentences; he has rales to midlung field and +3 pitting edema in the bilateral lower extremities. His ECG is unchanged from prior. The patient is placed in observation.
> - 99224 — physicians typically spend 15 minutes at the bedside and on a patient's hospital floor or unit.
> - 99225 — physicians typically spend 25 minutes at the bedside and on a patient's hospital floor or unit.
> - 99226 — physicians typically spend 35 minutes at the bedside and on a patient's hospital floor or unit.

### The observation discharge code (Current Procedural Terminology code 99217)

The discharge code 99217 (officially recognized in 1994) is used to report the work performed on the final day of a multiday observation stay. Observation care discharge management includes services on the date of observation discharge (can only be used on a calendar day other than the initial day of observation). The documentation for 99217 should include the following: a final examination, discussion of the observation stay, follow-up instructions, and documentation.

### Subsequent observation care (Current Procedural Terminology codes 99224, 99225, and 99226)

In 2011, the RUC published values for subsequent observation codes to represent the middle days of care provided to patients staying in observation status for multiple days (see **Table 2**), likely driven with the advent of the two-midnight rule and changes in the delivery of observation services. Although available, they are less frequently used in an EDOU setting where stays rarely cross 3 days. The codes include reviewing the medical record and the results of diagnostic studies and changes in a patient's status since the last assessment by the physician. Because they are subsequent visit codes, based on *CPT* principles, only 2 of the 3 key components of history, physical examination, and medical decision making are required to be satisfied.

### Physician documentation requirements

Although several different coding and documentation paradigms exist, the Medicare 1995 documentation guidelines represent a set of concrete guidelines for history,

**Table 3**
*Current Procedural Terminology* documentation-level requirements

|  | Detailed | Comprehensive |
|---|---|---|
| Documentation Level Required | | |
| Observation *CPT* codes | 99218, 99234 | 99219, 99220 99235, 99236 |
| Documentation Elements Required | | |
| History of present illness | 4 elements | 4 elements |
| Past, family, or social history | 1 area | 3 areas |
| Review of systems | 2–9 systems | 10 systems |
| Physical examination | 5–7 organ systems | 8 organ systems |

physical examination, and the intensity of medical decision making required to support a given observation code choice. Although CPT identifies 7 elements contributing to the potential scoring of cases, observation cases are scored primarily based on the key elements of the history, physical examination, and medical decision making. Except for the lowest level of service, observation services typically require a complex history and physical examination (**Table 3**).

**Table 4**
*Current Procedural Terminology* code comparisons

| Service | Current Procedural Terminology | Documentation Requirements | | | 2017 Work Relative Value Units | 2017 Total Relative Value Units |
|---|---|---|---|---|---|---|
| | | History | Physical | Medical Decision Making | | |
| Emergency level 3 | 99283 | EPF | EPF | M | 1.34 | 1.75 |
| Emergency level 4 | 99284 | D | D | M | 2.56 | 3.32 |
| Emergency level 5 | 99285 | C | C | H | 3.80 | 4.90 |
| Obs + same day disch — low | 99234 | D or C | D or C | L | 2.56 | 3.77 |
| Obs + same day disch — mod | 99235 | C | C | M | 3.24 | 4.78 |
| Obs + same day disch — high | 99236 | C | C | H | 4.20 | 6.16 |
| Observation initial day — low | 99218 | D or C | D or C | L | 1.92 | 2.82 |
| Observation initial day — mod | 99219 | C | C | M | 2.60 | 3.84 |
| Observation initial day — high | 99220 | C | C | H | 3.56 | 5.25 |
| Obs subsequent day — low | 99224 | PF | PF | L | 0.76 | 1.13 |
| Obs subsequent day — mod | 99225 | EPF | EPF | M | 1.39 | 2.06 |
| Obs subsequent day — high | 99226 | D | D | H | 2.00 | 2.97 |
| Observation discharge day | 99217 | + | + | + | 1.28 | 2.06 |

*Abbreviations:* C, comprehensive; D, detailed; EPF, expanded problem focused; H, high; L, low; M, moderate; Obs, observation; PF, problem focused.

## THE RELATIVE VALUE UNIT VALUATION PROCESS

Physician services are reported using the *CPT* coding system. When the *CPT* committee approves a new code, the next step is assigning an RVU valuation to that service. The new code is sent to the RUC where members review detailed information, including physician survey data, to aid in assigning an appropriate relative value to the service. For each *CPT* code, RVU valuations are calculated for physician work, practice expense, and liability expense. Each of these 3 components is assigned an RVU value and the sum represents the total RVUs for that *CPT* code (**Table 4**).

## SUMMARY

Independent of US policy history, observation units have been described in every major continent and country around the world. Policy shifts have contributed to the observation pendulum swinging between encouraging inpatient admission at one time, then observation at another. Patients who fall into the 6-hour to 24-hour category, will always exist. Observation patients need protocol-driven observation units, as do EDs.[23,64] Just as EDs have become the safety net of the health system, observation units have become the safety net of EDs —preventing inappropriate discharges or admissions while improving health care resource utilization. Observation medicine research will continue to refine and improve this well-established service, to the benefit of ED patients and their health care system.

## REFERENCES

1. Rupke J. Twenty-five years on the front line. Dallas (TX): American College of Emergency Physicians; 1993.
2. Boose L. The use of observation beds in emergency service units. Hosp Forum 1965;30–2.
3. Ross MA, Aurora T, Graff L, et al. State of the art: emergency department observation units. Crit Pathw Cardiol 2012;11(3):128–38.
4. Rao MN, Raj S, Reddi YR. Working of a short stay unit in an outpatient department. Indian Pediatr 1973;10(4):241–4.
5. Goldman L, Cook EF, Brand DA, et al. A computer protocol to predict myocardial infarction in emergency department patients with chest pain. N Engl J Med 1988; 318(13):797–803.
6. Rouan GW, Hedges JR, Toltzis R, et al. A chest pain clinic to improve the follow-up of patients released from an urban university teaching hospital emergency department. Ann Emerg Med 1987;16(10):1145–50.
7. Henneman PL, Marx JA, Cantrill SC, et al. The use of an emergency department observation unit in the management of abdominal trauma. Ann Emerg Med 1989; 18(6):647–50.
8. Harrop SN, Morgan WJ. Emergency care of the elderly in the short-stay ward of the accident and emergency department. Arch Emerg Med 1985;2(3):141–7.
9. Zwicke DL, Donohue JF, Wagner EH. Use of the emergency department observation unit in the treatment of acute asthma. Ann Emerg Med 1982;11(2):77–83.
10. Yealy DM, De Hart DA, Ellis G, et al. A survey of observation units in the United States. Am J Emerg Med 1989;7(6):576–80.
11. Graff LG 4th, Radford MJ, Gunning MA, et al. The observable patient in the DRG era. Am J Emerg Med 1988;6(2):93–103.

12. Rydman RJ, Isola ML, Roberts RR, et al. Emergency department observation unit versus hospital inpatient care for a chronic asthmatic population: a randomized trial of health status outcome and cost. Med Care 1998;36(4):599–609.
13. Rydman RJ, Zalenski RJ, Roberts RR, et al. Patient satisfaction with an emergency department chest pain observation unit. Ann Emerg Med 1997;29(1): 109–15.
14. Roberts RR, Zalenski RJ, Mensah EK, et al. Costs of an emergency department-based accelerated diagnostic protocol vs hospitalization in patients with chest pain: a randomized controlled trial. JAMA 1997;278(20):1670–6.
15. Rydman RJ, Roberts RR, Albrecht GL, et al. Patient satisfaction with an emergency department asthma observation unit. Acad Emerg Med 1999;6(3):178–83.
16. Shen WK, Decker WW, Smars PA, et al. Syncope evaluation in the emergency department study (SEEDS): a multidisciplinary approach to syncope management. Circulation 2004;110(24):3636–45.
17. Ross MA, Compton S, Medado P, et al. An emergency department diagnostic protocol for patients with transient ischemic attack: a randomized controlled trial. Ann Emerg Med 2007;50(2):109–19.
18. Decker WW, Smars PA, Vaidyanathan L, et al. A prospective, randomized trial of an emergency department observation unit for acute onset atrial fibrillation. Ann Emerg Med 2008;52(4):322–8.
19. Alpern ER, Calello DP, Windreich R, et al. Utilization and unexpected hospitalization rates of a pediatric emergency department 23-hour observation unit. Pediatr Emerg Care 2008;24(9):589–94.
20. Rentz AC, Kadish HA, Nelson DS. Physician satisfaction with a pediatric observation unit administered by pediatric emergency medicine physicians. Pediatr Emerg Care 2004;20(7):430–2.
21. Ross MA, Compton S, Richardson D, et al. The use and effectiveness of an emergency department observation unit for elderly patients. Ann Emerg Med 2003; 41(5):668–77.
22. Baugh CW, Bohan JS. Estimating observation unit profitability with options modeling. Acad Emerg Med 2008;15(5):445–52.
23. Ross MA, Hockenberry JM, Mutter R, et al. Protocol-driven emergency department observation units offer savings, shorter stays, and reduced admissions. Health Aff (Millwood) 2013;32(12):2149–56.
24. Wiler JL, Ross MA, Ginde AA. National study of emergency department observation services. Acad Emerg Med 2011;18(9):959–65.
25. Baugh CW, Venkatesh AK, Hilton JA, et al. Making greater use of dedicated hospital observation units for many short-stay patients could save $3.1 billion a year. Health Aff (Millwood) 2012;31(10):2314–23.
26. Mahler SA, Riley RF, Hiestand BC, et al. The HEART pathway randomized trial: identifying emergency department patients with acute chest pain for early discharge. Circ Cardiovasc Qual Outcomes 2015;8(2):195–203.
27. American College of Emergency Physicians. Emergency department observation services. Ann Emerg Med 2008;51(5):686.
28. Ross MA, Amsterdam E, Peacock WF, et al. Chest pain center accreditation is associated with better performance of centers for medicare and medicaid services core measures for acute myocardial infarction. Am J Cardiol 2008;102(2):120–4.
29. Zalenski RJ, Rydman RJ, Ting S, et al. A national survey of emergency department chest pain centers in the United States. Am J Cardiol 1998;81(11):1305–9.
30. Care SoCP. 2016; Available at: http://www.scpc.org/index.aspx. Accessed September 9, 2016.

31. Weiss AJ, Elixhauser A. Overview of hospital stays in the United States, 2012: statistical brief #180. Healthcare Cost and Utilization Project (HCUP) Statistical Briefs. Rockville (MD); 2014.

32. National Hospital Ambulatory Medical Care Survey: 2012 Emergency department summary tables. In: Center for Disease Control NCfHS, ed. 2012.

33. Center for Medicare and Medicaid Services HHS. Recovery auditing in medicare for fiscal year 2014-FY 2014 Report to Congress as Required by Section 1893(h) of the Social Security Act. In: Center for Medicare and Medicaid Services HHS, ed. CMS.gov2014.

34. Center for Medicare and Medicaid Services HHS. Medicare claims processing manual, Chapter 4-Part B Hospital (Including Inpatient Hospital Part B and OPPS), Section 290 outpatient observation services. (Rev. 3556, 07-01-16) ed2016.

35. Ross MA, Graff LG. Principles of observation medicine. Emerg Med Clin North Am 2001;19(1):1–17.

36. Center for Medicare and Medicaid Services HHS. NHE Fact Sheet, 2014. Office of the Actuary; 2016.

37. CMS.gov. CMS Regional Offices. 2016. Available at: https://www.cms.gov/About-CMS/Agency-Information/RegionalOffices/index.html?redirect=/regionaloffices/. Accessed September 9, 2016.

38. Medicare.gov. What's Medicare? 2016. Available at: https://www.medicare.gov/sign-up-change-plans/decide-how-to-get-medicare/whats-medicare/what-is-medicare.html. Accessed September 9, 2016.

39. CMS.gov. Medicare Program - General Information. 2016; https://www.cms.gov/Medicare/Medicare-General-Information/MedicareGenInfo/index.html. Accessed November 16, 2016.

40. Center for Medicare and Medicaid Services HHS. Medicare & Medicaid Milestones 1937-2015. https://www.cms.gov/About-CMS/Agency-Information/History/Downloads/Medicare-and-Medicaid-Milestones-1937-2015.pdf. July 2015. Accessed September 9, 2016.

41. Health Care Financing Administration HHS. Medicare program; prospective payment system for hospital outpatient services proposed rule. In: Health Care Financing Administration HHS, ed. vol. 63, No. 173 Tuesday September 8, 1998 Federal Register: Federal Register; 1998:47570.

42. Health Care Financing Administration HHS. Medicare program prospective payment system for hospital outpatient services; final rule. In: Health Care Financing Administration HHS, ed. vol. 65, No. 68 Friday, April 7, 2000. Federal Register: Federal Register; 2000:18443, 18448, 18450.

43. Office of the Inspector General OoAS, H.H.S. Audit of Observation Service Billing by PPS Hospitals. Common Identification Number A-06-01-00028. Available at: https://oig.hhs.gov/oas/reports/region6/60100028.pdf2002. Accessed September 9, 2016.

44. Center for Medicare and Medicaid Services HHS. Medicare program; changes to the hospital outpatient prospective payment system for calendar year 2008; final rule. In: Center for Medicare and Medicaid Services HHS, ed. vol. 72, No. 227, Tuesday November 27 2007. Federal Register2007:66646–66652.

45. Feng Z, Wright B, Mor V. Sharp rise in medicare enrollees being held in hospitals for observation raises concerns about causes and consequences. Health Aff (Millwood) 2012;31(6):1251–9.

46. Zuckerman RB, Sheingold SH, Orav EJ, et al. Readmissions, observation, and the hospital readmissions reduction program. New Engl J Med 2016;374(16): 1543–51.
47. Venkatesh AK, Wang C, Ross JS, et al. Hospital use of observation stays: cross-sectional study of the impact on readmission rates. Med Care 2016;54(12): 1070–7.
48. Hockenberry JM, Mutter R, Barrett M, et al. Factors associated with prolonged observation services stays and the impact of long stays on patient cost. Health Serv Res 2014;49(3):893–909.
49. National Hospital Ambulatory Medical Care Survey: 2011 Emergency Department Summary Tables. Table 27. Hospital and emergency department characteristics, by emergency department visit volume and metropolitan status: United States, 2011. In: Center for Disease Control NCfHS, ed. Available at: http://www.cdc. gov/nchs/data/ahcd/nhamcs_emergency/2011_ed_web_tables.pdf: Center for Disease Control; 2011:Table 27. Accessed September 9, 2016.
50. Wright B, Jung HY, Feng Z, et al. Hospital, patient, and local health system characteristics associated with the prevalence and duration of observation care. Health Serv Res 2014;49(4):1088–107.
51. Office of the Inspector General OoAS, H.H.S. Memorandum Report: Hospitals' Use ofObservation Stays and Short Inpatient Stays for Medicare Beneficiaries, OEI-02-12-00040. Available at: https://oig.hhs.gov/oei/reports/oei-02-12-00040. pdf2013. Accessed September 9, 2016.
52. Baugh CG, M. New CMS Rules Introduce Bundled Payments for Observation Care. ACEP Now. Available at: http://www.acepnow.com/article/new-cms-rules-introduce-bundled-payments-for-observation-care/2/: American College of Emergency Physicians; 2016. Accessed September 9, 2016.
53. Kangovi S, Cafardi SG, Smith RA, et al. Patient financial responsibility for observation care. J Hosp Med 2015;10(11):718–23.
54. Doyle BJ, Ettner SL, Nuckols TK. Supplemental insurance reduces out-of-pocket costs in medicare observation services. J Hosp Med 2016;11(7):502–4.
55. Center for Medicare and Medicaid Services HHS. Medicare Benefit Policy Manual Chapter 8-Coverage of Extended Care (SNF) Services Under Hospital Insurance. CMSgov. 2016;(Rev. 228, 10-13-16). Available at: https://www.cms. gov/Regulations-and-Guidance/Guidance/Manuals/downloads/bp102c08.pdf. Accessed September 9, 2016.
56. Centers for Medicare and Medicaid Services HHS. Your Medicare Coverage - Skilled nursing facility (SNF) care. In: Center for Disease Control NCfHS, ed. Available at: https://www.medicare.gov/coverage/skilled-nursing-facility-care. html: Medicare.gov; 2016. Accessed September 9, 2016.
57. Feng Z, Jung HY, Wright B, et al. The origin and disposition of Medicare observation stays. Med Care 2014;52(9):796–800.
58. Grebla RC, Keohane L, Lee Y, et al. Waiving the three-day rule: admissions and length-of-stay at hospitals and skilled nursing facilities did not increase. Health Aff (Millwood) 2015;34(8):1324–30.
59. Center for Medicare and Medicaid Services HHS. Fact Sheet: Two-Midnight Rule. 2016; Available at: https://www.cms.gov/Newsroom/MediaReleaseDatabase/Fact-sheets/2015-Fact-sheets-items/2015-07-01-2.html. Accessed November 20, 2016.
60. Congress.gov. Summary H.R.876-NOTICE ACT - 114th Congress (2015-2016). 2015-2016. Available at: https://www.congress.gov/bill/114th-congress/house-bill/876. Accessed November 20, 2016.

61. Center for Medicare and Medicaid Services HHS. Beneficiary Notices Initiative (BNI) - Medicare Outpatient Observation Notice (MOON). 2016; Available at: https://www.cms.gov/Medicare/Medicare-General-information/Bni/index.html. Accessed November 20, 2016.
62. CMS Manual System Pub 100-04 Medicare Claims Processing Transmittal 2282 August 26, 2011; pages 8-9. Available at: https://www.cms.gov/Regulations-and-Guidance/Guidance/Transmittals/downloads/R2282CP.pdf2011. Accessed September 9, 2016.
63. American Medical Association. Medicare RBRVS: the physicians' guide 2017. Chicago: American Medical Association, 2012; 2017.
64. Ross MA, Hockenberry JM. Dedicated observation unit for patients with "observation status". JAMA Intern Med 2014;174(2):301.

# The Establishment and Management of an Observation Unit

Jared Conley, MD, PhD, MPH[a,b,]*, J. Stephen Bohan, MD, MS[b],
Christopher W. Baugh, MD, MBA[b]

## KEYWORDS

- Observation unit • Observation medicine • Clinical management
- Clinical workflow and design

## KEY POINTS

- Careful design of the observation unit (OU) process, location, and layout enables optimal clinical care and finances.
- Several acute medical and surgical conditions are amenable to the OU clinical pathway; developing and maintaining protocols to guide patient selection and clinical care are critical to successful management of these conditions.
- Ongoing OU management requires a strong, collaborative leadership model; appropriate staffing; and a robust monitoring system for quality, safety, and finances.

## ESTABLISHING AN OBSERVATION UNIT

Creating a dedicated area within a hospital to cohort observation patients is an essential best practice that enables safe and efficient care. As national and local trends continue to increase demand for observation services, clinicians increasingly understand the benefits of an OU. Accordingly, OUs are becoming increasingly common in larger hospitals in the United States. This article explores the key elements to consider when establishing an OU, such as location, size, staffing, and workflows. Common areas of debate, such as open versus closed design, alternative uses for OU beds, and the care of behavioral health patients, are also discussed. With a better understanding of these considerations, department and hospital leaders can establish and sustain service excellence for their observation patient population.

---

Disclosure Statement: The authors have no conflicts of interest.
[a] Department of Emergency Medicine, Massachusetts General Hospital, Harvard Medical School, 55 Fruit Street, Boston, MA 02114, USA; [b] Department of Emergency Medicine, Brigham and Women's Hospital, Harvard Medical School, 75 Francis Street, Boston, MA 02115, USA
* Corresponding author. Department of Emergency Medicine, Massachusetts General Hospital, Harvard Medical School, 55 Fruit Street, Boston, MA 02114.
E-mail address: jconley@mgh.harvard.edu

Emerg Med Clin N Am 35 (2017) 519–533
http://dx.doi.org/10.1016/j.emc.2017.03.002
emed.theclinics.com

### Observation Unit Design and Layout

Keen attention to designing the optimal structure for an OU is critical to ensure clinical effectiveness and financial viability. Several design components merit attention.

#### Type 1 observation unit

As characterized by Ross and colleagues,[1] there are 4 main types of observation care, depending on the use of a dedicated space for observation and protocols to guide clinical care. Type 1 settings are dedicated OUs that are managed through protocol-driven care. Type 2 settings are dedicated OUs but clinical management is done at the discretion of each individual clinician (without the use of protocols). Type 3 settings involve observation care that occurs in any hospital bed but care is driven by protocols. Lastly, type 4 settings consist of discretionary, nonprotocolized observational care that happens in any hospital bed. The primary focus of this article is on type 1 OUs. Research has demonstrated this structure as superior to other types of OUs. Prospective randomized studies of patients with chest pain, asthma, transient ischemic attack, syncope, and atrial fibrillation managed in an emergency department OU (EDOU) have shown improved patient satisfaction, shorter lengths of stay (LOSs), lower costs, and comparable or improved clinical outcomes relative to similar patients admitted to an inpatient floor.[2–13]

#### Open unit versus closed unit

An important element of OU structure is whether to establish an open unit versus closed unit. In closed units, the management of patient care is under the direction of a single physician group or specialty, such as emergency medicine. On the other hand, open OUs grant more than 1 group of physicians the opportunity to place a patient in the unit; as such, patient care is generally driven by the discretion of individual clinicians. As alluded to previously, evidence demonstrates the superiority of a closed, protocol-driven unit, which is the most common design. With more unified leadership in closed units, condition-specific protocols are used that incorporate inclusion/exclusion criteria, typical interventions performed, and specific criteria for discharge or inpatient admission. There is also greater consistency in ensuring appropriate patients are placed in the unit and better adherence to the specific endpoints of time-conscious protocols.[14,15] In addition, as a result of a smaller and more consistent clinician group, individual clinicians themselves acquire more expertise and efficiency in managing patients in the OU setting. These closed unit settings make it easier to provide targeted feedback and education as well as enforce accountability and ensure quality control.

#### Hybrid unit

For smaller hospitals and those just starting an OU, 1 of the initial challenges becomes justifying the ongoing costs of maintaining nursing and ancillary support staff salaries while the fledgling unit is not consistently operating at full capacity. In these instances, creating a hybrid OU may seem desirable. Hybrid units essentially allow the dedicated space of an OU to be used by both observation patients and other patient populations, such as recovering elective procedure patients. A study by Ross and colleagues[16] revealed that such a design demonstrated a complementary diurnal occupancy pattern, which improved both hourly census and nurse resource use. It also had the added benefit of more efficient management of scheduled procedure patients—without resulting in any adverse effects on the LOS or discharge rate of OU patients.

The appeal of hybrid functioning OUs to maximize operational capacity also pertains to hold or boarder patients who are awaiting transfer to an inpatient bed or another facility. Although including these patients in a hybrid design seems enticing in the afternoon hours (when OU occupancy reliably drops due to the efficiency of morning discharges and an expected arrival peak in the late afternoon and evening), it must be avoided—except perhaps in cases of extreme hospital census when ED waiting room conditions become unsafe due to a lack of acute care bed capacity. Avoidance of this practice is due to the reality that the hold or boarding time frames are unknown and often longer than expected. Thus, when patients in an ED need OU beds in the evening hours, capacity is lacking. A vicious cycle may ensue wherein patients eligible for shorter observation stays must be managed by less efficient inpatient teams due to a lack of OU capacity, further exacerbating the lack of inpatient capacity. The default policy should be no boarding within an OU; the rare practice of OU boarding can be justified at times, although strong leadership is required to ensure it does not become the norm.

### Location
From both patient care and logistics perspectives, location is a critical design component of OU development. The highest potential for patient comfort, hospital bed use efficiency, and cost savings stems from the creation of a dedicated physical space for observation patients. Locating this dedicated space within or immediately adjacent to the emergency department (ED) aids in the success of such units, because processes are minimally disrupted and close proximity to clinicians, supplies, and equipment enables safe and efficient care. The placement of the unit at a significant distance from the ED might not change the internal dynamic but results in a loss of efficiency in clinical re-evaluation, transport, and communication.[17] As distance from the ED increases, patient expectations of a brief hospitalization and manifestation of the ED culture of rapid throughput and continuous rounding may become more difficult to maintain. At the same time, for those hospitals with crowded EDs and limited department space, it likely does not make sense to undersize the ED to generate a close-proximity OU. In these cases, it may be more amenable to have a remote OU—remembering that the OU is only 1 resource among competing interests.

### Volume capacity
Another important step in the establishment of an OU is understanding the projected daily volume capacity and thus the ideal number of beds contained within the unit. Studies have demonstrated that approximately 5% to 10% of all ED patients may be good candidates for observation care.[18–20] Facilities opening a new unit can expect to start closer to 5% and increase over time as new protocols are implemented and staff comfort rises. Another metric used is to estimate OU volume as approximately 2 beds per every 10,000 ED visits. At the same time, the minimum recommended size for a dedicated unit is 5 beds to 8 beds, which allows for an efficient nurse-to-patient staffing ratio of 1:5 or 1:4. Based on an average LOS of 15 hours and a size of 5 OU beds, the expected average daily volume is 8 patients (assuming full occupancy and perfect matching of arrivals and departures). Therefore, the minimum ED volume to support 8 OU patients/d in a 5-bed unit is 80 ED visits/d (10% of ED volume) or approximately 29,000 ED visits per year. As a result, most hospitals do not consider opening an OU until ED annual visit volume rises well above 30,000.

### Physical space layout
Careful thought is required in designing the physical space of a new OU. Ideally, the OU is set up in such a way to optimize clinical care—with primary considerations centering around space usage, the patient-clinician relationship, and allocated funds. Generating a design that maximizes the use of space with an eye toward balancing

patient comfort and clinician workflow is critical. It is necessary to be attentive upfront to the planned nurse-to-patient ratio (1:4–1:6), because it has an impact on the number of beds included in the OU. Whether the location is built within new or renovated space also has an impact on decision making regarding OU design. Local factors, such as state and city departments of public health regulations, may also heavily influence OU design.

In addressing the patient-clinician relationship, a key design element that requires attention pertains to providing structure to the patient space within an OU. Variations in such structure exist within current OUs, with some possessing curtained cubicles and others using closed-walled rooms—both have advantages and disadvantages. Structuring the physical space in such a way that it promotes the patient-clinician relationship is equally important. One option includes having nursing stations that face all patient rooms/cubicles. At one of the authors' institutions (Brigham and Women's Hospital), this is done with a semicircular nursing station that enables direct visualization of all patients, allowing patients to feel better cared for during their stay. Other design considerations include creating a patient nourishment station, medication preparation area, workstations for consultants and other staff (pharmacy, physical therapy, and care coordination), and space and accommodation for visitors.

### Time cutoff

Establishing an LOS time cutoff is another relevant consideration for determining how to structure an OU. Traditionally, most EDOUs used a 24-hour maximum cutoff; however, on October 1, 2013, the Centers for Medicare & Medicaid Services (CMS) introduced the Two-Midnight Rule, wherein all Medicare patients with an expected hospital LOS of less than 2 midnights should be classified as observation patients. Although the application of this rule has undergone several revisions,[21] it continues as standard CMS policy.[22] Depending on the hour of patient arrival for initial ED evaluation, observation patients can spend well over 24 hours in the hospital. These recent changes, however, do not remove the need for prospective, explicit endpoints to determine either a safe discharge to home or further inpatient hospitalization.

### Conditions of Interest and Protocol Development

Successful establishment of an OU requires the determination of which acute medical and surgical conditions are appropriate for this clinical pathway, leading to the development of protocols that aid clinicians to select appropriate patients and manage them with evidence-based diagnostics and interventions. This process is outlined in 5 main phases: (1) choosing the condition(s), (2) initial protocol development, (3) drafting of protocol with key components, (4) protocol verification and implementation, and (5) protocol maintenance (**Fig. 1**).

### Amenable conditions

In the past few decades, several conditions have been studied and found amenable for OU management. Chest pain was the initial focus of such efforts.[3,10,12,23] Further research, however, has shown the efficacy of treating several other conditions, including asthma, atrial fibrillation, transient ischemic attack, syncope, acute decompensated heart failure, and pulmonary embolism.[2,4–9,24,25] Other conditions have been managed in an OU as well (eg, abdominal pain, dehydration, renal colic, cellulitis, back pain, headache, pyelonephritis, chronic obstructive pulmonary disease exacerbation, community-acquired pneumonia, metabolic derangement, deep vein thrombosis, and psychiatric emergency) but limited to no formal assessment of their efficacy has been published to date.[26,27]

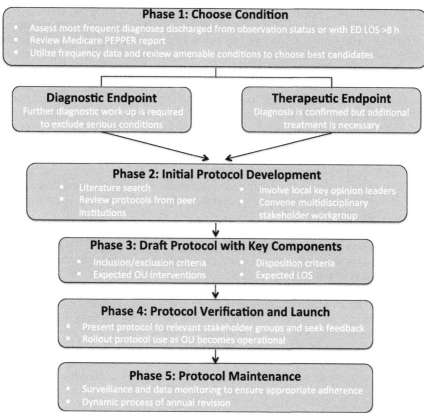

**Fig. 1.** Phases of OU protocol development.

Once a survey of these potential conditions of interest is complete, the determination of optimal conditions for a new OU can be performed through data analysis and discussions with key leadership. Important areas of analysis include internal hospital data (ie, most frequent diagnoses discharged from inpatient teams in observation status or those with ED LOS greater than 8 hours) as well as using external resources, such as Medicare reports (eg, Program for Evaluating Payment Patterns Electronic Report [PEPPER] report, https://www.pepperresources.org/). This work to identify those conditions with the highest volume opportunity to manage in an OU, in combination with leadership approval, guides decision making. Often, however, when starting an OU, it is wise to start with more widely established pathways, such as chest pain. Over time, successful implementation of this protocol builds consensus and enables development of the additional amenable conditions discovered through analysis.

*Inclusion of patients with mental illness*
An additional consideration in the establishment of an OU is whether to include the population of behavioral health patients. At the core of this debate is whether care of this population fits with the definition of the purpose of observation care, which is to determine if inpatient admission is necessary. Some OU leaders argue that a behavioral health patient, such as one with suicidal ideation who is held for placement in an

inpatient psychiatric facility, is inappropriate for OU care, because the disposition is not in doubt and the delay in care is related to a bed search alone. The counterargument is that some of these patients improve with new or resumed medical therapy while in observation status and, on re-evaluation, can be discharged back into the community with a safe outpatient follow-up plan; accordingly, there is legitimate uncertainty around the need for inpatient admission in many cases and observation care is justified. Nevertheless, each institution should examine its own patient populations and resources; discuss options with psychiatry, security, and compliance colleagues; and determine the practice that is most appropriate. For those who proceed with the care of this special population, the OU must be adequately equipped with resources to meet the needs of this patient population. For example, the rooms need to be made safe for patients at risk for self-harm, security should be near the unit, and the unit's atmosphere should be calm and supportive. Patients requiring physical or chemical restraints, or those with evidence of acute intoxication, should not be managed in an OU.

### Diagnostic versus therapeutic endpoints

Once the best candidate conditions have been chosen, the next branch point in this process is the selection of diagnostic versus therapeutic endpoints for these conditions of interest. Diagnostic protocols, as their name suggests, focus on using time in the OU to obtain a necessary diagnosis (or more likely, sufficiently exclude life-threatening diagnoses, such as acute coronary syndrome in patients with chest pain). Therapeutic protocols, on the other hand, concentrate on providing appropriate time-sensitive therapies (medications, fluids, and so forth) where a diagnosis has already been obtained or will be sought after in the outpatient setting (ie, a patient with asthma who needs more time for steroids and albuterol to control symptoms).

### Protocol development

Once conditions of interest have been chosen and diagnostic versus therapeutic endpoints selected, the next phase is protocol development. As referenced previously, type 1 OUs use protocol-driven care to assist in achieving superior clinical outcomes, patient satisfaction, and efficiency. Generating protocols has a unique ability to enable clinicians choosing patients for OU management, as well as OU staff, to have a clear sense of patient selection and planned management. The process of protocol development commences with a thorough literature review. Then, because many institutions have a long history of OU practice and freely share protocols, gathering existing protocols may be a useful early step in the process. Discussion with local and national content experts may also inform best practices and evidence-based care. Once this is complete, enlisting all relevant stakeholders (OU leadership and appropriate consultants) allows for the joint creation of an OU pathway. A multidisciplinary approach is often best, including not only physician staff but also nurses, advanced practice providers (APPs), and all other staff who may be impacted by the protocol.

The key areas of discussion and subsequent protocol development are (1) inclusion/exclusion criteria, (2) expected OU interventions, and (3) disposition criteria. Additional considerations for the protocol include expected LOS and considerations for the medical record. Inclusion/exclusion criteria establish clinical variables for each condition of interest that enables work-up that is suitable for an OU while maintaining a reasonable discharge-to-home rate. Avoidance of patients who clearly require inpatient management or would be better managed by discharge home with clinic follow-up should be emphasized in patient selection. Expected OU interventions outline diagnostic and/or therapeutic activities that are typically done within the unit and provide a template to guide clinicians rather than a prescriptive to-do list, given the variability between patients. Disposition criteria facilitate appropriate patient flow and efficiency within the OU as well as assist in the sometimes difficult decision to admit a patient to the hospital. LOS often varies for each condition; generating an overall sense of expected LOS for each respective condition assists clinicians to make the optimal use of OU resources. Lastly, outlining specific considerations for the medical record (ie, contact with primary care provider or outpatient follow-up plan) can aid clinicians in navigating the nuances of OU medical documentation.

### Protocol verification, implementation, and maintenance

With the key components identified, the next phase involves protocol verification and launch. During this time, the protocol is vetted by the relevant stakeholder groups and feedback is obtained. Once sufficient review and editing have been performed, the protocol for the condition of interest can become operational in the OU. The implementation process requires intense surveillance and solicitation of feedback in the critical period after launch. Typically, a new protocol may take several months from inception to implementation.

The final phase in this process involves protocol maintenance. Protocol development is not a static but a dynamic process. Once a set of protocols is developed, updating and/or retiring the algorithms is necessary. In the authors' practice, this is done every year at a minimum to ensure optimal use of the OU management pathway.

## OBSERVATION UNIT MANAGEMENT
### Leadership

Strong leadership is critical to the successful management of an OU.[28–31] The ideal OU leadership model is a triad consisting of a physician director, a nurse director, and an administrative operations director who can ensure excellent and efficient patient care through collaboration and accountability. This leadership triad is responsible for the key functions of the OU, which include monitoring utilization and quality, implementing protocols, and overseeing research/educational activities as indicated. In addition, the physician director takes primary responsibility over interdepartment relations, developing protocols for new conditions, and monitoring physician activities and workflow. The nurse director specifically oversees all nursing interventions, care coordination, and case management. The administrative operations director is responsible for managing the finances, interfacing with hospital administration, workflow metric reporting, compiling the annual report, and assessment of overall return on investment of the OU.

The American College of Emergency Physician's policy on EDOUs also recommends that the OU leadership develop guidelines for admission/discharge criteria, a clear statement delineating which physician and nurse are responsible for each patient throughout the day, how documentation and transfer of care will occur, timing of physician notification, maximum allowable LOS in the unit, and means of addressing conflicts and outliers.[32] Another important role for OU leadership is to establish and maintain a strong commitment from hospital leadership and foster collaboration. This executive sponsorship can be accomplished, in part, through quarterly meetings with the hospital vice president, ED chair or vice chair, and chief nursing officer as well as the chief compliance officer where the annual report (discussed later) can be reviewed.

### Communication plan

In an effort to establish a new OU, creating and executing a solid communication plan is paramount. The groundwork for an OU is complex, involving multiple hospital entities; thus, communication across multiple channels of leadership and frontline staff is necessary to ensure success. The conveyance of critical information regarding the structure, patient populations, and function of the OU should be done both by the unified leadership triad (discussed previously) and individually in their respective domains (physicians, nurses, and administrative/operations). Involving consultant services early on in the discussions enable a more smooth process of consensus building and implementation planning.

### Timeline

Ideally, an institution allocates approximately 6 months to 9 months for the development and opening of an OU. This time allows for the key phases of planning, construction, staffing, and protocol development to be accomplished in a smooth manner. Most new OUs do not require a significant level of new staffing but rather a repurposing of existing staff given the expected shift of patients from inpatient beds into a dedicated unit managed. For the limited amount of new staff who are necessary, hiring, credentialing, and enrolling them with payers typically requires a minimum of 6 months. Additionally, creation and implementation of new protocols ideally take several months. Formation of the OU team and development of protocols can be done in parallel if needed. Finally, there are dozens of clinical and ancillary departments and staff who will be impacted by the creation of an OU. Meeting with these stakeholders in advance of opening the OU to explain its purpose and gain their support is a key activity, and, for some stakeholders, several meetings are needed.

### Staffing

#### Clinicians

Appropriate staffing is essential to effective OU management.[33] Clinician staffing for OUs generally consists of physicians, APPs (eg, physician assistants or nurse practitioners), nurses, and medical assistants. Each fulfills a unique role in the care of OU patients and the optimal combination of these individuals differs by institution, based on unique patient needs, available resources, and billing requirements (especially for physician staffing).

Two primary models of clinical care exist. The first is that of an attending physician-nurse team that assumes all care responsibilities for each OU patient. The second involves an APP-nurse team with attending physician oversight. In 2003, only 21.4% of OUs reported using APPs[20]; however, there is a growing trend of increased APP involvement.[34] By maintaining a presence in the physical space of the OU, an APP can rapidly evaluate patients, respond to nursing questions or suggestions, and ensure laboratory and imaging results are followed-up and completed. At the same time, even with the use of APPs, supervising physicians should be immediately available to come to the OU and evaluate patients given their ultimate responsibility for each patient's clinical care. Critical decisions (ie, overall OU management plan and endpoints for successful discharge) are typically made by the supervising physician and then subsequently managed by the APP. If a patient decompensates or if test/imaging results are concerning, the supervising physician should be re-engaged to address them as clinical management necessitates. Nonetheless, an experienced APP should be capable of handling much of the hands-on work needed to care for observation patients safely.[35]

From a nursing perspective, OUs are typically staffed by registered nurses who possess the clinical skills and experience to care for this patient population. The degree of nursing intensity in an OU is usually less than or similar to that provided on an inpatient hospital floor. Approximately 1 nurse is needed per shift for every 4 patients to 6 patients in an OU, compared with 1 nurse for every 4 patients (or even 1 nurse for every 3 patients) on an average inpatient floor.[17,20,36] In general, an OU has a fixed number of beds, which determines the number of nurses needed based on staffing ratios. One characteristic of observation care is that for a majority of patients, the medical decision making may be straightforward, but the accompanying nursing care required may be complex. Thus, inpatient admission should strongly be considered for patients who likely require more nursing care than can be adequately provided in the OU—this is informed by both the number of patients in the unit and their relative demand on nursing resources. One final consideration for nurse staffing is the use of float pool nurses versus dedicated observation or emergency nurses. Given the incredible impact of nursing care on the timeliness of patient care, whenever possible, float nurses should be avoided in the OU due to their lack of familiarity with the standard protocols and the unique needs of the observation patient population.[31] Because increased efficiency is a major hallmark of OU-based care, any factor that diminishes this capacity for efficiency undoubtedly threatens the value proposition of an OU.

### Support staff

Beyond physicians, APPs, and nurses, additional support staff play a crucial role in facilitating excellent patient care within the OU, including a care coordinator, a unit clerk, and a medical assistant.[35] The care coordinator (often a nurse by training) can enable key disposition decisions to maintain good flow through the OU—particularly for those patients going to a rehabilitation facility, nursing home, or requiring home services. The authors recommend having 1 clerk and 1 nursing assistant for a 10-bed OU. Care coordination should be available from approximately 7:00 AM until at least the early evening each day and there should be adequate time to prioritize OU patients.

### Ancillary Support

### Consultants

Consulting services are a key resource to ensure optimal care for patients with more complex medical and surgical needs.[35] As alluded to previously, establishing strong relationships with consulting services early enables smooth delivery of care processes and management—both within the OU and afterward in the outpatient setting. It is, thus, advisable upfront to establish clear clinical pathways for each condition of interest with consideration of priority access to consultants seeing patients, preferred testing resources, and appropriate follow-up. The primary consulting services used by an OU include cardiology, neurology, general surgery, urology, and gastroenterology—although this might differ depending on an OU's conditions of interest and patient population.

Physical therapy and social work are additional key consultant services. Physical therapy can assist in the safe and efficient disposition of many OU patients who have mobility needs and need assessment before discharge. The OU also functions more optimally with a motivated, accessible social worker who can assist with patient needs regarding home situation, medication dispensing, transportation, and follow-up.[37]

It is also important to develop a mutually respectful, working relationship with utilization management (UM). A majority of institutions require a utilization review of all OU patients and inform whether inpatient criteria are met. Conflict may transpire when UM recommends an inpatient upgrade, yet the patient is clinically improving with discharge imminent. An alternative scenario can also occur when a patient seems to require more time and resources than the OU is equipped to provide and UM is not supportive of conversion to inpatient admission.[37] It is important to recognize, however, that UM relies on third-party decision-making tools that do not always capture important considerations for each individual patient or the attendant local resources. Ultimately, it is up to the attending physician to navigate the best disposition for each patient in the OU.

### Imaging modalities
Ease of access to key imaging modalities is a critical management feature and enables an OU to provide efficient and effective care. Upfront conversations and agreements with radiology and cardiology should be the focus of efforts. Imaging studies with priority attention include CT, MRI, echocardiogram, and various stress testing modalities.

## Workflow

There are several key factors in OU workflow and each assists in optimizing the patient care experience.

### Length of stay
Most studies of OU patients have shown the expected average LOS to be approximately 15 hours.[20,30,38] When an OU complaint-specific LOS frequently exceeds 24 hours, it is likely there is an opportunity for more efficient management or this group of patients might require inpatient admission. Patient populations with LOS between 8 hours to 15 hours are more favorable. If LOS is approached from a financial perspective alone using Medicare billing requirements, the ideal stay is just over 8 hours for each patient, because no significant extra reimbursement is obtained for additional hours of care in the OU payment model once this minimum threshold is met.[17] Caution should be exercised for short OU stays, however, because the risks of handoffs, additional work of observation documentation, and logistics of moving patients may not justify observation care if the anticipated LOS is less than or equal to 8 hours.

### Rounds and in-person coverage
Rounding on OU patients is an important aspect of clinical re-evaluation and management. Quality standards and payer requirements generally dictate that an attending physician perform both an observation admission and discharge assessment.[35,39] (One alternative in many states, however, is for APPs to evaluate and manage patients on their own without physician involvement but bill at a reduced rate.) From the authors' experience, rounding with a resident physician or APP should comprise communication and re-examining that last a total of 6 minutes to 9 minutes per patient. Ideally, an uninterrupted minimum of 1 hour is generally needed to round on a traditional 10-bed OU when taking over for another physician. Once rounds are complete, the attending physician need only be available, not physically present, for the care of OU patients. This enables cross-coverage of other areas in the hospital, including the acute care arena of the ED.[31] Nonetheless, the distribution of patients assigned to any single physician must acknowledge the demands of both patient volume and complexity, not only at the averages but also at peak times.

### Communication and documentation
Communication and documentation of care in the OU begin with the traditional pass-off and documentation of the initial evaluation and management in the ED. At minimum, these should include initial decision making, results of tests/imaging, and plans

for care in the OU. The ED documentation needs to be in a patient's chart or within the mutually accessible electronic health record on arrival to the OU. An order to place a patient in the OU must be entered to enable hospital billing capabilities for appropriate observation services. OU orders are a requisite; there is often opportunity to generate protocol-driven order sets for specific conditions.[40] Progress notes are done as needed for optimal patient care and a final discharge summary should always be written. The discharge summary includes a patient's clinical course while in the OU, the final physical examination and diagnosis, a preparation of discharge or admission records, and instructions for continuing beyond the OU environment—as required for optimal patient care and billing for observation services. If physicians from the same practice and specialty provide both emergency and observation services on the same day, then the observation *Current Procedural Terminology* (*CPT*) codes are to be used for billing.[41] Both generate similar relative value units for the initial evaluation and subsequent management in the ED. Yet, unlike the emergency *CPT* codes, observation *CPT* codes additionally reimburse for the work of discharging a patient.[40] As a result, there are significantly higher relative value units associated with an observation visit versus a similarly complex ED visit.

## Quality Assurance Process and Metrics

### Key metrics to maximize safety and efficiency
In an effort to optimize the use of an OU, several key performance indicators should garner the full attention of OU leadership. Principal metrics of focus include LOS, occupancy rate, discharge to home and inpatient conversion rate, ED revisit rates, and patient satisfaction.[17] The national benchmark LOS mean for OUs is 15 hours[20,30]; it is recommended to also track outliers (LOS <6 hours, LOS >24 hours, LOS >36 hours, and LOS >2 midnights) and assess LOS by condition. For occupancy rate, it is estimated that an appropriate standard is 60% to 75%,[20] although this is likely increasing in recent years with the additional patient volume burdens on EDs and hospital inpatient services. The midnight census should nearly always be 100% occupancy for an OU operating at peak efficiency. For the discharge to home and inpatient conversion rate, evidence suggests the appropriate rates to be 80% and 20%, respectively.[17,20,30]

Close monitoring of these indicators enables effective patient flow through the OU and generates a more robust disposition option from the ED, while also redirecting patients away from inappropriate inpatient admission—lessening both ED and inpatient crowding. This critical work helps hospitals deliver an appropriate intensity of care to each patient by better matching resources to patient needs. Although such efforts are important, it must be emphasized that patient care is paramount and that an effective OU is ultimately designed to prioritize serving patients and not management or finance concerns.

### Dashboards
Synthesizing operations data in an easy-to-read and interpretable manner is critical to the successful management of an OU. Dashboards enable this continuous quality improvement and have been used throughout health care for this purpose. Data are pulled from multiple sources and summarized into a succinct visual representation of key performance indicators. When designing an OU dashboard, the focus should be on choosing the best data, optimizing presentation design and layout, and deciding on the best timing frequency for updating information. Actionable data on volume, LOS, inpatient conversion rate, quality, and finances are ripe for inclusion (**Fig. 2**). Designing the information layout in such a way to maximize understanding and drive

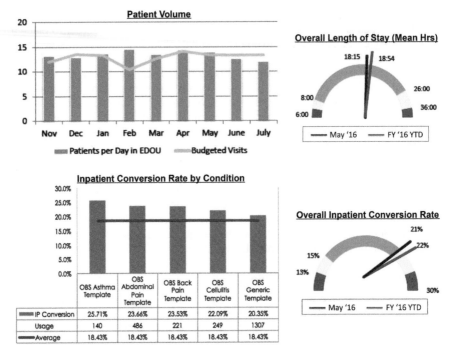

**Fig. 2.** OU data dashboard. FY, fiscal year; IP, inpatient; OBS, observation unit.

discussion is crucial. Updating the data every month enables continuous, thoughtful improvement. It is also important to recognize that dashboards should be initially created during the planning process (not once operations have begun), tailored to each audience, and further refined over time.

### Policy manual
Generating and maintaining an OU policy manual strengthens best practices within a unit and promotes a joint conversation between staff members to address key issues. Within the policy manual, a unified approach is condoned for each issue of interest. Policy manuals also greatly assist with the daily function of the OU by preventing communication errors and having oft-encountered problems already addressed and with a clear path for resolution. In addition, they aid in promoting a culture of safety and in allowing staff to feel more secure in the discharge of their respective responsibilities. Specific processes, such as documentation expectations, patient handoff logistics, and electronic health record orders, should be explicitly detailed. The policy manual should be developed early in the management phase of the OU and then be updated every 6 months to 12 months.

### Annual report
Lastly, providing departmental and hospital leadership with a clear sense of the value creation the OU unit generates each year is an imperative. Such efforts should be done at the end of every fiscal or calendar year and assist in the appropriation of necessary resources as well as potentiating growth opportunities. It can be done through the preparation of a formal annual report. Such a document aims to highlight OU contributions, revenue generated, hospital bed hours saved, safety record, and patient satisfaction.

## SUMMARY

The current US health care landscape and evidence support the establishment of type 1 OUs to provide safe and efficient care for observation patients. Careful attention is required in the design of OU process, location, and layout to enable optimal care and finances. Several acute medical and surgical conditions are amenable to the OU clinical pathway; developing and maintaining protocols to guide patient selection and clinical care are critical. Ongoing OU management requires a strong, collaborative leadership model; appropriate staffing; and a robust monitoring system for quality, safety, and finances. With a better understanding of these principles of OU establishment and management, department and hospital leaders can generate and sustain service excellence for their observation patient population.

## REFERENCES

1. Ross MA, Hockenberry JM, Mutter R, et al. Protocol-driven emergency department observation units offer savings, shorter stays, and reduced admissions. Health Aff 2013;32(12):2149–56.
2. McDermott MF, Murphy DG, Zalenski RJ, et al. A comparison between emergency diagnostic and treatment unit and inpatient care in the management of acute asthma. Arch Intern Med 1997;157:2055–62.
3. Roberts RR, Zalenski RJ, Mensah EK, et al. Costs of an emergency department-based accelerated diagnostic protocol vs hospitalization in patients with chest pain: a randomized controlled trial. JAMA 1997;278:1670–6.
4. Ross MA, Compton S, Medado P, et al. An emergency department diagnostic protocol for patients with transient ischemic attack: a randomized controlled trial. Ann Emerg Med 2007;50(2):109–19.
5. Koenig BO, Ross MA, Jackson RE. An emergency department observation unit protocol for acute-onset atrial fibrillation is feasible. Ann Emerg Med 2002;39: 374–81.
6. Decker WW, Smars PA, Vaidyanathan L, et al. A prospective, randomized trial of an emergency department observation unit for acute onset atrial fibrillation. Ann Emerg Med 2008;52:322–8.
7. Shen WK, Decker WW, Smars PA, et al. Syncope Evaluation in the Emergency Department Study (SEEDS): a multidisciplinary approach to syncope management. Circulation 2004;110:3636–45.
8. Zwicke DL, Donohue JF, Wagner EH. Use of the emergency department observation unit in the treatment of acute asthma. Ann Emerg Med 1982;11:77–83.
9. O'Brien SR, Hein EW, Sly RM. Treatment of acute asthmatic attacks in a holding unit of a pediatric emergency room. Ann Allergy 1980;45:159–62.
10. Gomez MA, Anderson JL, Karagounis LA, et al. An emergency department-based protocol for rapidly ruling out myocardial ischemia reduces hospital time and expense: results of a randomized study (ROMIO). J Am Coll Cardiol 1996; 28:25–33.
11. Goodacre S, Nicholl J. A randomised controlled trial to measure the effect of chest pain unit care upon anxiety, depression, and health-related quality of life [ISRCTN85078221]. Health Qual Life Outcomes 2004;2:39.
12. Farkouh ME, Smars PA, Reeder GS, et al. A clinical trial of a chest-pain observation unit for patients with unstable angina. Chest Pain Evaluation in the Emergency Room (CHEER) Investigators. N Engl J Med 1998;339:1882–8.
13. Jagminas L, Partridge R. A comparison of emergency department versus inhospital chest pain observation units. Am J Emerg Med 2005;23(2):111–3.

14. Pena ME, Fox JM, Southall AC, et al. Effect on efficiency and cost-effectiveness when an observation unit is managed as a closed unit vs an open unit. Am J Emerg Med 2013;31(7):1042–6.

15. Pena ME. Open vs. Closed Units. American College of Emergency Physicians. Available at: https://www.acep.org/Physician-Resources/Practice-Resources/Administration/Observation-Services-Toolkit/. Accessed August 4, 2016.

16. Ross MA, Naylor S, Compton S, et al. Maximizing use of the emergency department observation unit: a novel hybrid design. Ann Emerg Med 2001;37(3):267–74.

17. Baugh CW, Venkatesh AK, Bohan JS. Emergency department observation units: A clinical and financial benefit for hospitals. Health Care Manage Rev 2011;36(1):28–37.

18. Graff LG. Observation medicine: The healthcare system's tincture of time. 2009. Available at: https://www.acep.org/Physician-Resources/Practice-Resources/Administration/Observation-Services-Toolkit/. Accessed August 10, 2016.

19. Wiler JL, Ross MA, Ginde AA. National study of emergency department observation services. Acad Emerg Med 2011;18(9):959–65.

20. Mace SE, Graff L, Mikhail M, et al. A national survey of observation units in the United States. Am J Emerg Med 2003;21(7):529–33.

21. Cassidy A. The Two-Midnight Rule. Health Affairs 2015. Available at: http://www.healthaffairs.org/healthpolicybriefs/brief.php?brief_id=133. Accessed October 5, 2016.

22. Center for Medicare & Medicaid Services. Inpatient Hospital Reviews. Available at: https://www.cms.gov/Research-Statistics-Data-and-Systems/Monitoring-Programs/Medicare-FFS-Compliance-Programs/Medical-Review/InpatientHospitalReviews.html. Accessed September 16, 2016.

23. Goodacre SW. Should we establish chest pain observation units in the UK? a systematic review and critical appraisal of the literature. J Accid Emerg Med 2000;17(1):1–6.

24. Collins SP, Pang PS, Fonarow GC, et al. Is hospital admission for heart failure really necessary? The role of the emergency department and observation unit in preventing hospitalization and rehospitalization. J Am Coll Cardiol 2013;61(2):121–6.

25. Stewart M, Bledsoe J, Madsen T, et al. Utilization and Safety of a pulmonary embolism treatment protocol in an emergency department observation unit. Crit Pathw Cardiol 2015;14(3):87–9.

26. Ross MA, Hemphill RR, Abramson J, et al. The recidivism characteristics of an emergency department observation unit. Ann Emerg Med 2010;56(1):34–41.

27. Bohan J. Brigham and Women's Hospital Observation Protocols. American College of Emergency Physicians. Available at: https://www.acep.org/content.aspx?id=46142. Accessed July 9, 2016.

28. Crenshaw LA, Lindsell CJ, Storrow AB, et al. An evaluation of emergency physician selection of observation unit patients. Am J Emerg Med 2006;24(3):271–9.

29. Burkhardt J, Peacock WF, Emerman CL. Predictors of emergency department observation unit outcomes. Acad Emerg Med 2005;12(9):869–74.

30. Ross MA, Compton S, Richardson D, et al. The use and effectiveness of an emergency department observation unit for elderly patients. Ann Emerg Med 2003;41(5):668–77.

31. Brillman J, Mathers-Dunbar L, Graff L, et al. Management of observation units. American College of Emergency Physicians. Ann Emerg Med 1995;25(6):823–30.

32. ACEP Emergency Medicine Practice Committee. Emergency department observation services. Ann Emerg Med 2008;51:686.
33. Ross MA, Graff LG. Principles of Observation Medicine. Emerg Med Clin North Am 2001;19(1):1–17.
34. Osborne A, Weston J, Wheatley M, et al. Characteristics of hospital observation services: a society of cardiovascular patient care survey. Crit Pathw Cardiol 2013; 12(2):45–8.
35. Baugh CW, Graff LG. Management – Staffing. In: Graff LG, editor. Observation medicine: The healthcare system's tincture of time. 2009. Available at: https://www.acep. org/Physician-Resources/Practice-Resources/Administration/Observation-Services-Toolkit/. Accessed August 10, 2016.
36. Greene J. Nurse groups, administrators battle over mandatory nursing ratios: california law debated on national stage. Ann Emerg Med 2009;54:31–3.
37. Bennett RS. Development and maintenance of key partnerships in the ED observation unit. American College of Emergency Physicians. Available at: https://www. acep.org/Physician-Resources/Practice-Resources/Administration/Observation-Services-Toolkit/. Accessed August 4, 2016.
38. Hostetler B, Leikin JB, Timmons JA, et al. Patterns of use of an emergency department-based observation unit. Am J Ther 2002;9(6):499–502.
39. Centers for Medicare & Medicaid Services (CMS). CMS Manual System: Pub 100–04 Medicare Claims Processing. 2008.
40. American College of Emergency Physicians. State of the Art: Observation Units in the Emergency Department. 2011. Available at: https://www.acep.org/Physician-Resources/Practice-Resources/Administration/Observation-Services-Toolkit/. Accessed July 28, 2016.
41. Mace SE. An analysis of patient complaints in an observation unit. J Qual Clin Pract 1998;18:151–8.

# Care of the Patient with Chest Pain in the Observation Unit

Joseph B. Borawski, MD, MPH[a],*, Louis G. Graff, MD[b],
Alexander T. Limkakeng, MD, MHS[a]

## KEYWORDS

• Chest pain • Emergency department • Observation unit

## KEY POINTS

• Increases in emergency department (ED) use by patients presenting with chest pain has led to the development of short-term observation units to facilitate an expedited and accurate assessment of their symptoms.
• Clinical decision rules have evolved to help clinicians assess risk of acute coronary syndrome (ACS) in patients presenting with chest pain and play an integral role in determining whether a patient should be a candidate for placement in an observation unit.
• Several provocative testing modalities are available to clinicians to help determine the extent, if any, of symptomatic coronary artery disease.

---

### Case Study

Lucy Epstein is a 63-year-old woman with a history of hypothyroidism, hypertension and breast cancer (now in remission after treatment). Over the past 3 weeks, she has noticed increased dyspnea on exertion. This morning she felt a 4/10 substernal chest pressure in the shower. The pain did not radiate; it was nonpleuritic and spontaneously resolved after approximately 20 minutes. She denies diaphoresis or nausea. Two hours after the chest pain episode, she arrives in an ED where she has an ECG that shows normal sinus rhythm with no new T-wave inversions or ST-segment depressions or elevations. Her physical examination, a chest radiograph and an initial troponin assay are normal. She is placed in an observation unit and repeat ECG and troponin at 6 hours are unchanged; the next day she receives a stress echo that is reassuring and is discharged home with instructions to follow-up with her primary care doctor within the next week.

---

Disclosures: None.
[a] Division of Emergency Medicine, Duke University Medical Center, 2424 Erwin Road, Suite 504, Durham, NC 27705, USA; [b] Department of Emergency Medicine, The Hospital of Central Connecticut, New Britain, CT, USA
* Corresponding author.
*E-mail address:* joseph.borawski@duke.edu

Emerg Med Clin N Am 35 (2017) 535–547
http://dx.doi.org/10.1016/j.emc.2017.03.003
0733-8627/17/© 2017 Elsevier Inc. All rights reserved.

## INTRODUCTION

The evaluation of ACS in EDs remains diagnostically challenging. On a yearly basis it is estimated that more than 6 million people visit an ED for the evaluation of chest pain or other symptoms that are concerning for myocardial ischemia.[1] The differential diagnosis of chest pain is broad and includes many organ systems. In addition to ACS, there are other immediately life-threatening diseases, such as pulmonary embolism, tension pneumothorax, cardiac tamponade, and aortic dissection, that also need to be considered.[2] In several cases, a diagnosis can be made quickly based on initial screening ECG with detection of ST-segment elevation myocardial infarction (STEMI).[3] Patients who present de novo to an ED with STEMI, however, are by far the minority compared with all-comers with a chief complaint of chest pain. Clinical decision rules and accelerated diagnostic protocols help with timely and accurate risk assessment but do not allow for immediate discharge of a majority of patients.

Apprehension about preventable sudden death drives most physicians to err conservatively on the side of admission.[4] The cost of these admissions, however, remains high. As early as 1997 in the United States, hospitalization for more than 3 million patients cost approximately $3 billion to 4 billion annually for those who ultimately are determined disease-free.[5,6] Furthermore, despite diagnostic advances in recent years, missed acute myocardial infarction (AMI) and ACS remain problematic, with estimates ranging between 2% and 10%.[7] Missed AMI remains one of the leading causes of malpractice suits against emergency physicians.[7]

These factors combined to produce the development of a safe, effective, and efficient manner of assessing risk of ACS in ED patients.[8] The use of observation units

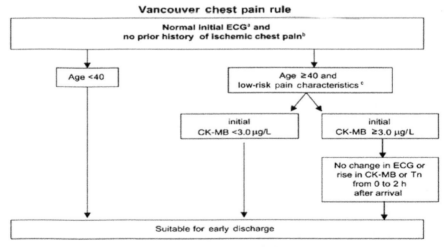

**Fig. 1.** Vancouver Chest Pain Rule algorithm for early discharge of very-low-risk patients with chest pain. CK-MB, creatine kinase–myocardial band isoenzyme. Note: patients with suspicion of other causes for chest pain (eg, pulmonary embolus, aortic dissection) should be investigated independent of this clinical prediction rule. [a] T-wave flattening is the only acceptable ST-T abnormality. [b] Prior ischemic chest pain is defined as a past known diagnosis of MI or angina, previously prescribed nicroglycerin or a clear history of effort-related angina. [c] Low-risk Pain Characteristics is defined as pain not radiating (arm/neck/jaw) OR increasing with a deep breath OR increasing with palpation. MI, myocardial infarction; Tn, troponin. (*From* Christenson J, Innes G, McKnight D, et al. A clinical prediction rule for early discharge of patients with chest pain. Ann Emerg Med 2006;47(1):6; with permission from Elsevier.)

dates back to the late 1980s as EDs began to struggle with growing waiting room numbers, hospital crowding, and overall lack of available inpatient beds. The popularity of ED-based observation units (EDOUs) has increased in recent years and is likely to continue, given policy pressures to reduce hospitalizations, in particular short-terms hospitalizations.[9] EDOUs afford institutions the ability to perform serial cardiac biomarker testing and a wide array of stress testing modalities to identify those patients who would benefit from timely intervention to reduce their risk of a major adverse cardiac event (MACE). EDOUs have been associated with significant reductions in patient-related costs.[10,11] Furthermore, this model has been shown safe and cost-effective and has a high sensitivity for diagnosis of ACS.[11,12]

There are many methods for identifying appropriate EDOU patients.[13] Typically, patients who are selected for observation for this indication receive serial cardiac biomarkers, telemetry monitoring, and some form of objective cardiac testing, such as stress testing. Some units variably incorporate other elements of patient cardiac risk reduction education (smoking cessation, for example) or other further risk stratification care, such as measuring of serum lipids. This article reviews tenets of observation medicine for ED patients with symptoms suggestive of ACS.

## PATIENT SELECTION

In patients with ACS presenting with significant ECG changes, such as STEMI and/or increased levels of cardiac biomarkers, the disposition is often straightforward. Absence of such abnormalities, however, does not exclude ACS.[3] Several clinical risk scores have been proposed and validated in ED patients with symptoms suggestive of ACS.

### HEART Risk Score

The HEART risk score was developed specifically for patients presenting to an ED with undifferentiated chest pain.[14,15] This score is composed of 5 parameters: history, ECG, age, risk factors, and troponin. The provider attributes a score (0–2) within each category to calculate a total of 0 to 10 (**Table 1**). The risk of MACE in patients with a HEART score less than or equal to 3 is 0.9%, 12% in patients with HEART score 4 to 6, and 65% in patients with HEART score greater than or equal to 7.[15] The HEART score was consecutively validated in a single-center retrospective study in 122 patients[14] and a multicenter retrospective investigation in 880 patients.[15] Mahler and colleagues[16] conducted a randomized trial of implementing a pathway incorporating the HEART score, finding a 12.1% reduction in objective testing and a 21.3% increase in early discharges without any MACE in discharged patients. The lead author's institution (JBB, Duke University Medical Center) currently advises routine cardiology admission for patients with HEART scores greater than 7.

### Thrombolysis in Myocardial Infarction

The Thrombolysis in Myocardial Infarction (TIMI) investigators, led by Antman and colleagues,[17] developed and validated a 7-point risk score (**Table 2**) to predict the risk of an adverse cardiac outcome (death, [re]infarction, or recurrent severe ischemia requiring revascularization) within 14 days of presentation for patients with unstable angina or non-STEMI.

The TIMI risk score is derived from the TIMI 11B trial, a multinational, randomized clinical trial, comparing unfractionated heparin to enoxaparin, which included all patients with confirmed ACS.[16] Pollack and colleagues[18] tested the score in an undifferentiated ED population and showed that the risk of 30-day adverse events ranged

**Table 1**
**Composition of the HEART score for chest pain patients in an emergency department**

| HEART score for Chest Pain Patients | | |
|---|---|---|
| History | Highly suspicious | 2 |
| | Moderately suspicious | 1 |
| | Slightly suspicious | 0 |
| ECG | Significant ST depression | 2 |
| | Nonspecific repolarization disturbance | 1 |
| | Normal | 0 |
| Age | ≥65 y | 2 |
| | 45–65 | 1 |
| | ≤45 y | 0 |
| Risk factors | ≥3 risk factors of history of atherosclerotic disease | 2 |
| | 1 or 2 risk factors | 1 |
| | No risk factors known | 0 |
| Troponins | ≥3× normal limit | 2 |
| | 1–3× normal limit | 1 |
| | ≤ normal limit | 0 |

from 2.1% for patients with TIMI score of 0 or 1 to 45% to 100% for patients with a TIMI score of 6 or 7. Furthermore, the utility of this score was confirmed specifically in an EDOU population.[19]

### ADAPT Study

In 2012, Than and colleagues[20] published a new accelerated diagnostic protocol (ADAPT) to identify low-risk ED chest pain patients suitable for early discharge. With the use of this ADP, a large group of patients (20%) presenting with possible ACS was identified as suitable for outpatient care.[21] The ADAPT study team later validated this tool and demonstrated the ability to discharge patients safely with short ED

**Table 2**
**Thrombosis in Myocardial Infarction score for unstable angina/Non–ST-segment Elevation Myocardial Infarction**

| Historical | |
|---|---|
| Age ≥65 y | 0 |
| | 1 |
| ≥3 risk factors for coronary artery disease | 0 |
| | 1 |
| Known coronary artery disease (stenosis ≥50%) | 0 |
| | 1 |
| Acetylsalicylic acid use in the past 7 d | 0 |
| | 1 |
| **Presentation** | |
| Recent (≤24 h) severe angina | 0 |
| | 1 |
| Positive cardiac biomarkers | 0 |
| | 1 |
| ST deviation ≥0.5 mm | 0 |
| | 1 |

stays.[22] This group also derived and validated a second tool called the Emergency Department Assessment of Chest Pain Score accelerated diagnostic pathway that identified half of a large validation cohort as low risk, with 100% sensitivity. An external validation of this rule failed, however, to identify 2 of 17 patients with ACS.

### Vancouver Chest Pain Rule

Like the risk stratification scores discussed previously, the Vancouver Chest Pain Rule sought to identify patients with chest pain who are safe for discharge after 2 hours of ED evaluation. The rule missed fewer than 2% of ACS patients and allowed for discharge within 2 to 3 hours of at least 30% of patients without ACS.[23]

Using this decision-making tree (**Fig. 1**), the Vancouver Chest Pain Rule was 98% sensitive and 32.5% specific for prediction of adverse cardiac events within 30 days of presentation. Jalili and colleagues[24] later validated this decision rule in a prospective cohort study.

In summary, numerous risk stratification tools exist to screen patients who have too low a risk for observation unit care. These seem to improve on clinician gestalt in identifying patients who require further care. A further advance has been the development of shared decision-making tools for ACS work-up.[25] These tools have been shown to decrease testing without any increase in adverse cardiac events.

## CARDIAC BIOMARKERS

Concurrent with the evolution of EDOUs has been the adoption of cardiac troponin assays. In 2000, the American College of Cardiology (ACC), American Heart Association (AHA), and European Society of Cardiology officially advanced the definition of an AMI to the troponin standard.[26,27] This move was made in recognition of troponin's prognostic value and impact on therapeutic decision making, which was demonstrated in numerous studies.[28] A major limitation of cardiac troponin assays is the delay between onset of symptoms and elevation of serum levels.[29] As such, the diagnosis of AMI may require prolonged monitoring and serial blood sampling over a period of up to 3 hours to 12 hours.[30]

An important consideration is that performing a rule out with only cardiac markers is often insufficient.[31] There remains a subset of patients with serial negative troponin assays who remain at short-term risk for MACE. Limkakeng and colleagues[32] evaluated the use of a single cardiac troponin I value in conjunction with a Goldman risk score[33] of less than or equal to 4%, with the hope of identifying patients at low enough risk to immediately be discharged from EDs. The results indicated that even with the combination of a low clinical risk and a negative initial troponin I, the risk for AMI was still present (2.3% at 30 days). The risk stratification tools, discussed previously, have reduced the need for provocative testing and some investigators postulate other technological advances may obviate it (discussed later). For the near future, however, there remains a population of patients who benefit from further objective cardiac testing beyond serial cardiac markers.

## STRESS TESTING

Stress tests attempt to briefly induce myocardial ischemia by means of a stressor and to identify that regional malperfusion through some form of myocardial imaging. To date, there have been many algorithms to determine which patients require further testing before discharge.[34,35] Selected recommendations based on the ACC/AHA guidelines for ECG stress testing (**Box 1**) are discussed.

---

**Box 1**
**American College of Cardiology/American Heart Association recommendations for ECG stress testing**

*Class I (evidence or agreement that the test is indicated)*

1. To diagnose CAD in adult patients with intermediate pretest probability of CAD based on gender, age, and symptoms (specific exceptions noted in class II and III)

2. In patients with suspected or known CAD, previously evaluated, who present with significant change in clinical status

3. Low-risk unstable angina patients 8 hours to 12 hours after presentation who are symptom-free and without signs of heart failure

*Class II (evidence or consensus is conflicted on whether the test is indicated: class IIa – evidence or agreement leans more toward indicated; class IIb – evidence or agreement is inconclusive)*

Class IIa
1. To diagnose CAD in patients with vasospastic angina
2. Evaluation of intermediate-risk unstable angina patients with normal cardiac markers initially and 6 hours to 12 hours after onset of symptoms, repeat ECG without significant changes, and no other evidence of ischemia
3. Evaluation of patients with known or suspected exercise-induced arrhythmias

Class IIb
1. To diagnose CAD in patients with high or low pretest probability based on age, symptoms, and gender

*Class III (evidence or agreement that the test is not indicated)*

1. To diagnose CAD in patients with the following ECG abnormalities: Wolff-Parkinson-White syndrome, electronically paced ventricular rhythm, >1 mm of resting ST depression, or complete LBBB

2. To diagnose CAD in patients with a documented myocardial infarction or prior coronary angiography demonstrating significant disease (however, test can determine ischemia and risk)

*Abbreviation:* CAD, coronary artery disease.

---

Although stress testing is a noninvasive and generally safe procedure, there are patients who have absolute contraindications. Ideally, the clinician, together with the patient, should discuss the appropriate risk/benefit analysis before proceeding with stress testing. **Box 2** outlines those patients in whom stress testing is contraindicated.

### Stressors – Exercise

At the authors' institutions, exercise is preferred whenever possible as the stressor for the stress tests. The reason is that additional prognostic information is gleaned from the test beyond imaging. Prestress test evaluation should assess exercise tolerance as well as look for ECG abnormalities that would confound the exercise ECG interpretation (ST/T changes, left ventricular hypertrophy, left bundle branch block [LBBB], ventricular pre-excitation, and paced ventricular rhythm).[36–38]

The Bruce protocol has become the most widely used treadmill protocol. There are 3 separate stages separated by 3-minute periods. Patients must reach 85% of their age-predicted maximum heart rate, attain more than 5 metabolic equivalents workload, and exercise for at least 3 minutes to complete stage 1 of the standard Bruce protocol.[39] It is common to terminate tests when patients reach 85% of their targeted

Box 2
Stress testing contraindications

*Absolute*

- AMI within 2 days
- High-risk unstable angina
- Uncontrolled cardiac arrhythmia with hemodynamic compromise
- Uncontrolled arrhythmias causing symptoms or hemodynamic compromise
- Symptomatic severe aortic stenosis
- Uncontrolled symptomatic heart failure
- Acute pulmonary embolism or pulmonary infarction
- Acute myocarditis or pericarditis
- Endocarditis
- Acute aortic dissection
- Acute noncardiac issue (sepsis and toxicologic)

*Relative*

- Left main coronary artery stenosis
- Moderate to severe aortic stenosis
- Electrolyte abnormalities
- Severe arterial hypertension (>200/110 mm Hg)
- Tachyarrhythmias or bradyarrhythmias
- Hypertrophic cardiomyopathy or other forms of outflow tract obstruction
- Mental or physical impairment leading to inability to exercise adequately
- High-degree atrioventricular block

heart rate based on age.[39,40] Additionally, the ACC/AHA have set forth guidelines that specify other reasons for termination of exercise testing (**Table 3**).[41]

### Stressors – Pharmacologic

Invariably, there is a portion of patients unable to complete exercise testing. In these instances, pharmacologic testing with vasodilators is recommended. Vasodilator agents are classified by their action on the adenosine receptor. There are 4 types of adenosine receptors: A1, A2A, A2B, and A3. Stimulation of the A2A receptor causes coronary artery dilation, whereas the other receptors cause side effects. There are nonselective agents, such as adenosine and dipyridamole, and there are selective agents, namely binodenoson, regadenoson, and apadenoson.[42] Currently, regadenoson is the only US Food and Drug Administration–approved selective adenosine receptor agonist agent and is the most commonly used vasodilator agent for myocardial perfusion imaging (MPI). In comparison to adenosine, it is less rapidly metabolized, allowing it to be given as a bolus rather than an intravenous infusion.[35]

There is a subset of patients for whom these agents are contraindicated. Specifically, those with reactive airway disease (RAD) or high-grade heart block should not be given these agents. Furthermore, patients must have abstained from caffeine, β-blockers, nitrates, and methylxanthine-containing medications for 24 hours prior to

**Table 3**
**Reasons for termination of a stress test**

| Absolute Indications for Termination of Testing | Relative Indications for Termination of Testing |
|---|---|
| • Drop in SBP of more than 10 mm Hg from baseline, despite an increase in workload, when accompanied by other evidence of ischemia<br>• Moderate to severe angina<br>• Increasing nervous system symptoms (eg, ataxia, dizziness, and near-syncope)<br>• Signs of poor perfusion (cyanosis or pallor)<br>• Technical difficulties in monitoring ECG tracings or SBP<br>• Subject's desire to stop<br>• Sustained ventricular tachycardia<br>• ST elevation (>1 mm) in leads without diagnostic Q waves (other than V1 or aVR) | • Drop in SBP of 10 mm Hg or more from baseline, despite an increase in workload, in the absence of other evidence of ischemia<br>• ST or QRS changes, such as excessive ST depression (horizontal or down-sloping ST-segment depression >2 mm) or marked axis shift<br>• Arrhythmias other than sustained ventricular tachycardia, including multifocal PVCs, triplets of PVCs, supraventricular tachycardia, heart block, or bradyarrhythmias<br>• Fatigue, shortness of breath, wheezing, leg cramps, or claudication<br>• Development of bundle branch block or intraventricular conduction delay that cannot be distinguished from ventricular tachycardia<br>• Increasing chest pain<br>• Hypertensive response (SBP of 250 mm Hg, DBP higher than 115 mm Hg, or both) |

*Abbreviations:* DBP, diastolic blood pressure; PVC, premature ventricular contraction; SBP, systolic blood pressure.

the study. Medications containing dipyridamole and verapamil should be stopped 48 hours prior to the test.[43,44]

Another stressor agent is the positive inotropic agent, dobutamine. Although this agent does have a higher side-effect profile, if the patient is extremely exercise limited, has RAD, and/or has consumed caffeine in the last 24 hours, this modality may be the stressor of choice.[31] **Table 4** outlines specific dobutamine contraindications.

There are several articles that outline the specific details regarding the administration and timing of stressor agent.[45–47]

### Assessments

Most centers have added imaging components to ECG during stress testing due to the increased diagnostic and prognostic information that is gained.[48] Stress echocardiography is a noninvasive technology that images the heart using ultrasound.[49] Baseline images at rest are compared with those obtained during or immediately after

**Table 4**
**Contraindications to dobutamine use**

| | |
|---|---|
| Recent AMI | Unstable angina |
| Aortic stenosis | Atrial tachycardias |
| Uncontrolled hypertension | Thoracic aortic aneurysm |
| LBBB | History of ventricular tachycardia |

stress. Areas of wall motion abnormality (induced by stress) are evidence of myocardial ischemia.

An alternative modality is MPI, which uses a radiopharmaceutical tracer to evaluate the changes in myocardial perfusion at rest and after stress. At the authors' institutions, the most commonly used MPI modality is single photon-emission CT (SPECT) with technetium TC 99m Tc stestamibi. There are few contraindications to MPI apart from optimizing patient selection based on pretest probability.[50] Because MPI does involve exposure to radioactive materials, patients who have received prior nuclear medicine agents for tests, such as ventilation/perfusion scans, should not receive MPI for at least 24 hours. Furthermore, patients weighing more than 400 pounds may require a 2-day protocol in which resting and stress images are obtained separately due to the maximum safe amount of radioactive tracer that can be administered in 1 dose.[35,49]

### Test Selection

In practice, local standards, resources, and preference often drive stress test modality selection. This discussion reflects the approach taken by the authors' institutions' emergency medicine, cardiology, and nuclear cardiology divisions. Exercise should be included when possible because of the additional prognostic information provided.[48,51] At the authors' institutions, the preferred modality is stress echocardiography. This was chosen due to technical experience, lack of radiation, and evidence of modestly higher specificity.[38] For those who require pharmacologic testing, dobutamine SPECT or PET is typically done. Lastly, for those that cannot have either echocradiogram or SPECT, who have prior equivocal stress test results, or who have known coronary artery disease, cardiac MRI is also an option.

### CONTROVERSIES

One common difficult scenario for ED physicians is patients with recurrent or persistent symptoms who recently had a normal stress test. It has been noted in contemporary practice that stress testing did not decrease subsequent recurrent testing in such patients.[38] A guide in such scenarios is that the overall incidence rate of MACE after a normal, adequate stress test is less than 1% per patient per year. That said, it is incumbent on ED physicians to ascertain patients' prior stress testing results and to risk-stratify them based on their current symptoms and ECG. If a patient's recurrent presentation is still low risk for ACS, it is the authors' practice to consider other causes for the patients' symptoms, particularly if the stress test was performed within the past year. For patients whose recurrent presentation is thought to be at high risk for ACS, cardiac MRI and/or cardiology consultation is considered, regardless of when the last stress test occurred.

Some investigators have suggested that the growing prevalence of chest pain observation units has contributed to an increasingly overconservative approach to ACS evaluation. In 1 study, up to 15% to 20% of stress tests that were ordered did not meet appropriate use guidelines.[48] Blecker and colleagues[52] recently posited that observation units may create a supply-induced demand. They estimated that approximately half of ED visits that resulted in observation unit care for chest pain would have been discharged home had the observation unit not been available.

Some investigators have questioned the utility of routine stress testing, arguing that the risks from stress testing outweigh any benefit.[53,54] The authors agree that careful selection of patients is important, as discussed previously. There have been some investigators, for example, who have found low utility of stress testing in patients under the age of 40 years.[55] Furthermore, it is important to recognize that the purpose of stress testing is to provide an estimate of a patient's risk of having significant coronary artery disease; it, therefore, does not need to be repeated reflexively at every ED visit or ordered for patients judged at very low risk for this disease.

A recent development has been the introduction of high-sensitivity cardiac troponin assays. Such assays have a much lower (as much as 10-fold) limit of detection and higher precision at lower concentrations. Although these assays represent a technological advance, they cannot obviate continued observation for a portion of patients. Reichlin and colleagues[56] reported that up to only 25% of patients would be affected by the implementation of their high-sensitivity cardiac troponin T–1-hour algorithm. Patients in the observational zone would still need to go on to further diagnostic (including stress) testing to complete their evaluation. Given that there will be an increasing proportion of patients with an initially detectable troponin level using these assays, observation units may see an increase in volumes.

## SUMMARY

Observation units have been developed to improve care of patients who do not have an obvious clinical condition after their ED evaluation. Selected people with chest pain are one of the most prominent groups of such patients. They benefit from observation unit care with standardizing timely and accurate risk assessment, implementation of clinical decision rules, and use of accelerated diagnostic protocols. They are a modern structure for cost-effective, high-quality outpatient/in-hospital patient care.

## REFERENCES

1. Bhiuya FA, Pitts SR, McCaig LF. Emergency department visits for chest pain and abdominal pain: United States, 1999-2008. NCHS Data Brief. 2010 (43). Hyattsville (MD): Nation Center for Health Statistics; 2010.
2. Swap CJ, Nagurney JT. Value and limitations of chest pain history in the evaluation of patients with suspected acute coronary syndromes. JAMA 2005;294(20): 2623–9.
3. Backus BE, Six AJ, Kelder JH, et al. Risk scores of patients with chest pain: evaluation in the emergency department. Curr Cardiol Rev 2011;7:2–8.
4. Wears RL, Li S, Hernandez JD, et al. How many myocardial infarctions should we rule out? Ann Emerg Med 1989;18:953–63.
5. McCarthy BD, Wong JB, Selker HP. Detecting acute ischemia in the emergency department: a review of the literature. J Gen Intern Med 1990;5:365–73.
6. Lambrew CT. Chest pain evaluation: through a glass darkly. Ann Emerg Med 1997;29:116–25.
7. McCarthy BD, Beshansky JR, D'Agostino RB, et al. Missed diagnoses of acute myocardial infarction in the emergency department: results from a multi-center study. Ann Emerg Med 1993;22:579–82.
8. Ross MA, Aurora T, Graff L, et al. State of the art: emergency department observation units [review]. Crit Pathw Cardiol 2012;11(3):128–38.
9. Sheehy AM, Caponi B, Gangireddy S, et al. Observation and inpatient status: clinical impact of the 2-midnight rule. J Hosp Med 2014;9:203–9.
10. Roberts RR, Zalenski RJ, Mensah EK, et al. Costs of an emergency department-based accelerated diagnostic protocol vs hospitalization in patients with chest pain: a randomized controlled trial. JAMA 1997;278:1670–6.

11. Gomez MA, Anderson JL, Karagounis LA, et al. An emergency department-based protocol for rapidly ruling out myocardial ischemia reduces hospital time and expense: results of a randomized study (ROMIO). J Am Coll Cardiol 1996; 24:1249–59.

12. Graff L, Delera J, Ross M, et al. Chest pain evaluation registry (CHEPER) study: impact on the care of the emergency department chest pain patient. Am J Cardiol 1997;80:563–8.

13. Wilkerson K, Severance H. Identification of chest pain patients appropriate for an emergency department observation unit. Emerg Med Clin North Am 2001;19(1): 35–66.

14. Six AJ, Backus BE, Kelder JC. Chest pain in the emergency room: value of the HEART score. Neth Heart J 2008;16:191–6.

15. Backus BE, Six AJ, Kelder JC, et al. Chest pain in the emergency room: a multi-center validation of the HEART score. Crit Pathw Cardiol 2010;9:164–9.

16. Mahler SA, Riley RF, Hiestand BC, et al. The HEART Pathway randomized trial: identifying emergency department patients with acute chest pain for early discharge. Circ Cardiovasc Qual Outcomes 2015;8(2):195–203.

17. Antman EM, Cohen M, Bernink PJ, et al. The TIMI risk score for unstable angina/non-ST elevation MI: a method for prognostication and therapeutic decision making. JAMA 2000;101:835–42.

18. Pollack CV, Sites FD, Shofer FS, et al. Application of the TIMI risk score for unstable angina and non-ST-elevation acute coronary syndrome to an unselected emergency department chest pain population. Acad Emerg Med 2006;13(1): 13–8.

19. Chavez J, Srinivasan A, Ely S, et al. Thrombolysis in myocardial infarction risk score in an observation unit setting. Crit Pathw Cardiol 2013;12(3):137–40.

20. Than M, Cullen L, Aldous S, et al. A 2-hour accelerated diagnostic protocol to assess patients with chest pain symptoms using contemporary troponins as the only biomarker: the ADAPT trial. J Am Coll Cardiol 2012;59:2091–8.

21. Than M, Aldous S, Lord SJ, et al. A 2-hour diagnostic protocol for possible cardiac chest pain in the emergency department: a randomized clinical trial. JAMA Intern Med 2014;174:51–8.

22. Than MP, Pickering JW, Aldous SJ, et al. Effectiveness of EDACS versus ADAPT accelerated diagnostic pathways for chest pain: a pragmatic randomized controlled trial embedded within practice. Ann Emerg Med 2016;68(1): 93–102.e1.

23. Christenson J, Innes G, McKnight D, et al. A clinical prediction rule for early discharge of patients with chest pain. Ann Emerg Med 2006;47(1):1–10.

24. Jalili M, Hejripour Z, Honarmand A, et al. Validation of the Vancoouver Chest Pain Rule: a prospective cohort study. Acad Emerg Med 2012;19(7):837–42.

25. Hess EP, Knoedler MA, Shah ND, et al. The chest pain choice decision aid: a randomized trial. Circ Cardiovasc Qual Outcomes 2012;5(3):251–9.

26. Newby LK, Kaplan AL, Granger BB, et al. Comparison of cardiac troponin T versus creatine kinase-MB for risk stratification in a chest pain evaluation unit. Am J Cardiol 2000;85:801–5.

27. Alpert JS, Thygesen K, Antman E, et al. Myocardial infarction redefined–a consensus document of The Joint European Society of Cardiology/American College of Cardiology Committee for the redefinition of myocardial infarction. J Am Coll Cardiol 2000;36:959–69.

28. Hamm CW, Heeschen C, Goldmann B, et al. Benefit of abciximab in patients with refractory unstable angina in relation to serum troponin T levels. c7E3 Fab

Antiplatelet Therapy in Unstable Refractory Angina (CAPTURE) Study Investigators. N Engl J Med 1999;340:1623–9.

29. Hamm CW, Goldmann BU, Heeschen C, et al. Emergency room triage of patients with acute chest pain by means of rapid testing for cardiac troponin T or troponin I. N Engl J Med 1997;337:1648–53.

30. Fesmire FM, Decker WW, Diercks DB, et al. American College of Emergency Physicians Clinical Policies Subcommittee (Writing Committee) on Non-ST-Segment Elevation Acute Coronary Syndromes. Clinical policy: critical issues in the evaluation and management of adult patients with non-ST-segment elevation acute coronary syndromes. Ann Emerg Med 2006;48(3):270–301.

31. Miyamoto MI, Vernotico SL, Majmundar H, et al. Pharmacologic stress myocardial perfusion imaging: a practical approach. J Nucl Cardiol 2007;14(2):250–5.

32. Limkakeng A, Gibler W, Pollack C, et al. Combination of Goldman Risk and initial cardiac troponin I for emergency department chest pain patient risk stratification. Acad Emerg Med 2001;8(7):696–702.

33. Goldman L, Weinberg M, Weisberg M, et al. A computerderived protocol to aid in the diagnosis of emergency room patients with acute chest pain. N Engl J Med 1982;307:588–96.

34. Wright RS, Anderson JL, Adams CD, et al. 2011 ACCF/AHA focused update incorporated into the ACC/AHA 2007 Guidelines for the Management of Patients with Unstable Angina/Non-ST-Elevation Myocardial Infarction: a report of the American College of Cardiology Foundation/American Heart Association Task Force on Practice Guidelines developed in collaboration with the American Academy of Family Physicians, Society for Cardiovascular Angiography and Interventions, and the Society of Thoracic Surgeons. J Am Coll Cardiol 2011;57(19):e215–367.

35. Borges-Neto S, Coleman RE, Jones RH. Perfusion and function at rest and treadmill exercise using technetium-99m-sestamibi: comparison of one- and two-day protocols in normal volunteers. J Nucl Med 1990;31(7):1128–32.

36. Fihn SD, Gardin JM, Abrams J, et al. 2012 ACCF/AHA/ACP/AATS/PCNA/SCAI/STS Guideline for the diagnosis and management of patients with stable ischemic heart disease: a report of the American College of Cardiology Foundation/American Heart Association Task Force on Practice Guidelines, and the American College of Physicians, American Association for Thoracic Surgery, Preventive Cardiovascular Nurses Association, Society for Cardiovascular Angiography and Interventions, and Society of Thoracic Surgeons. J Am Coll Cardiol 2012;60(24):e44–164.

37. Patel RN, Arteaga RB, Mandawat MK, et al. Pharmacologic stress myocardial perfusion imaging. South Med J 2007;100(10):1006–14 [quiz: 4].

38. Fleischmann KE, Hunink MG, Kuntz KM, et al. Exercise echocardiography or exercise SPECT imaging? A meta-analysis of diagnostic test performance. JAMA 1998;280(10):913–20.

39. Shah BN. On the 50th anniversary of the first description of a multistage exercise treadmill test: re-visiting the birth of the 'Bruce protocol'. Heart 2013;99(24):1793–4.

40. Tanaka H, Monahan KD, Seals DR. Age-predicted maximal heart rate revisited. J Am Coll Cardiol 2001;37(1):153–6.

41. Hlatky MA, Pryor DB, Harrell FE Jr, et al. Factors affecting sensitivity and specificity of exercise electrocardiography. Multivariable analysis. Am J Med 1984;77(1):64–71.

42. Rakesh N, Patel M, Roque B, et al. Pharmacologic stress myocardial perfusion imaging. South Med J 2007;100(10):1006–14.

43. Underwood SR, Anagnostopoulos C, Cerqueira M, et al. Myocardial perfusion scintigraphy: the evidence. Eur J Nucl Med Mol Imaging 2004;31(2):261–91.
44. Committee OHTA. Single photon emission computed tomography for the diagnosis of coronary artery disease: an evidence-based analysis. Ont Health Technol Assess Ser 2010;10(8):1–64.
45. Ficaro EP. Imaging guidelines for nuclear cardiology procedures. J Nucl Cardiol 2006;13(6):888.
46. Thomas GS, Prill NV, Majmundar H, et al. Treadmill exercise during adenosine infusion is safe, results in fewer adverse reactions, and improves myocardial perfusion image quality. J Nucl Cardiol 2000;7(5):439–46.
47. Iskandrian AE, Bateman TM, Belardinelli L, et al. Adenosine versus regadenoson comparative evaluation in myocardial perfusion imaging: results of the ADVANCE phase 3 multicenter international trial. J Nucl Cardiol 2007;14(5):645–58.
48. Johnson TV, Rose GA, Fenner DJ, et al. Improving appropriate use of echocardiography and single-photon emission computed tomographic myocardial perfusion imaging: a continuous quality improvement initiative. J Am Soc Echocardiogr 2014;27(7):749–57.
49. Committee OHTA. Stress echocardiography for the diagnosis of coronary artery disease: an evidence-based analysis. Ont Health Technol Assess Ser 2010;10(9): 1–61.
50. Hendel RC, Berman DS, Di Carli MF, et al. ACCF/ASNC/ACR/AHA/ASE/SCCT/SCMR/SNM 2009 Appropriate use criteria for cardiac radionuclide imaging: a report of the American College of Cardiology Foundation Appropriate Use Criteria Task Force, the American Society of Nuclear Cardiology, the American College of Radiology, the American Heart Association, the American Society of Echocardiography, the Society of Cardiovascular Computed Tomography, the Society for Cardiovascular Magnetic Resonance, and the Society of Nuclear Medicine. J Am Coll Cardiol 2009;53(23):2201–29.
51. Iskander S, Iskandrian AE. Risk assessment using single-photon emission computed tomographic technetium-99m sestamibi imaging. J Am Coll Cardiol 1998;32(1):57–62.
52. Blecker S, Gavin N, Park H, et al. Observation units as substitutes for hospitalization or home discharge. Ann Emerg Med 2016;67(6):706–13.e2.
53. Foy AJ, Liu G, Davidson WR Jr, et al. Comparative effectiveness of diagnostic testing strategies in emergency department patients with chest pain: an analysis of downstream testing, interventions, and outcomes. JAMA Intern Med 2015; 175(3):428–36.
54. Hermann LK, Newman DH, Pleasant WA, et al. Yield of routine provocative cardiac testing among patients in an emergency department-based chest pain unit. JAMA Intern Med 2013;173(12):1128–33.
55. Hermann LK, Weingart SD, Yoon YM, et al. Comparison of frequency of inducible myocardial ischemia in patients presenting to emergency department with typical versus atypical or nonanginal chest pain. Am J Cardiol 2010;105(11):1561–4.
56. Reichlin T, Cullen L, Parsonage WA, et al. Two-hour algorithm for triage toward rule-out and rule-in of acute myocardial infarction using high-sensitivity cardiac troponin T. Am J Med 2015;128(4):369–79.e4.

# Cardiovascular Conditions in the Observation Unit

## Beyond Chest Pain

Jeremiah D. Gaddy, MD[a], Kathleen T.P. Davenport, MD[b],
Brian C. Hiestand, MD, MPH[a],*

### KEYWORDS

- Emergency department • Observation unit • Cardiovascular conditions
- Atrial fibrillation • Syncope • Heart failure • Venous thromboembolism

### KEY POINTS

- The first emergency department observation units (EDOUs) focused on chest pain and potential acute coronary syndromes.
- Most EDOUs now cover multiple other conditions that lend themselves to protocolized, aggressive diagnostic and therapeutic regimens.
- We discuss 4 cardiovascular conditions that have been successfully deployed in EDOUs around the country.

## INTRODUCTION

The first emergency department (ED) observation units (EDOUs) focused on chest pain and potential acute coronary syndromes. However, most EDOUs now cover multiple other conditions that lend themselves to protocolized, aggressive diagnostic and therapeutic regimens. In this article, the authors discuss the management of 4 cardiovascular conditions that have been successfully deployed in EDOUs around the country.

## ATRIAL FIBRILLATION
### Epidemiology and Disease Burden

Atrial fibrillation (AF) is the most common clinically significant cardiac arrhythmia, affecting more than 2 million people in the United States and more than 46 million people worldwide.[1–3] The incidence of new-onset AF increases with age and is estimated

[a] Department of Emergency Medicine, Wake Forest School of Medicine, Medical Center Boulevard, Winston-Salem, NC 27157, USA; [b] Department of Emergency Medicine, Brigham and Women's Hospital, Harvard Medical School, 75 Francis Street, Boston, MA 02115, USA
* Corresponding author. Medical Center Boulevard, Winston-Salem, NC 27157.
E-mail address: bhiestan@wakehealth.edu

Emerg Med Clin N Am 35 (2017) 549–569
http://dx.doi.org/10.1016/j.emc.2017.03.004
0733-8627/17/© 2017 Elsevier Inc. All rights reserved.
emed.theclinics.com

to occur in 1% of persons aged 60 to 68 years and in 5% of persons aged 69 years and older.[4]

AF is a significant contributor to the national health care expenditure. Currently, AF accounts for 1% of total ED visits and the rate is increasing.[5] From 1993 to 2004, the number of ED visits for AF increased by 88%; of those patients, approximately 65% were hospitalized.[2,3,6] The rate of hospitalization has increased by 66% over the last 2 decades because of both the growth in the aging population and the increased prevalence of chronic heart disease.[7]

The ever-growing prevalence of AF, hospital overcrowding, and the increasing cost of inpatient admissions have spurred the development of new and innovative management strategies to safely and efficiently care for these patients.[5,8] In the United States, most (70%) patients presenting to the ED with a primary diagnosis of AF are admitted to the hospital.[9] This finding contrasts with the experience in Canada, where studies have demonstrated that 85% of ED patients with AF can be safely discharged home.[1,10] This practice variation has sparked interest in the use of the EDOU for rapid management of patients with AF.[1] Decker and colleagues[4] established that new-onset AF managed in an EDOU, compared with the inpatient setting, can result in a decreased median length of stay (10 hours vs 25 hours) with similar rates of rate and rhythm control. These studies and others have formed the basis for the successful implementation of safe, efficient, and cost-effective EDOU protocols.

## PATIENT SELECTION

A successful EDOU protocol for AF relies on an expedited algorithm incorporating anticoagulation, rate and rhythm control, and mechanisms to ensure rapid outpatient follow-up. Managing patients with AF in the EDOU relies on appropriate patient selection. The ideal patients are stable, without cardiac ischemia, and with onset of AF of less than 48 hours duration.[2] The systolic blood pressure (SBP) should be 90 mm Hg or greater and heart rate less than 110 beats per minute (bpm) at the time of disposition to the EDOU, after administration of any required intravenous medications for rate control.[1] Patients with AF secondary to an underlying cause, such as sepsis, pulmonary embolism, gastrointestinal (GI) bleed, or other life-threatening conditions that require hospital admission, are not candidates for EDOU management.[11] Other relative contraindications to placing patients in the EDOU include acute renal insufficiency, pregnant patients, patients with an unknown time of AF onset, and patients with an expected length of stay of greater than 36 hours due to other comorbidities or socioeconomic considerations complicating their care.[6] Additionally, patients who have poor health literacy, lack close follow-up, or who are unable to adhere to their treatment plan are not appropriate EDOU patients because they will require more intensive hospital and case management resources.[2]

## PATIENT MANAGEMENT

The management of patients with unstable AF is not appropriate for the EDOU and is not reviewed here. After initial ED evaluation, the next step is to decide whether to control the heart rate or convert patients to a normal sinus rhythm. In patients 65 years of age and older, there is no difference in 5-year outcomes of stroke or death with rate versus rhythm control.[11] Therefore, in this age group, rate control and anticoagulation, if indicated, should generally be the EDOU goal.[12]

Younger patients (aged <65 years) have been shown to benefit from rhythm control and should be considered for cardioversion.[11] The risk factors for immediate stroke following cardioversion include an unknown time from onset, a history of transient ischemic attack (TIA) or stroke in the last 6 months, and valve disease.[12] The focus in these patients should be on rate rather than rhythm control.[11] Also, patients with electrolyte abnormalities, such as hypokalemia, or with digoxin toxicity are at higher risk of poor outcomes with immediate rhythm control and should be managed with rate control.[11] If patients are deemed low risk for stroke, with an AF onset of 48 hours ago or less or if patients have been on anticoagulation for 3 weeks or more, then cardioversion can be considered.[6,12] This low-risk group of patients can be ideally managed in the EDOU.

When controlling rate, the two most commonly used pharmacologic agents are β-blockers (commonly metoprolol) and nondihydropyridine calcium channel blockers (commonly diltiazem).[11] There is no solid evidence of one agent being superior to the other. However, the authors do suggest providers avoid crossing classes; if patients are already taking an oral β-blocker, for example, a parenteral β-blocker should be considered for first-line therapy as opposed to initiating a calcium channel blocker. Following administration of the intravenous agent, patients should be started on the equivalent oral dose of the medication to maintain adequate rate control.[5] The goal heart rate, before EDOU placement, should be less than 100 bpm while at rest and less than 120 bpm when ambulatory.[6] These acceptable rates vary, and some guidelines suggest adequate rate control is achieved at less than 110 bpm while at rest and less than 130 bpm while ambulatory.[11]

The availability of procedural sedation in the EDOU may dictate whether cardioversion occurs in the ED before observation placement. If planning a synchronized electrical cardioversion, it is recommended to use an initial 150 to 200 J of energy with anterior-posterior pad electrical placement using a biphasic waveform device.[12,13] This method has been shown to successfully convert patients 90% of the time.[11] For patients who are poor sedation candidates, chemical cardioversion may be preferred. The most common pharmacologic agents include intravenous procainamide (Vaughan Williams class Ia), oral flecainide (class Ic), or intravenous ibutilide (class III).[6,11] Procainamide is not the preferred method in the United States and is not included in the American Heart Association's (AHA) guidelines.[2] If anticoagulation is going to be used, it is generally advised to start as soon as possible.[12]

In some systems, rapid transesophageal echocardiography (TEE) may be available for patients with unclear or prolonged duration of their AF. These patients, if otherwise appropriate for EDOU management, could receive rate control, anticoagulation, and TEE to evaluate for cardiac thrombi. Cardioversion immediately after TEE could occur during the same procedural sedation. Local resources will dictate the feasibility of that particular strategy.

Following cardioversion or rate control, the provider must determine the need for long-term anticoagulation.[2] The most commonly used and validated clinical tool for stroke and thromboembolism risk stratification is the $CHA_2DS_2$-VASc (congestive HF, hypertension, age, diabetes mellitus, prior stroke or TIA or thromboembolism, vascular disease, age, sex) score (**Table 1**).[2,14] The AHA recommends oral anticoagulation for a score of 2 or greater, whereas European guidelines recommend oral anticoagulation for scores of one or greater.[11] The Canadian guidelines suggest giving aspirin to patients with a score of zero but with known coronary artery disease.[12] Providers must also assess patients' bleeding risk. One validated scheme is the HAS-BLED score. This scoring system applies one point for each of the following risk factors: *H*ypertension, *A*bnormal liver or kidney dysfunction, *S*troke, *B*leeding predisposition, *L*abile international normalized ratio (INR), *E*lderly (older than 65 years), and *D*rugs (use of antiplatelet medications, such as clopidogrel (Plavix) or aspirin, or alcohol consumption >8 drinks per week). A score of 3 or greater indicates a high

| Table 1 | |
|---|---|
| CHA$_2$DS$_2$-VASc scoring system | |
| **CHA$_2$DS$_2$-VASc** | **Score** |
| Congestive heart failure | 1 |
| Hypertension | 1 |
| Age $\geq$75 y | 2 |
| Diabetes mellitus | 1 |
| Stroke/TIA/thromboembolism | 2 |
| Vascular disease | 1 |
| Age 65–74 y | 1 |
| Sex category (ie, female sex) | 1 |
| Total maximum score | 9 |

*From* Peacock WF, Clark CL. Short stay management of atrial fibrillation. Switzerland: Springer International Publishing; 2016; with permission.

risk of bleeding.[11] If patients are at high risk of bleeding and have a high stroke risk, then the decision to prescribe anticoagulation should be made with patients weighing the risk and benefits of anticoagulation and using shared decision-making to come to a conclusion.[13]

Historically, warfarin was the most commonly used anticoagulation agent; however, it requires blood levels to be drawn and interacts with many foods and medications. The non–vitamin K direct oral anticoagulants (NOACs, formerly novel oral anticoagulants, sometimes called target-specific oral anticoagulants or direct oral anticoagulants [DOACs], the term that is used through the remainder of this work) have become increasingly popular in recent years and are generally preferred over warfarin in patients with nonvalvular AF. These medications are more convenient for patients and have proven to be equally safe and effective.[2,12] Additionally, there is no requirement to bridge with unfractionated heparin (UFH) or low-molecular-weight heparin (LMWH) with rivaroxaban or apixaban, as there is with warfarin. DOACs are also preferred in situations whereby patients cannot reliably get their INR blood levels checked or adhere to the diet restrictions required when taking warfarin.[2,11] If patients have renal failure or new acute renal insufficiency or hepatic disease, then consultation or discussion with cardiology regarding appropriate anticoagulation is recommended.

If at any point patients become unstable or the EDOU treatment protocol fails, patients should be formally admitted to the hospital for further management and evaluation.

## EDUCATION

Admission to the EDOU provides a unique opportunity to educate patients on their diagnosis of AF. The discussion should focus on determining patients' AF symptoms and identifying their specific triggers.[2] If patients are started on anticoagulation, they should be educated about bleeding risks and potential bleeding complications. They should also be instructed to carry a medication card in their wallet or wear a medical alert bracelet that informs emergency medical services and other providers that they are on an anticoagulation medication.[2] Additionally, if patients are being discharged on rate or rhythm control medications, they should be educated about the common side effects of the medications and the importance of taking the medications as prescribed.[2] The most important aspect of patient education is emphasizing the importance of early outpatient follow-up.

## DISCHARGE AND FOLLOW-UP

In order for patients to be discharged from the EDOU, they must demonstrate clinical stability with either their AF rate controlled or their rhythm converted to normal sinus for at least 1 to 2 hours.[1] Most EDOU protocols also require negative serial cardiac biomarker tests before discharge if ACS is suspected as a contributory factor.[1] Outpatient follow-up in 3 to 5 days following discharge should be established before patients leave the EDOU. Additionally, a 30-day prescription for the selected method of anticoagulation, if indicated, should be given before discharge.[8] If patients were not cardioverted and are being discharged on rate control medications, they should be prescribed the lowest long-acting oral dose equivalent to what they received in the EDOU.[6] Finally, patients and their families should be provided with strict return precautions so that they understand when to return to the ED or hospital for care. Following these guidelines will allow for a successful EDOU visit and early discharge, thus, minimizing the burden of an AF diagnosis on patients' daily life.

## ACUTE HEART FAILURE
### Epidemiology and Disease Burden

Heart failure (HF) is a substantial public health problem with an ever-increasing incidence and prevalence. According to community surveillance reports, there are 915,000 new HF cases annually, resulting in an estimated 5.7 million Americans with chronic HF.[15] As a result of the epidemiologic burden, HF is the single most costly diagnosis in the US health care system.[16] In the United States, acute HF currently results in 676,000 annual ED visits, with more than 80% of patients requiring hospitalization.[15,17] As a result, emergency physicians serve as the primary gate keeper for one of the costliest decisions for patients with acute HF: admission versus outpatient care.

EDOUs have been established as excellent alternatives for patients who are not stable for immediate discharge from the ED but may not need greater than 24 hours of care. EDOUs provide a cost-effective alternative to admission that has been shown to offer savings, shorter stays, and reduced admissions.[18–23] With proper patient selection and risk stratification, EDOU care can be a valuable tool in the management of patients with acute HF.

## PATIENT SELECTION

Obviously, not all patients with acute HF are appropriate for observation care. Patients at high risk for inpatient morbidity or mortality, those who will require inpatient procedures or critical care acuity, or those with socioeconomic challenges that would preclude safe disposition within 48 and, ideally, 24 hours will not be good candidates for observation management. Multiple risk stratification schemes have been published that identify high-risk patients. Therefore, it is cognitively simple to identify those patients who are completely inappropriate for observation care. It is important to realize, however, that the absence of a high risk for mortality does not mean that patients are considered low risk and, therefore, appropriate for rapid disposition from an EDOU.

The Society of Chest Pain Centers (now the Society for Cardiovascular Patient Care) published recommendations on risk stratification as well as EDOU management of acute HF syndrome,[24] which were later validated in an external data set.[25] However, the strength of evidence for most of these recommendations was based on expert consensus. At that time, a definitive evidence base for patient risk stratification from the ED for acute HF was lacking. This evidence deficit continues to the current era.[26–28] The literature base on ED risk stratification and the specific identification of low-risk, short-stay-appropriate patients continues to evolve[29–32]; but further work is needed to define a broadly applicable, validated decision tool that adds to physician decision-making. Therefore, the statements that follow are based on the best available evidence but should be considered recommendations, as opposed to rigid guidelines, in most cases.

Most patients with newly diagnosed HF presenting with acute symptoms should be admitted to an inpatient unit. The initial workup and management required will generally surpass the recommended 24-hour observation time. Mild cases of new-onset HF could conceivably be referred for outpatient management, but this may not be typical of patients' acuity presenting to the ED. Likewise, access to appropriate outpatient follow-up in a timely fashion from the ED may be difficult for many patients.[33]

Any new ischemic changes noted in the electrocardiogram (EKG) should be exclusion criteria for EDOU management, as should an unstable cardiac arrhythmia.[24] Hypotension is less clear. Patients presenting with a SBP less than 120 mm Hg have been shown to have increased inpatient mortality.[34,35] However, given the adverse effects of increased afterload in chronic HF, target blood pressures for outpatient management are frequently lower than this.[36] Therefore, it is more useful to recommend that poor perfusion, or symptomatic hypotension, serve as the criterion for EDOU exclusion as opposed to an absolute number.

Dyspnea is one of the most common presenting symptoms of acute HF. After initial treatment, respiratory rate and oxygen requirements should be taken into account when deciding on EDOU versus inpatient admission. Although noninvasive ventilatory support (NIV) may reduce respiratory distress and improve physiologic parameters,[37] patients who are unable to be weaned in the ED should be admitted to the hospital and are not appropriate for EDOU management. However, the patient response to initial management should be considered as well. Flash pulmonary edema may initially require aggressive management with afterload reduction and NIV. Frequently, though, these patients quickly respond and no longer require intensive care unit–level interventions within hours of treatment initiation. If patients are rapidly improving and have successfully been weaned from NIV and parenteral vasodilators, EDOU management may be considered if respiratory distress has resolved with initial treatment. If patients require more than minimal oxygen supplementation, are not improving with ED treatment, or have substantial persistent respiratory distress, they should be admitted to the inpatient setting.

Troponin elevation is associated with inpatient mortality,[38,39] and patients with normal troponin levels on presentation have a greater likelihood of successful discharge from the EDOU within 24 hours[30] and lower adverse event rates at 30 days.[29] However, many patients with stable chronic HF have detectable or elevated troponin levels at baseline, although these patients do have poorer long-term survival.[40] If the physician has access to previous troponin measurements that show chronic mild elevation, a trial of observation with serial biomarker measurement may be reasonable if the presenting troponin level is not elevated beyond the baseline. However, if these previous data are not available or if patients present with symptoms of angina concomitant with acute HF, troponin elevation should prompt an inpatient admission.

Multiple studies have evaluated the prognostic value of natriuretic peptides (NP), most commonly B-type natriuretic peptide (BNP) or its biological precursor N-terminal pro-BNP (NT-proBNP). The authors acknowledge that there are many nuances that apply to the interpretation of NP testing, including the effect of age, adiposity, renal clearance, and preserved versus reduced ejection fraction. In general, though, the higher the NP level, the more specific the diagnosis of acute HF[41] and the higher the risk of mortality.[32,42–44] There is insufficient evidence to define an explicit NP level that delineates admission from observation with certainty, although a BNP greater than 1000 pg/mL or NT-proBNP greater than 5000 pg/mL has been suggested as the threshold for admission.[24,45] When available, outpatient or discharge dry-weight NP levels may aid in the interpretation of the test obtained in the ED.

Patients who experience acute kidney injury and decreased renal function have been shown to have increased in-hospital mortality and postdischarge mortality. Fonarow and colleagues[34] showed that both serum urea nitrogen (BUN) greater than 43 mg/dL and serum creatinine greater than 2.75 mg/dL were markers of increased inpatient mortality. Other studies have shown that elevated creatinine greater than 3.0 mg/dL and BUN greater than 40 mg/dL are strongly correlated to mortality.[46] In addition to being a poor prognostic factor, impaired renal function complicates rapid, aggressive diuresis that may be required to successfully discharge patients from the EDOU within 24 hours.[47]

## PATIENT MANAGEMENT

The goal of therapy in the EDOU should be to reduce symptoms, continue risk stratification, avoid unnecessary admission to the hospital, provide patient education and link follow-up after discharge.

Patients should have a recorded weight and oxygen requirement on arrival to the unit. Strict input and output measurement should be initiated at the start of their EDOU stay. Low urine output may indicate a need for higher loop diuretic doses, the addition of synergistic thiazide diuretics, or worsening renal failure necessitating admission. Given the high rate of malignant atrial and ventricular arrhythmias in patients with HF,[48–52] cardiac monitoring is required.

Electrolytes should be measured to ensure that hypokalemia or hypomagnesemia is not induced with aggressive diuresis. The authors recommend serial troponin measurements for all patients being treated in an EDOU for HF, regardless of cause. Elevated troponin is a marker of worsening prognosis in both ischemic and nonischemic cardiomyopathy.[39] In patients with ischemic cardiomyopathy, increasing troponins may indicate a need for admission and revascularization.[53] The practice of following serial NP levels to assess response to therapy and readiness for discharge has not been validated in the literature.[54]

Patients will need fluid restriction (<2000 mL/d) and to be placed on a 1500-mg sodium diet. Home medications should be restarted in the absence of intolerance or contraindication. Ideally, this will consist of an angiotensin-converting enzyme inhibitor (ACE) or angiotensin receptor blocker as well as a β-blocker. Contraindications to ACE include previous angioedema, pregnancy, hypotension, renal artery stenosis, creatinine levels greater than 3 mg/dL, and hyperkalemia (serum levels >5.0 mEq/L).[36] To date, there are no clinical trials evaluating the initiation of an angiotensin receptor-neprilysin inhibitor in the setting of acute HF in the ED or EDOU.

Most patients with acute HF present acutely and typically have an SBP greater than140 mm Hg.[55] These patients often present with greater initial symptoms but the potential for overall shorter length of stay and lower mortality.[35] These patients are often in afterload crisis, with a fluid distribution problem to the lungs but not total body fluid overload.[56] There may be benefit from a strategy of emphatic afterload reduction and modest diuresis.[57,58]

Those patients who are normotensive tend to experience a gradual accumulation of total body fluid and present with milder dyspnea and greater peripheral edema compared with hypertensive patients.[58] Because total body fluid is often the cause of their presentation, these patients can be more aggressively diuresed. Patients who are compliant with their diuretic medication but still presenting with volume overload should receive an initial intravenous dose that is at least equal to or exceeds their usual oral daily dose,[36] followed by initiation or escalation of their outpatient regimen. Felker and colleagues[59] found no benefit to administering diuretics in continuous infusion as opposed to bolus dosing in the DOSE (Diuretic Optimization Strategies Evaluation) trial. Escalation of vasodilators should be used with caution as these patients can become hypotensive quickly and must be reassessed after initial diuresis. Initiation of a synergistic thiazide diuretic should be considered if there is inadequate response to the initial intravenous diuretic dose.

## EDUCATION

EDOUs provide clinicians more time to not only treat symptoms but to take a more in depth look at what lead to the HF exacerbation. The EDOU also allows a better environment for patient education.

Many hospitalizations could be avoided with adherence to medication and diet and by monitoring developing symptoms.[60,61] As the evidence base for HF therapy grows, polypharmacy is a frequent consequence. Providers should look for common precipitants of medication noncompliance, including financial barriers, depression, forgetfulness, real or perceived side effects, and understanding the importance of the medication. For those who are unable to afford medications, many pharmaceutical companies offer assistance programs; consultation with the social work or case management teams may provide an important contribution to the patients' care.

Dietary nonadherence can also contribute to acute HF exacerbations. The AHA currently advocates restriction of sodium intake to 1500 mg per day,[62] compared with the daily American average of greater than 3400 mg per day.[63] It is important to teach each patient how to read nutrition labels and to provide common low-sodium options for dining out and cooking at home using spices and herbs. Every attempt should be made to include family and friends in regard to education of diet and medication adherence.

Self-care education has been associated with decreased HF readmission rates.[61] Educating patients about signs and symptoms associated with worsening HF along with their families will provide an opportunity to have multiple people watching for changes in patients' physical status. Signs and symptoms of increasing dyspnea, increase in weight gain, and increasing fatigue should be stressed to both patients and families.

## DISPOSITION AND FOLLOW-UP

There is scant evidence defining when patients are ready for discharge after an EDOU stay for acute HF. Often, patients who are discharged are done so based on resolution dyspnea and peripheral edema. The amount of improvement required to avoid a revisit to the ED has not been quantified. If fluid balance, weight, oxygen requirement, and vital signs have not improved during the observation period or if patients have a decline in cardiac, pulmonary, or renal function, they should be admitted to the hospital for further management.

Before discharge, patients should receive education regarding medication and diet compliance as well as education of signs and symptoms of early HF exacerbation. It is appropriate to collaborate with the primary physician or cardiologist regarding adjustments to the medication regimen at discharge. A recent meta-analysis evaluated home-health visits, HF multidisciplinary clinic referral, and telephone follow-up; all reduced mortality and HF readmissions.[64] Early physician follow-up, regardless of whether with cardiology or primary care, also reduces HF recidivism.[65] Early on in the EDOU stay, case management should be engaged to begin discharge planning to include specialty clinic referral, physician follow-up, and home health services when appropriate. Even if patients do not improve substantially and require admission from the EDOU, they will still require outpatient care; early initiation of discharge planning has been shown to improve postdischarge outcomes.[66]

## SYNCOPE
### Epidemiology and Disease Burden

Syncope, a transient loss of consciousness due to cerebral hypoperfusion, remains a significant challenge. Syncope accounts for approximately 740,000 annual visits to the ED, representing 0.8% of all ED visits.[67] The causes of syncope can range from fatal to relatively benign, although even vasovagal syncope is associated with increased morbidity and decreased quality of life.[68,69] Because syncopal episodes can represent a precursor to sudden cardiac death, patients with cardiovascular history or worrisome presentations are frequently admitted to the hospital. The annual cost of hospitalization is substantial, with conservative estimates of inpatient costs approaching approximately $2.4 billion.[70]

Despite the high frequency of hospitalization and subsequent consumption of health care resources, there is no current literature to suggest that this current practice improves long-term quality of life or mortality. As the utilization of EDOUs continues to grow in the United States, there has been an increased interest in using them for patients with syncope.[71,72]

## PATIENT SELECTION

It should be clear that the authors are discussing the management of patients without a clear cause for syncope after the initial ED evaluation. When a clear cause, such as subarachnoid hemorrhage, pulmonary embolism, acute GI bleeding, hypovolemia, or malignant arrhythmia, is diagnosed during the initial ED course, the underlying condition should be addressed. Although certain conditions may lend themselves to observation management (dehydration secondary to gastroenteritis, for example), severe disease will merit inpatient admission.

Multiple risk stratification rules have been published for syncope, but none have demonstrated an improvement in outcome over physician judgment.[73,74] Published studies have suggested a range of markers of both high and low risk for poor outcomes, resulting in nebulously defined and inconsistent recommendations from various specialty society guidelines and invalidated decision rules.[71,72,75–80] The most commonly cited markers of risk center on cardiac dysfunction and include family history of sudden cardiac death, severe cardiac disease (including dilated cardiomyopathy, aortic stenosis, hypertrophic cardiomyopathy, or left ventricular [LV] outflow disease), EKG abnormalities (such as preexcitation syndrome, Brugada syndrome, QT interval abnormalities, or conduction blocks), or exertional syncope.

Patients who are considered low risk should usually be discharged. If all of the following characteristics apply, admission or observation is not likely to be value added: age less than 50 years, clear vasovagal cause, no history of cardiovascular disease, normal EKG, and a normal cardiovascular examination.[71,76]

Specialty society guidelines have indicated that the history of cardiovascular disease should be considered a marker of high risk.[77–79] However, Numeroso and colleagues[76] recently published research suggesting that the simple history of cardiovascular disease (known chronic HF or known coronary artery disease), unless presenting with an acute exacerbation, does not convey elevated risk for adverse outcomes. Likewise, increasing age was associated with more high-risk features but was not independently predictive of adverse outcomes. Although requiring external validation and confirmation, this would suggest that patients with clinical stability but a history of cardiac disease who would otherwise not meet high-risk criteria, or those with advanced age but no other high-risk features, could potentially be managed in an EDOU.[81]

## MANAGEMENT

As indicated earlier, patients who present with active exacerbations of cardiac disease and syncope (acute HF, ongoing angina), electrophysiologic instability, or syncope associated with other severe disease should be admitted; those who have clear vasovagal syncope should more than likely be discharged from the ED. EDOU management is an excellent option for patients at intermediate risk.

EDOU management starts with a baseline set of vitals and cardiac monitoring. The time frame that patients should be observed on monitoring varies, but most experts agree monitoring should last at least 3 hours.[75] The further course of EDOU management should center on the suspected cause of syncope. If patients are suspected to have occult GI bleed, serial hemoglobin monitoring would be suggested. If dehydration is the primary cause, rehydration with fluids and reassessment including repeat basic metabolic panel may be appropriate for these patients. As most patients will have a suspected cardiac cause, serial troponin measurements, BNP measurement, and continuous cardiac monitoring may be appropriate. The role of echocardiography in the evaluation of acute syncope has been recently challenged; in 2 studies, the rate of pathologic findings on echocardiography was quite low in patients with normal physical examinations and normal EKGs.[82,83] Tilt table testing is not helpful in the EDOU. Although there may be a role for tilt table testing in the outpatient arena,[77] there is not a definitive need to make a diagnosis of neuromediated syncope acutely.

## DISPOSITION

Given that the primary role of the EDOU is to rule out severe disease, as opposed to ruling in a diagnosis, the unsatisfying truth is that many patients presenting with syncope will be discharged without a clear diagnosis. If a diligent evaluation of potentially dangerous causes has failed to reveal an urgent underlying etiology, these patients remain suitable for discharge and follow-up with their physician.

If cardiac arrhythmia is suspected but not confirmed during the EDOU stay, outpatient cardiac monitoring may be considered. The diagnostic yield of Holter monitoring and loop recording (external or internal) is higher in patients with preexisting cardiac disease, the association of palpitations before syncope, and presence of EKG abnormalities.[84] Outpatient Holter monitoring is widely available, but its utility depends on the arrhythmia occurring within a time frame of 24 to 72 hours. Other EKG recording devices, such as external loop recorders and implantable loop recorders, may be more appropriate but should be managed in consultation with cardiology.

## VENOUS THROMBOEMBOLISM
### Epidemiology and Disease Burden

Acute venous thromboembolic disease (VTE), which includes deep venous thrombosis (DVT) and pulmonary embolism (PE), is a frequent reason for patients to present to the ED and require hospitalization. The annual incidence of VTE in the United States is estimated at 1 to 2 per 1000 patients, or approximately 300,000 to 600,000 cases per year, resulting in an estimated 60,000 to 100,000 deaths each year.[85] The therapeutic strategy for VTE has remained unchanged for decades: anticoagulation to prevent clot propagation, new or recurrent PE, secondary pulmonary hypertension, and, in the case of DVT, to mitigate longer-term and nonlethal complications, such as postthrombotic syndrome.

Historically, treatment of VTE mandated hospital admission for UFH infusion while vitamin K antagonists (VKAs) were administered. The availability of LMWH, which can be administered subcutaneously with a predictable therapeutic effect, shifted the initial management of uncomplicated DVT toward the outpatient setting. The diagnosis of PE, however, remained a reason for hospital admission for anticoagulation and monitoring for hemodynamic compromise. This practice largely remains the standard in the United States.[86] For both DVT and PE, ongoing treatment with VKAs, and the consequent requisite monitoring of prothrombin time/INRs while on therapy, remained the mainstay of long-term treatment.

The introduction of DOACs has expanded our therapeutic options. Currently, one direct thrombin inhibitor (dabigatran) and 3 factor Xa inhibitors (apixaban, edoxaban, and rivaroxaban) are approved in the United States for the treatment of acute VTE.[87–91] In a recent systematic review, the only treatment strategy less efficacious than LMWH/VKA was UFH/VKA combination therapy.[92] Therefore, the advent of the DOAC class of medication has the potential to transform the acute (ED, observation, and hospital based) management of VTE.

## PATIENT SELECTION

The first consideration in risk stratification for patients is hemodynamic status. On one end of the spectrum are patients with substantial hemodynamic instability: hypotension, shock, or acute cardiac arrest. Obviously, these patients are not candidates for observation management, requiring admission to a monitored bed or critical care setting. However, in stable patients, one may consider further studies that may predict mortality and can assist with risk stratification in PE.

Recent meta-analyses suggest an approximate 2-fold increase in adverse outcomes if right ventricular (RV) dysfunction is seen on echocardiography; however, when hemodynamically unstable patients were excluded, the prognostic accuracy was not as clear because of the heterogeneity of the included studies.[93,94] Likewise, in another meta-analysis, an increased RV/LV ratio or septal bowing on computed tomography pulmonary angiography (92% sensitive for the presence of RV dysfunction on echocardiogram)[95] demonstrated an increased 30-day mortality in all patients with PE (odds ratio [OR] 2.08; 95% confidence interval [CI] 1.63–2.66) with a weaker risk association in hemodynamically stable patients (OR 1.64; 95% CI 1.06–2.52).[96] Trujillo-Santos and colleagues[97] found similar results in a separate meta-analysis. The presence of RV dysfunction may suggest admission is warranted in otherwise hemodynamically stable patients.

Plasma levels of BNP and NT-proBNP are elevated in patients experiencing increased myocardial stretch, such as patients with hemodynamically significant PE. Although elevated levels are independently associated with mortality risk,[98] this is likely a proxy effect that is confounded by hemodynamic stability. In other words, patients clinically at high risk for adverse outcomes are more likely to have elevated levels of BNP and NT-proBNP.[99] Those patients who are hemodynamically stable but have elevated biomarker levels are not at substantially higher risk for immediate compromise. This idea was demonstrated by den Exter and colleagues,[100] who randomized patients with low-risk PE to immediate discharge or measurement of NT-proBNP, with hospitalization for those patients with elevated natriuretic peptides. There was no statistical difference in 30-day event rates between groups, and the event rate was 0% in those low-risk patients hospitalized only because of elevated NT-proBNP.

Troponin elevation is not uncommon in the setting of acute PE. A meta-analysis by Becattini and colleagues[101] demonstrated elevated troponins in approximately 50% of patients with acute PE, with an associated increase in mortality (OR 5.24; 95% CI 3.28–8.38). The relationship was preserved in patients who were hemodynamically stable (OR 4.98; 95% CI 2.64–9.39). In a more recent meta-analysis, however, Jimenez and colleagues[102] found that in hemodynamically stable patients, elevated troponin did not substantially affect mortality prediction. The use of high-sensitivity troponins has been reported to be perfectly sensitive at a threshold of 14 pg/mL for the detection of adverse events in patients with hemodynamically stable PE; however, this comes at the cost of poor specificity (8%; 95% CI 3.5%–15.0%).[103]

Patient comorbidities can also influence the need for inpatient care by limiting the patients' physiologic reserve or by complicating the decision of anticoagulation. Patients with underlying HF, pulmonary disease, or active cancer have significantly higher mortality rates in the setting of acute PE[104,105] and may, therefore, require higher levels of care than patients without such comorbidities. Scoring systems, such as the Pulmonary Embolism Severity Index (PESI),[106] the Simplified Pulmonary Embolism Severity Index (sPESI),[107] the Hestia score,[108,109] and the Geneva score,[110] incorporate medical history and clinical criteria into a score that establishes patients at either low or very low risk for adverse outcomes. Both the PESI and sPESI have demonstrated sufficient sensitivity to indicate outpatient or observation management in patients with low scores.[108,111–114] Likewise, a Hestia score of zero indicates low risk. The elements of the PESI and sPESI scores are listed in **Table 2** and the Hestia score in **Box 1**.

**Table 2**
**Pulmonary Embolism Stratification Score and Simplified Pulmonary Embolism Stratification Score**

| Characteristic | PESI[106] | sPESI[107] |
|---|---|---|
| Age | One point per y of age | 1 point if aged >80 y |
| Male sex | 10 points | — |
| Cancer | 30 points | 1 point |
| History of HF | 10 points | 1 point if either/both |
| Chronic pulmonary disease | 10 points | |
| Heart rate >100 | 20 points | 1 point |
| SBP <100 mm Hg | 30 points | 1 point |
| Respiratory rate >30 | 20 points | — |
| Temperature <36.0°C/96.8°F | 20 points | — |
| Altered mental status | 60 points | — |
| Oxygen saturation <90% | 20 points | 1 point |

Patients are considered to be low risk if the sPESI is 0. Patients with a PESI score of less than 65 are considered to be at very low 30-day mortality risk (class I); class II patients are considered to be at low mortality risk with a score between 66 and 85 points.

---

**Box 1**
**Characteristics comprising the Hestia risk stratification score**

Hemodynamically unstable

Indication for fibrinolysis or thrombectomy

At high risk for bleeding[a]

Supplemental oxygen required for oxygen saturation greater than 90%

PE occurred while on anticoagulation

Parenteral pain medication required[b]

Medical or social reason necessitating inpatient admission

Creatinine clearance less than 30 mL/min

Severe hepatic impairment

Pregnant

History of heparin-induced thrombocytopenia

Any positive response requires inpatient management.
[a] GI bleeding within the last 14 days, stroke within 4 weeks, surgery within 2 weeks, bleeding diathesis, thrombocytopenia (<75 × 10$^9$/L), uncontrolled hypertension (SBP >180 mm Hg, diastolic blood pressure >110 mm Hg).
[b] In the original derivation study,[109] parenteral pain medications needed for greater than 24 hours.
*Data from* Zondag W, den Exter PL, Crobach MJ, et al. Comparison of two methods for selection of out of hospital treatment in patients with acute pulmonary embolism. Thromb Haemost 2013;109:47–52; and Zondag W, Mos IC, Creemers-Schild D, et al. Outpatient treatment in patients with acute pulmonary embolism: the Hestia Study. J Thromb Haemost 2011;9:1500–7.

---

There are fewer indications for admission of uncomplicated DVT. Critical limb ischemia caused by high tissue pressures (phlegmasia cerulea dolens) requires hospitalization and urgent vascular surgery consultation. Similarly, large, iliac, or pelvic DVTs (proximal to the inguinal ligament) may benefit from direct thrombectomy or a pharmacomechanical approach[115] as an inpatient procedure. Patients with decompensated comorbidities that require inpatient management and patients with unsuitable home or socioeconomic conditions will likely require inpatient admission. Those patients with strong contraindications to anticoagulation may require an inferior vena cava filter for PE prophylaxis in acute DVT. However, most patients with DVT can be managed primarily in the outpatient setting.[116]

## PATIENT MANAGEMENT

For stable patients without comorbidities, there is a trend toward managing low-risk acute PE with a rapid transition to outpatient care. As stated earlier, both the PESI and sPESI scores (see **Table 2**) as well as the Hestia score[108,109] (see **Box 1**) have been shown to be effective in identifying patients as potentially appropriate for early outpatient management.[108,111–114,117,118] The literature base remains sparse with regard to prospective randomized studies of inpatient versus outpatient care for low-risk PE. Multiple small outpatient feasibility studies have been published, using various scoring criteria and treatment algorithms.[108,114,117,119] At the current time, the MERCURY PE (Multicenter Trial of Rivaroxaban for Early Discharge of Pulmonary Embolism from the Emergency Department) trial is randomizing Hestia-negative patients to standard care versus early ED discharge with home treatment with rivaroxaban[120]; however, current clinical practice may outpace the development of the scientific rationale.

Currently there are four DOACs available for treatment of VTE in the United States. In the trials leading to the approval for these agents, edoxaban and dabigatran used a study design that required at least 5 days of parenteral anticoagulation (UFH or LMWH) before the initiation of the DOAC.[88,90] As a result of this study design, the US Food and Drug Administration labeling for these agents requires similar up-front parenteral anticoagulation. It should be noted that this is not bridging or overlapping therapy as seen with UFH/LMWH and VKA; rather, it is more accurately described as lead-in therapy. In contrast, the apixaban and rivaroxaban studies allowed for immediate initiation of oral anticoagulation therapy without required parenteral bridging or lead in.[87,89,91] However, this apparent advantage is offset in part by the requirement for a change in dosing regimen downstream. Initial treatment with rivaroxaban is 15 mg twice daily for 21 days and then 20 mg once daily for the duration of therapy. Apixaban begins at 10 mg twice daily for 7 days and is then given 5 mg twice daily for the duration of treatment. These different strategies (up-front parenteral anticoagulation vs higher oral dosing initially) are both designed to mitigate the increased risk of recurrent or worsening VTE due to the active prothrombotic state that is highest in the first 2 weeks after the index VTE event, with a more aggressive initial approach.[121] In low-risk patients with no anticipated need for inpatient treatment, the use of immediate DOAC-based treatment would obviate home-administered parenteral therapy with LMWH.

## DISPOSITION AND FOLLOW-UP

Economic considerations frequently influence treatment options. In the United States, insurance coverage (or lack thereof) may have more effect on which drug regimen will be used than the scientific evidence. Determining which medication is cost-feasible, cross-checking payer formularies, and establishing follow-up with a physician willing to manage either a DOAC-based regimen or take responsibility for VKA monitoring is difficult to execute in the typical overcrowded ED.

The EDOU is an ideal setting to address outpatient care planning while providing ongoing monitoring and treatment. Although medication is administered and reaching therapeutic levels (which with DOACS are attained within a few hours of the first dose), social work or case management personnel can work with patients to ensure medication availability and engage in follow-up planning. Education of patients and their caregivers regarding their disease, management options, and bleeding risk can also take place in the observation setting. When VKA agents are the selected strategy, patients and caregivers can receive education about dietary restrictions and medication interactions as well.

## REFERENCES

1. Koenig BO, Ross MA, Jackson RE. An emergency department observation unit protocol for acute-onset atrial fibrillation is feasible. Ann Emerg Med 2002;39: 374–81.
2. Peacock WF, Clark CL. Short stay management of atrial fibrillation. Switzerland: Springer International Publishing; 2016.
3. Barrett TW, Martin AR, Storrow AB, et al. A clinical prediction model to estimate risk for 30-day adverse events in emergency department patients with symptomatic atrial fibrillation. Ann Emerg Med 2011;57:1–12.
4. Decker WW, Smars PA, Vaidyanathan L, et al. A prospective, randomized trial of an emergency department observation unit for acute onset atrial fibrillation. Ann Emerg Med 2008;52:322–8.

5. Elmouchi DA, VanOosterhout S, Muthusamy P, et al. Impact of an emergency department-initiated clinical protocol for the evaluation and treatment of atrial fibrillation. Crit Pathw Cardiol 2014;13:43–8.

6. Baugh CW, Epstein LM, Schuur JD, et al. Atrial fibrillation emergency department observation protocol. Crit Pathw Cardiol 2015;14:121–33.

7. Stiell IG, Clement CM, Brison RJ, et al. Variation in management of recent-onset atrial fibrillation and flutter among academic hospital emergency departments. Ann Emerg Med 2011;57:13–21.

8. Bellew SD, Bremer ML, Kopecky SL, et al. Impact of an emergency department observation unit management algorithm for atrial fibrillation. J Am Heart Assoc 2016;5.

9. Lin MP, Ma J, Weissman JS, et al. Hospital-level variation and predictors of admission after ED visits for atrial fibrillation: 2006 to 2011. Am J Emerg Med 2016;34:2094–100.

10. Scheuermeyer FX, Grafstein E, Stenstrom R, et al. Thirty-day and 1-year outcomes of emergency department patients with atrial fibrillation and no acute underlying medical cause. Ann Emerg Med 2012;60:755–65.e2.

11. Atzema CL, Barrett TW. Managing atrial fibrillation. Ann Emerg Med 2015;65: 532–9.

12. Verma A, Cairns JA, Mitchell LB, et al. 2014 focused update of the Canadian Cardiovascular Society Guidelines for the management of atrial fibrillation. Can J Cardiol 2014;30:1114–30.

13. Atzema CL. Atrial fibrillation: would you prefer a pill or 150 joules? Ann Emerg Med 2015;66:655–7.

14. Freedman B, Potpara TS, Lip GY. Stroke prevention in atrial fibrillation. Lancet 2016;388:806–17.

15. Mozaffarian D, Benjamin EJ, Go AS, et al. Executive summary: heart disease and stroke statistics–2016 update: a report from the American Heart Association. Circulation 2016;133:447–54.

16. Heidenreich PA, Albert NM, Allen LA, et al. Forecasting the impact of heart failure in the United States: a policy statement from the American Heart Association. Circ Heart Fail 2013;6:606–19.

17. Collins SP, Schauer DP, Gupta A, et al. Cost-effectiveness analysis of ED decision making in patients with non-high-risk heart failure. Am J Emerg Med 2009; 27:293–302.

18. Ross MA, Hockenberry JM, Mutter R, et al. Protocol-driven emergency department observation units offer savings, shorter stays, and reduced admissions. Health Aff (Millwood) 2013;32:2149–56.

19. Collins SP, Pang PS, Fonarow GC, et al. Is hospital admission for heart failure really necessary?: the role of the emergency department and observation unit in preventing hospitalization and rehospitalization. J Am Coll Cardiol 2013;61: 121–6.

20. Pang PS, Jesse R, Collins SP, et al. Patients with acute heart failure in the emergency department: do they all need to be admitted? J Card Fail 2012;18:900–3.

21. Peacock WF, Young J, Collins S, et al. Heart failure observation units: optimizing care. Ann Emerg Med 2006;47:22–33.

22. Schrager J, Wheatley M, Georgiopoulou V, et al. Favorable bed utilization and readmission rates for emergency department observation unit heart failure patients. Acad Emerg Med 2013;20:554–61.

23. Storrow AB, Collins SP, Lyons MS, et al. Emergency department observation of heart failure: preliminary analysis of safety and cost. Congest Heart Fail 2005; 11:68–72.

24. Peacock WF, Fonarow GC, Ander DS, et al. Society of Chest Pain Centers recommendations for the evaluation and management of the observation stay acute heart failure patient-parts 1-6. Acute Card Care 2009;11:3–42.

25. Collins SP, Lindsell CJ, Naftilan AJ, et al. Low-risk acute heart failure patients: external validation of the Society of Chest Pain Center's recommendations. Crit Pathw Cardiol 2009;8:99–103.

26. Miro O, Peacock FW, McMurray JJ, et al. European Society of Cardiology-Acute Cardiovascular Care Association position paper on safe discharge of acute heart failure patients from the emergency department. Eur Heart J Acute Cardiovasc Care 2016. [Epub ahead of print].

27. Collins SP, Storrow AB, Levy PD, et al. Early management of patients with acute heart failure: state of the art and future directions–a consensus document from the SAEM/HFSA acute heart failure working group. Acad Emerg Med 2015;22: 94–112.

28. Collins S, Hiestand B. Confounded by hospitalization: risk stratification and admission decisions in emergency department patients with acute heart failure. Acad Emerg Med 2013;20:106–7.

29. Collins SP, Jenkins CA, Harrell FE Jr, et al. Identification of emergency department patients with acute heart failure at low risk for 30-day adverse events: the STRATIFY decision tool. JACC Heart Fail 2015;3:737–47.

30. Diercks DB, Peacock WF, Kirk JD, et al. ED patients with heart failure: identification of an observational unit-appropriate cohort. Am J Emerg Med 2006;24: 319–24.

31. Lee DS, Stitt A, Austin PC, et al. Prediction of heart failure mortality in emergent care: a cohort study. Ann Intern Med 2012;156:767–75. W-261, W-262.

32. Stiell IG, Clement CM, Brison RJ, et al. A risk scoring system to identify emergency department patients with heart failure at high risk for serious adverse events. Acad Emerg Med 2013;20:17–26.

33. Cheung PT, Wiler JL, Lowe RA, et al. National study of barriers to timely primary care and emergency department utilization among Medicaid beneficiaries. Ann Emerg Med 2012;60:4–10.e2.

34. Fonarow GC, Adams KF Jr, Abraham WT, et al. Risk stratification for in-hospital mortality in acutely decompensated heart failure: classification and regression tree analysis. JAMA 2005;293:572–80.

35. Gheorghiade M, Abraham WT, Albert NM, et al. Systolic blood pressure at admission, clinical characteristics, and outcomes in patients hospitalized with acute heart failure. JAMA 2006;296:2217–26.

36. Yancy CW, Jessup M, Bozkurt B, et al. 2013 ACCF/AHA guideline for the management of heart failure: a report of the American College of Cardiology Foundation/American Heart Association Task Force on practice guidelines. Circulation 2013;128:e240–327.

37. Gray AJ, Goodacre S, Newby DE, et al. A multicentre randomised controlled trial of the use of continuous positive airway pressure and non-invasive positive pressure ventilation in the early treatment of patients presenting to the emergency department with severe acute cardiogenic pulmonary oedema: the 3CPO trial. Health Technol Assess 2009;13:1–106.

38. Moe GW, Howlett J, Januzzi JL, et al, Canadian Multicenter Improved Management of Patients With Congestive Heart Failure Study Investigators. N-terminal

pro-B-type natriuretic peptide testing improves the management of patients with suspected acute heart failure: primary results of the Canadian prospective randomized multicenter IMPROVE-CHF study. Circulation 2007;115:3103–10.

39. Peacock WFT, De Marco T, Fonarow GC, et al. Cardiac troponin and outcome in acute heart failure. N Engl J Med 2008;358:2117–26.

40. Miller WL, Hartman KA, Burritt MF, et al. Profiles of serial changes in cardiac troponin T concentrations and outcome in ambulatory patients with chronic heart failure. J Am Coll Cardiol 2009;54:1715–21.

41. Martindale JL, Wakai A, Collins SP, et al. Diagnosing acute heart failure in the emergency department: a systematic review and meta-analysis. Acad Emerg Med 2016;23:223–42.

42. Fonarow GC, Peacock WF, Horwich TB, et al. Usefulness of B-type natriuretic peptide and cardiac troponin levels to predict in-hospital mortality from ADHERE. Am J Cardiol 2008;101:231–7.

43. Fonarow GC, Peacock WF, Phillips CO, et al. Admission B-type natriuretic peptide levels and in-hospital mortality in acute decompensated heart failure. J Am Coll Cardiol 2007;49:1943–50.

44. Harrison A, Morrison LK, Krishnaswamy P, et al. B-type natriuretic peptide predicts future cardiac events in patients presenting to the emergency department with dyspnea. Ann Emerg Med 2002;39:131–8.

45. Peacock WF, Cannon CM, Singer AJ, et al. Considerations for initial therapy in the treatment of acute heart failure. Crit Care 2015;19:399.

46. Formiga F, Chivite D, Manito N, et al. Predictors of in-hospital mortality present at admission among patients hospitalised because of decompensated heart failure. Cardiology 2007;108:73–8.

47. Burkhardt J, Peacock WF, Emerman CL. Predictors of emergency department observation unit outcomes. Acad Emerg Med 2005;12:869–74.

48. MERIT-HF Study Group. Effect of metoprolol CR/XL in chronic heart failure: metoprolol CR/XL Randomised Intervention Trial in Congestive Heart Failure (MERIT-HF). Lancet 1999;353:2001–7.

49. Myerburg RJ. Sudden cardiac death: exploring the limits of our knowledge. J Cardiovasc Electrophysiol 2001;12:369–81.

50. Ip JE, Cheung JW, Park D, et al. Temporal associations between thoracic volume overload and malignant ventricular arrhythmias: a study of intrathoracic impedance. J Cardiovasc Electrophysiol 2011;22:293–9.

51. Moore HJ, Peters MN, Franz MR, et al. Intrathoracic impedance preceding ventricular tachyarrhythmia episodes. Pacing Clin Electrophysiol 2010;33:960–6.

52. Perego GB, Landolina M, Vergara G, et al. Implantable CRT device diagnostics identify patients with increased risk for heart failure hospitalization. J Interv Card Electrophysiol 2008;23:235–42.

53. Braga JR, Tu JV, Austin PC, et al. Outcomes and care of patients with acute heart failure syndromes and cardiac troponin elevation. Circ Heart Fail 2013; 6:193–202.

54. Singer AJ, Birkhahn RH, Guss D, et al. Rapid Emergency Department Heart Failure Outpatients Trial (REDHOT II): a randomized controlled trial of the effect of serial B-type natriuretic peptide testing on patient management. Circ Heart Fail 2009;2:287–93.

55. Horton CF, Collins SP. The role of the emergency department in the patient with acute heart failure. Curr Cardiol Rep 2013;15:365.

56. Cotter G, Felker GM, Adams KF, et al. The pathophysiology of acute heart failure–is it all about fluid accumulation? Am Heart J 2008;155:9–18.

57. Cotter G, Metzkor E, Kaluski E, et al. Randomised trial of high-dose isosorbide dinitrate plus low-dose furosemide versus high-dose furosemide plus low-dose isosorbide dinitrate in severe pulmonary oedema. Lancet 1998;351:389–93.

58. Collins S, Storrow AB, Kirk JD, et al. Beyond pulmonary edema: diagnostic, risk stratification, and treatment challenges of acute heart failure management in the emergency department. Ann Emerg Med 2008;51:45–57.

59. Felker GM, Lee KL, Bull DA, et al. Diuretic strategies in patients with acute decompensated heart failure. N Engl J Med 2011;364:797–805.

60. Fitzgerald AA, Powers JD, Ho PM, et al. Impact of medication nonadherence on hospitalizations and mortality in heart failure. J Card Fail 2011;17:664–9.

61. Jovicic A, Holroyd-Leduc JM, Straus SE. Effects of self-management intervention on health outcomes of patients with heart failure: a systematic review of randomized controlled trials. BMC Cardiovasc Disord 2006;6:43.

62. Lloyd-Jones DM, Hong Y, Labarthe D, et al. Defining and setting national goals for cardiovascular health promotion and disease reduction: the American Heart Association's strategic Impact Goal through 2020 and beyond. Circulation 2010; 121:586–613.

63. Antman EM, Appel LJ, Balentine D, et al. Stakeholder discussion to reduce population-wide sodium intake and decrease sodium in the food supply: a conference report from the American Heart Association Sodium Conference 2013 Planning Group. Circulation 2014;129:e660–79.

64. Feltner C, Jones CD, Cene CW, et al. Transitional care interventions to prevent readmissions for persons with heart failure: a systematic review and meta-analysis. Ann Intern Med 2014;160:774–84.

65. Hernandez AF, Greiner MA, Fonarow GC, et al. Relationship between early physician follow-up and 30-day readmission among Medicare beneficiaries hospitalized for heart failure. JAMA 2010;303:1716–22.

66. Fox MT, Persaud M, Maimets I, et al. Effectiveness of early discharge planning in acutely ill or injured hospitalized older adults: a systematic review and meta-analysis. BMC Geriatr 2013;13:70.

67. Sun BC, Emond JA, Camargo CA Jr. Characteristics and admission patterns of patients presenting with syncope to U.S. emergency departments, 1992-2000. Acad Emerg Med 2004;11:1029–34.

68. Rose MS, Koshman ML, Spreng S, et al. The relationship between health-related quality of life and frequency of spells in patients with syncope. J Clin Epidemiol 2000;53:1209–16.

69. van Dijk N, Sprangers MA, Colman N, et al. Clinical factors associated with quality of life in patients with transient loss of consciousness. J Cardiovasc Electrophysiol 2006;17:998–1003.

70. Sun BC, Emond JA, Camargo CA Jr. Direct medical costs of syncope-related hospitalizations in the United States. Am J Cardiol 2005;95:668–71.

71. Shen WK, Decker WW, Smars PA, et al. Syncope Evaluation in the Emergency Department Study (SEEDS): a multidisciplinary approach to syncope management. Circulation 2004;110:3636–45.

72. Sun BC, McCreath H, Liang LJ, et al. Randomized clinical trial of an emergency department observation syncope protocol versus routine inpatient admission. Ann Emerg Med 2014;64:167–75.

73. Costantino G, Casazza G, Reed M, et al. Syncope risk stratification tools vs clinical judgment: an individual patient data meta-analysis. Am J Med 2014;127: 1126.e13–25.

74. Serrano LA, Hess EP, Bellolio MF, et al. Accuracy and quality of clinical decision rules for syncope in the emergency department: a systematic review and meta-analysis. Ann Emerg Med 2010;56:362–73.e1.

75. Costantino G, Sun BC, Barbic F, et al. Syncope clinical management in the emergency department: a consensus from the first international workshop on syncope risk stratification in the emergency department. Eur Heart J 2016;37: 1493–8.

76. Numeroso F, Mossini G, Giovanelli M, et al. Short-term prognosis and current management of syncopal patients at intermediate risk: results from the IRiS (Intermediate-Risk Syncope) Study. Acad Emerg Med 2016;23:941–8.

77. Moya A, Sutton R, Ammirati F, et al. Guidelines for the diagnosis and management of syncope (version 2009). Eur Heart J 2009;30:2631–71.

78. Huff JS, Decker WW, Quinn JV, et al. Clinical policy: critical issues in the evaluation and management of adult patients presenting to the emergency department with syncope. Ann Emerg Med 2007;49:431–44.

79. Sheldon RS, Morillo CA, Krahn AD, et al. Standardized approaches to the investigation of syncope: Canadian Cardiovascular Society position paper. Can J Cardiol 2011;27:246–53.

80. Thiruganasambandamoorthy V, Kwong K, Wells GA, et al. Development of the Canadian Syncope Risk Score to predict serious adverse events after emergency department assessment of syncope. CMAJ 2016;188:E289–98.

81. Nicks BA, Hiestand BC. Syncope risk stratification in the emergency department: another step forward. Acad Emerg Med 2016;23:949–51.

82. Anderson KL, Limkakeng A, Damuth E, et al. Cardiac evaluation for structural abnormalities may not be required in patients presenting with syncope and a normal ECG result in an observation unit setting. Ann Emerg Med 2012;60: 478–84.e1.

83. Chang NL, Shah P, Bajaj S, et al. Diagnostic yield of echocardiography in syncope patients with normal ECG. Cardiol Res Pract 2016;2016:1251637.

84. Ruwald MH, Zareba W. ECG monitoring in syncope. Prog Cardiovasc Dis 2013; 56:203–10.

85. Beckman MG, Hooper WC, Critchley SE, et al. Venous thromboembolism: a public health concern. Am J Prev Med 2010;38:S495–501.

86. Stein PD, Matta F, Hughes PG, et al. Home treatment of pulmonary embolism in the era of novel oral anticoagulants. Am J Med 2016;129:974–7.

87. Agnelli G, Buller HR, Cohen A, et al. Oral apixaban for the treatment of acute venous thromboembolism. N Engl J Med 2013;369:799–808.

88. Hokusai VTEI, Buller HR, Decousus H, et al. Edoxaban versus warfarin for the treatment of symptomatic venous thromboembolism. N Engl J Med 2013;369: 1406–15.

89. Investigators E-P, Buller HR, Prins MH, et al. Oral rivaroxaban for the treatment of symptomatic pulmonary embolism. N Engl J Med 2012;366:1287–97.

90. Schulman S, Kearon C, Kakkar AK, et al. Dabigatran versus warfarin in the treatment of acute venous thromboembolism. N Engl J Med 2009;361:2342–52.

91. Investigators E, Bauersachs R, Berkowitz SD, et al. Oral rivaroxaban for symptomatic venous thromboembolism. N Engl J Med 2010;363:2499–510.

92. Castellucci LA, Cameron C, Le Gal G, et al. Clinical and safety outcomes associated with treatment of acute venous thromboembolism: a systematic review and meta-analysis. JAMA 2014;312:1122–35.

93. Coutance G, Cauderlier E, Ehtisham J, et al. The prognostic value of markers of right ventricular dysfunction in pulmonary embolism: a meta-analysis. Crit Care 2011;15:R103.

94. Sanchez O, Trinquart L, Colombet I, et al. Prognostic value of right ventricular dysfunction in patients with haemodynamically stable pulmonary embolism: a systematic review. Eur Heart J 2008;29:1569–77.

95. Becattini C, Agnelli G, Vedovati MC, et al. Multidetector computed tomography for acute pulmonary embolism: diagnosis and risk stratification in a single test. Eur Heart J 2011;32:1657–63.

96. Becattini C, Agnelli G, Germini F, et al. Computed tomography to assess risk of death in acute pulmonary embolism: a meta-analysis. Eur Respir J 2014;43: 1678–90.

97. Trujillo-Santos J, den Exter PL, Gomez V, et al. Computed tomography-assessed right ventricular dysfunction and risk stratification of patients with acute non-massive pulmonary embolism: systematic review and meta-analysis. J Thromb Haemost 2013;11:1823–32.

98. Klok FA, Mos IC, Huisman MV. Brain-type natriuretic peptide levels in the prediction of adverse outcome in patients with pulmonary embolism: a systematic review and meta-analysis. Am J Respir Crit Care Med 2008;178:425–30.

99. Lankeit M, Jimenez D, Kostrubiec M, et al. Validation of N-terminal pro-brain natriuretic peptide cut-off values for risk stratification of pulmonary embolism. Eur Respir J 2014;43:1669–77.

100. den Exter PL, Zondag W, Klok FA, et al. Efficacy and safety of outpatient treatment based on the Hestia clinical decision rule with or without NT-proBNP testing in patients with acute pulmonary embolism: a randomized clinical trial. Am J Respir Crit Care Med 2016;194(8):998–1006.

101. Becattini C, Vedovati MC, Agnelli G. Prognostic value of troponins in acute pulmonary embolism: a meta-analysis. Circulation 2007;116:427–33.

102. Jimenez D, Uresandi F, Otero R, et al. Troponin-based risk stratification of patients with acute nonmassive pulmonary embolism: systematic review and meta-analysis. Chest 2009;136:974–82.

103. Lankeit M, Friesen D, Aschoff J, et al. Highly sensitive troponin T assay in normotensive patients with acute pulmonary embolism. Eur Heart J 2010;31:1836–44.

104. Monreal M, Munoz-Torrero JF, Naraine VS, et al. Pulmonary embolism in patients with chronic obstructive pulmonary disease or congestive heart failure. Am J Med 2006;119:851–8.

105. Chee CE, Ashrani AA, Marks RS, et al. Predictors of venous thromboembolism recurrence and bleeding among active cancer patients: a population-based cohort study. Blood 2014;123:3972–8.

106. Aujesky D, Obrosky DS, Stone RA, et al. Derivation and validation of a prognostic model for pulmonary embolism. Am J Respir Crit Care Med 2005;172: 1041–6.

107. Jimenez D, Aujesky D, Moores L, et al. Simplification of the pulmonary embolism severity index for prognostication in patients with acute symptomatic pulmonary embolism. Arch Intern Med 2010;170:1383–9.

108. Zondag W, den Exter PL, Crobach MJ, et al. Comparison of two methods for selection of out of hospital treatment in patients with acute pulmonary embolism. Thromb Haemost 2013;109:47–52.

109. Zondag W, Mos IC, Creemers-Schild D, et al. Outpatient treatment in patients with acute pulmonary embolism: the Hestia Study. J Thromb Haemost 2011;9: 1500–7.

110. Wicki J, Perrier A, Perneger TV, et al. Predicting adverse outcome in patients with acute pulmonary embolism: a risk score. Thromb Haemost 2000;84: 548–52.
111. Ferrer M, Morillo R, Elias T, et al. Validation of two clinical prognostic models in patients with acute symptomatic pulmonary embolism. Arch Bronconeumol 2013;49:427–31.
112. Lankeit M, Gomez V, Wagner C, et al. A strategy combining imaging and laboratory biomarkers in comparison with a simplified clinical score for risk stratification of patients with acute pulmonary embolism. Chest 2012;141:916–22.
113. Zhou XY, Ben SQ, Chen HL, et al. The prognostic value of pulmonary embolism severity index in acute pulmonary embolism: a meta-analysis. Respir Res 2012; 13:111.
114. Bledsoe J, Hamilton D, Bess E, et al. Treatment of low-risk pulmonary embolism patients in a chest pain unit. Crit Pathw Cardiol 2010;9:212–5.
115. Meissner MH, Gloviczki P, Comerota AJ, et al. Early thrombus removal strategies for acute deep venous thrombosis: clinical practice guidelines of the Society for Vascular Surgery and the American Venous Forum. J Vasc Surg 2012;55: 1449–62.
116. Douketis JD. Treatment of deep vein thrombosis: what factors determine appropriate treatment? Can Fam Physician 2005;51:217–23.
117. Agterof MJ, Schutgens RE, Snijder RJ, et al. Out of hospital treatment of acute pulmonary embolism in patients with a low NT-proBNP level. J Thromb Haemost 2010;8:1235–41.
118. Aujesky D, Roy PM, Verschuren F, et al. Outpatient versus inpatient treatment for patients with acute pulmonary embolism: an international, open-label, randomised, non-inferiority trial. Lancet 2011;378:41–8.
119. Beam DM, Kahler ZP, Kline JA. Immediate discharge and home treatment with rivaroxaban of low-risk venous thromboembolism diagnosed in two U.S. emergency departments: a one-year preplanned analysis. Acad Emerg Med 2015; 22:788–95.
120. Singer AJ, Xiang J, Kabrhel C, et al. Multicenter trial of rivaroxaban for early discharge of pulmonary embolism from the emergency department (MERCURY PE): rationale and design. Acad Emerg Med 2016;23(11):1280–6.
121. Authors/Task Force Management, Konstantinides SV, Torbicki A, et al. 2014 ESC guidelines on the diagnosis and management of acute pulmonary embolism: the Task Force for the Diagnosis and Management of Acute Pulmonary Embolism of the European Society of Cardiology (ESC) endorsed by the European Respiratory Society (ERS). Eur Heart J 2014;35(43):3033–69.

# Care of Acute Gastrointestinal Conditions in the Observation Unit

Jason J. Ham, MD[a],*, Edgar Ordonez, MD, MPH[b],
R. Gentry Wilkerson, MD[c]

## KEYWORDS

- Emergency Department Observation Unit • Acute gastrointestinal conditions
- Acute appendicitis • Gastrointestinal hemorrhage • Acute pancreatitis

## KEY POINTS

- The Emergency Department Observation Unit (EDOU) provides a viable alternative to inpatient admission for the management of many acute gastrointestinal conditions with additional opportunities of reducing resource utilization and reducing radiation exposure.
- Using available evidence-based criteria to determine appropriate patient selection, evaluation, and treatment provide higher-quality medical care and improved patient satisfaction.
- Descriptions of factors involved in creating an EDOU capable of caring for acute gastrointestinal conditions and clinical protocol examples of acute appendicitis, gastrointestinal hemorrhage, and acute pancreatitis provide a framework from which a successful EDOU can be built.

---

### Case study

Mr Smith is a 43-year-old man who presents to the emergency department with a complaint of "gnawing" epigastric pain associated with nonbloody, nonbilious vomiting. He admits to excessive alcohol intake the week prior. The current symptoms are similar to his 2 prior episodes of pancreatitis. Vital signs are normal except for mild tachycardia at 108 beats per minute. On examination, he is in obvious discomfort. He has tenderness in the epigastric region without rebound or guarding. Laboratory studies are significant only for a lipase level of 2200 U/L (normal <300). He is placed in the observation unit where he is treated with intravenous hydration and parenteral opioids. A right upper quadrant ultrasound is unremarkable. The following day his diet is advanced and he is transitioned to oral analgesics. Alcohol counseling is provided and he is discharged home to follow-up at his primary care provider 2 days later.

---

Disclosures: None.
[a] Department of Emergency Medicine, University of Michigan, 1500 East Medical Center Drive, Spc 5301, Ann Arbor, MI 48109, USA; [b] Department of Emergency Medicine, Baylor College of Medicine, 1 Baylor Plaza, Houston, TX 77030, USA; [c] Department of Emergency Medicine, University of Maryland School of Medicine, 110 South Paca Street, 6th Floor, Suite 200, Baltimore, MD 21201-1559, USA
* Corresponding author.
*E-mail address:* Jasham@med.umich.edu

Emerg Med Clin N Am 35 (2017) 571–587
http://dx.doi.org/10.1016/j.emc.2017.03.005
0733-8627/17/© 2017 Elsevier Inc. All rights reserved.

## INTRODUCTION

Gastrointestinal (GI) emergencies accounted for nearly 15 million of the 122 million emergency department (ED) visits in the United States in 2007 at a cost of $27.9 billion.[1] Traditionally, the care of a patient with abdominal pain was to perform a rapid diagnostic workup with efforts aimed at relief of symptoms. After the initial ED workup, patients would be either discharged home or admitted to a surgical or medical inpatient service. The ED provider, under pressure to rapidly and accurately diagnose and treat patients, has increasingly relied on early radiographic testing. The difference in imaging utilization for abdominal complaints rose from 19.9% in 1999 to 44.3% in 2008.[2] Some patients may benefit from a period of time during which they may undergo further diagnostic workup, risk stratification, and treatment before a final disposition. ED Observation Units (EDOUs) have the potential to improve diagnostic accuracy with more judicious use of imaging modalities, lower morbidity and mortality, improve the patient experience, and reduce health care expenditures.

The potential for EDOUs to reduce patient exposure to ionizing radiation deserves special emphasis. Recent studies in the trends of computed tomography (CT) use in the ED have revealed a tradeoff between the ability to diagnose high-risk conditions more rapidly at the expense of increased cost and increased exposure to radiation and iodinated contrast agents.[3] This is further compounded by the discovery of incidental findings that necessitate potentially needless additional diagnostic testing. The incidence of adrenal "incidentalomas," a term coined to denote the presence of an adrenal mass in an otherwise asymptomatic patient, found on CT scans approaches 9%.[4] The risk of ionizing radiation is dependent on the dose, tissue exposed, and age of the patient. A CT scan of the abdomen and pelvis exposes the patient to 10 mSv or 3 times the expected annual natural background radiation dose.[5] This exposure, especially when occurring earlier in life, has been associated with a small increase in interval development of cancer. This risk is small to the individual, but given the magnitude of the population that is exposed, the cumulative impact on increased cancer rates is significant.[6]

EDOUs balance the need to accurately and safely diagnose and treat patients with the pressure to do so rapidly but with judicious use of imaging. This balance is achieved by combining the ED assessment with standardized risk assessment tools and serial examinations, a core principle of observation medicine. For lower-risk cases for which no imaging has been performed as part of the initial ED evaluation, the period of observation provides the opportunity to perform repeat assessments of the patient's condition and to obtain imaging in the event of clinical worsening or failure to improve.

EDOU protocols pertaining to GI complaints will share many common themes. These include standard inclusion and exclusion criteria that exist to select for the most appropriate patient who would benefit from the time in the unit. These criteria must be individualized to local system needs and updated as systems change or new knowledge in the care of conditions evolves.

Inclusions and exclusions are considered on 3 levels: the health care system level, the general patient level, and within the specific patient protocol. Considerations at the level of the health care system include capacity constraints, availability of required resources, unit factors, and team factors. Risk tolerance is proportional to the ability of a system to provide the resources needed for a change in patient status. An example of a unit factor to consider is the presence of individual rooms versus a communal space that is set apart by curtains. The latter would not be conducive for the care of patients with communicable diseases, diarrhea, or those being prepared for a colonoscopy. The team treating the patients placed in the EDOU should have the required skills and expertise to care for the conditions that are likely to be encountered.

Abdominal pain has an exhaustive differential diagnosis that ranges from very low-risk conditions, such as constipation, to catastrophic conditions, such as a ruptured abdominal aortic aneurysm. General exclusion criteria include patients with unstable vital signs, presence of a surgical abdomen, or severe sepsis, or if the diagnostic workup reveals any emergent surgical condition. Patients who are immunocompromised are often not ideal candidates for placement in the EDOU. The severity of their condition is often not evident on initial evaluation and their care involves utilization of multiple resources. Patients with higher-risk immunosuppressive states, such as those who have received transplantation or those with malignancy undergoing chemotherapy, those with human immunodeficiency virus/AIDS, and those with rheumatologic conditions requiring immunosuppressive agents may have very atypical presentations of GI illnesses, such as peritonitis,[7] opportunistic infections, graft-versus-host-disease,[8] and neutropenic enterocolitis.[9] There are some disease-specific conditions that are not likely appropriate for the EDOU. These include conditions in which it is known that the patient will require a prolonged in-hospital stay, such as severe gastroparesis. High-risk conditions should be thoroughly considered in patients with risk factors before placement in the EDOU. One example is consideration of mesenteric ischemia in patients with a history of atrial fibrillation, cardiomyopathy, and other low-flow states.[10]

The provider should consider that several emergent conditions may initially appear to have a GI etiology. Misleading complaints include epigastric pain of an inferior wall acute myocardial infarction, right upper quadrant pain of hepatic congestion in congestive heart failure, generalized abdominal pain with nausea and vomiting in diabetic ketoacidosis, and back and flank pain in pulmonary embolism.[11]

Abdominal pain is the most common chief complaint among the elderly presenting to the ED. Patients older than 80 have nearly double the mortality of younger patients if the diagnosis is delayed.[8] Due to physiologic changes caused by lax abdominal wall musculature and increased use of medications, elderly individuals often have atypical or muted signs and symptoms, including lack of vital sign alteration, such as fever or tachycardia. Only 17% of elderly individuals with a perforated appendix have classic complaints.[12] Age-related physiologic changes may warrant exclusion of elderly individuals from some EDOU GI protocols.

Behavioral and social factors may preclude a reasonable safe disposition within the usual timeframe for EDOU care. For example, it may be unreasonable to perform an observation protocol for acute pancreatitis on a patient who also has symptoms of alcohol withdrawal due to ongoing behavior conditions that had previously occurred. This may affect the care of the patient, as well as the care of other patients in the EDOU.

Each health care system and ED team must consider a general approach to the patient with GI disorders that reflects the abilities of the system and all of its resources, including consultant availability and provider abilities and resources. General patient considerations of catastrophic conditions, immunosuppression, mimic condition considerations, elderly, and behavioral and social factors must be considered before consideration to place in an observation protocol.

Specific patient protocols use best clinical practices and available evidence to standardize care. EDOUs may be used for the evaluation and possible treatment of appendicitis, GI bleeding, and pancreatitis.

## APPENDICITIS
### Introduction/Epidemiology

Suspected appendicitis is a common diagnostic consideration in patients who present to the ED with abdominal pain and is the most common diagnosis of abdominal complaints that requires surgery. The lifetime risk of appendicitis is 8.6% for male individuals and 6.7% for female individuals.[13] The initial ED evaluation includes a thorough history and physical examination. Although laboratory evaluation may be undertaken, it is important to note that no single laboratory value can rule-in or rule-out the diagnosis of appendicitis. A retrospective review in 2015 showed that no single value of white blood cell count, C-reactive protein, or their combination resulted in a positive predictive value of greater than 80% or a negative predictive value of greater than 90%.[14] Thus, the diagnosis is considered based on the history, and physical and laboratory values can be used to support but not definitively rule-in or rule-out this diagnosis.

### Risk Scores/Imaging

Scoring systems have been developed to aid in the evaluation of patients with suspected appendicitis. These scores often use components of the history, physical, and laboratory values. The most commonly used is the Alvarado score, also known by its mnemonic, MANTRELS score.[15] This score uses 8 predictive factors (**Table 1**) that were given a point value of 1 or 2 based on diagnostic weight. Other scoring systems that may be used include the Pediatric Appendicitis Score,[16] Appendicitis Inflammatory Response Score,[17] Raja Isteri Pengiran Anak Saleha Appendicitis score,[18] and the Adult Appendicitis Score.[19] These clinical decision tools can be used to risk stratify patients into low, intermediate, and high risk for appendicitis.[20]

Imaging studies are obtained if the clinician has a high enough concern, especially if the clinical scoring system used places the patient in the moderate to high-risk group. CT imaging of the abdomen and pelvis with contrast is considered the most appropriate imaging modality by the American College of Radiology (ACR) for evaluation of adults

| Table 1 Alvarado scoring system for appendicitis | Points |
|---|---|
| **Symptoms** | |
| Nausea and/or vomiting | 1 |
| Anorexia | 1 |
| Migration of pain to the right lower quadrant | 1 |
| **Signs** | |
| Tenderness in the right lower quadrant | 2 |
| Rebound | 1 |
| Temperature $\geq$37.3°C (99.1°F) | 1 |
| **Laboratory tests** | |
| White blood cell count 10.0 $\times$ 10$^9$/L | 2 |
| Left shift | 1 |

Low Risk, 1 to 4; Intermediate Risk, 5 to 6; High Risk, 7 to 10.

with a classic clinical presentation for appendicitis.[21] CT findings of acute appendicitis include an enlarged, thickened (wall thickness >3 mm), fluid-filled appendix with or without an appendicolith with associated periappendiceal inflammatory changes. Other findings that may be associated with appendicitis include inflammatory changes of the adjacent bowel, enlarged mesenteric lymph nodes, and free fluid. A drawback to the use of CT scans is the exposure to ionizing radiation and iodinated contrast agents. Despite these concerns, the utilization of CT imaging has increased dramatically. In one single-center review, the utilization of CT before appendectomy increased from 1% in 1990 to 97.5% in 2007.[22] The classically accepted negative appendectomy rate, defined as the rate of pathologically normal appendices surgically removed in patients suspected of having appendicitis, was historically between 15% and 25%.[23] Recent data suggest that this has now decreased to less than 2%.[22]

Ultrasound is increasingly being used as the primary imaging modality in certain cases. The ACR recommends graded compression ultrasound as the initial imaging test in children younger than 14 and in pregnant patients.[24] This technique uses a high-resolution linear transducer placed at the site of maximal tenderness. Pressure is applied to compress and displace bowel loops to identify the appendix.[25] Normally, the appendix is a blind ending tubular structure that is compressible and may demonstrate peristalsis. In cases of appendicitis, the appendix becomes noncompressible and enlarges. Generally, it is considered abnormally large if the outer diameter is >6 mm although in one study of asymptomatic patients, 3.6% of visualized appendices exceeded this cutoff.[26]

Ultrasound is limited by availability and it is highly operator dependent and has lower sensitivity than CT.[27] Ultrasound, although recommended as the first-line imaging test for pregnant patients, has limited value during the second and third trimesters. Lehnert and colleagues[28] retrospectively evaluated 99 patients in the second and third trimesters who underwent sonographic evaluation for suspected appendicitis. The appendix was visualized in only 3 (3%) of the patients. Ultrasound detected an abnormal appendix in only 2 (27%) of the 7 cases that were surgically confirmed.

### Observation Unit Management

The benefit of active observation for pediatric patients with concern for appendicitis was demonstrated by White and colleagues in 1975.[29] They compared 2 groups of consecutive pediatric patients, the first receiving appendectomy and the second receiving a "protective approach" of active observation. The use of active observation reduced the negative appendectomy rate from 15.0% to 1.9% without a significant increase in the rate of perforation. This study was followed up in 1986 by a study by Thomson and Jones.[30] In this single-center study, there were 153 patients not treated with initial surgery who were placed in active observation where they underwent repeated examinations. Eighteen of these patients eventually had surgery, with 7 cases of appendicitis. The remaining 135 patients had no surgical intervention. Although the details reported are limited, the authors state that "no patient suffered as a result of this policy" and they were able to manage 88% of indeterminate cases nonoperatively.

Currently, the primary use of an observation unit for the care of a patient with suspected appendicitis is in cases of diagnostic uncertainty but lower risk using clinical decision tools. Some patients with a low score may benefit from being placed in observation and having serial clinical examinations and laboratory studies performed. This approach conforms to the radiological principle of ALARA (As Low As Reasonably Achievable) in which the providers reduce the exposure to radiation as much as possible. This may be especially beneficial in the pediatric population, which is more radiosensitive than their adult counterparts.[31] Another beneficial use of the observation unit is for patients who undergo imaging as part of their initial diagnostic workup but the results are either negative or indeterminate in a symptomatic patient. Wai and colleagues[32] performed a retrospective analysis of pediatric patients admitted to a single-center's EDOU. All patients placed in the EDOU had an initial evaluation that included nondiagnostic imaging. Of those, 16% were eventually admitted to the hospital, with 9% undergoing surgery. Of those who underwent surgery, more than half had appendectomies performed. The negative appendectomy rate in this group was 38%. The higher than traditional rate is likely due to preselection for a more diagnostically challenging population.

A retrospective study by Graff and colleagues[33] assessed the probability of appendicitis using the Alvarado score before placement in an observation unit compared with the score at the end of the observation period. Patients determined to have appendicitis had a change in average score from 6.8 to 7.8, whereas patients without appendicitis had a decrease from 3.8 to 1.6. Another study compared the use of an EDOU as compared with a Surgical Assessment Unit (SAU).[34] The time to decision for surgery and time to discharge from the hospital was not different between the EDOU and the SAU. This suggests that ED providers are as capable as surgeons at managing these indeterminate patients.

Recently, there has been debate about using a nonoperative, antibiotics-only approach for the treatment of select cases of appendicitis. The Non Operative Treatment for Acute Appendicitis (NOTA)[35] and Antibiotic Therapy versus Appendectomy for Treatment of Uncomplicated Acute Appendicitis (APPAC)[36] trials were published in 2014 and 2015, respectively. Nonoperative treatment of appendicitis remains controversial and would not currently be considered usual practice in a typical EDOU.

## GASTROINTESTINAL BLEEDING
### Introduction

Gastrointestinal bleeding (GIB) is usually categorized as upper gastrointestinal bleeding (UGIB) or lower gastrointestinal bleeding (LGIB), with the distinction made anatomically at the ligament of Treitz, the ligament that suspends the duodenojejunal flexure and inhibits the reflux of gastrointestinal contents distal to this site. Thus, hematemesis usually indicates bleeding from the upper GI tract. GIB can vary in clinical severity, risk of mortality, treatment requirements, length of stay, and cost. Several clinical risk scores have been developed to assist the provider in recognizing and managing these factors. GIB protocols with a standard approach to assessment and treatment occurring in an EDOU setting can improve these factors.

### Epidemiology

In the United States, 48 to 160 per 100,000 people have a UGIB annually,[37] whereas 20 per 100,000 have an LGIB.[38] Common causes of UGIB include peptic ulcer disease, erosive disease, variceal bleeding, esophagitis, and Mallory-Weis tear. Common causes of LGIB include diverticular bleeding, hemorrhoids, polyps, colorectal cancer, intestinal ischemia, angiodysplasia, and colitis.[39]

### Clinical Presentation

On presentation to the ED, the patient will undergo evaluation to determine the cause and severity of the GIB and urgent issues such as impending shock will be rapidly stabilized. A careful GIB history will include a description of hematemesis, stool color and frequency, symptoms of hepatic disease, and symptoms of blood loss, including syncope. Comorbid conditions must be noted, including previous GIB and endoscopy results, as well as use of nonsteroidal anti-inflammatory drugs (NSAIDs) and anticoagulants, as they are common causes of GIB.[40] Evaluation includes obtaining orthostatic vital signs, examination of any vomitus produced, and assessment of stool for evidence of blood. Signs of liver failure suggest the possibility of a variceal bleed and coagulopathy. Variceal bleeding is high risk and should be excluded from an EDOU GIB protocol. Nasogastric lavage can help identify UGIB when positive, but has not been found to exclude UGIB when negative.[41] Routine laboratory testing includes hemoglobin, blood urea nitrogen (BUN), creatinine (Cr), coagulation profile, and a type and screen. Blood transfusion should not be delayed for laboratory results in suspected impending shock. An elevated lactate greater than 2.5 mmol/L is associated with hypotension within 24 hours.[42]

When the source of GIB is not initially apparent, several factors may help increase the likelihood of correctly diagnosing the source. An upper GI source for bleeding is correlated with a history of passing black stool, presence of melena, history of prior UGIB, positive nasogastric tube aspirate and BUN to Cr ratio greater than 30. Factors reducing the likelihood of UGIB include presence of blood clots in stool, history of LGIB, and BUN to Cr ratio less than 30.[41]

Patients with GI bleeding can be successfully categorized into risk categories using clinical scores, such as the Clinical Rockall Score (CRS) and the Glasgow Blatchford Score (GBS), which can help define the likelihood of mortality, need for blood transfusion, risk for rebleeding and need of urgent endoscopy in UGIB.[43] In 2000, Blatchford and colleagues[44] identified clinical criteria that comprise the GBS, which correctly identified 99% of serious UGIB needing treatment. This study was validated in a multicenter trial showing that all patients sent home with a Blatchford Score of 0 had no need for intervention on follow-up. This validation study also showed a reduction in admission rate for UGIB from 96% to 71%.[45] A comparison of patients with low-risk scores by GBS or CRS showed the rate of rebleeding for both scoring systems to be 13%.[46] A retrospective analysis of patients placed in an EDOU found that only 5% of patients identified as low risk by GBS had a rebleeding episode within 90 days.[47] Thus, GBS and CRS can help stratify patients into low and high risk, but these should be used with caution when considering sending a patient directly home without endoscopy or further observation (**Table 2**).

In 1999, a treatment algorithm for patients 65 and older who presented with UGIB was evaluated.[40] Patients were initially risk stratified based on response to an intravenous fluid challenge. All patients had an upper endoscopy performed. Patients with

**Table 2**
**Clinical risk scores in upper gastrointestinal bleeding**

| Glasgow Blatchford Score: Low Risk | | Clinical Rockall Score: Low Risk | |
|---|---|---|---|
| BUN | <18.2 mg/dL | Age | <60 y |
| Hemoglobin men | >13 g/dL | SBP | ≥100 mm Hg |
| Hemoglobin women | >12 g/dL | Pulse | <100 beats per min |
| SBP | >109 mm Hg | | |
| Pulse | <100 beats per min | | |
| No syncope, melena, liver disease, heart failure | | No heart failure, ischemic heart disease, renal failure, liver failure, disseminated malignancy, or other major comorbidity | |

*Abbreviations:* BUN, blood urea nitrogen; SBP, systolic blood pressure.

low-risk lesions on endoscopy and no major criteria and fewer than 3 minor criteria for admission were treated as an outpatient. None of those treated as an outpatient had an episode of rebleeding. Of the 60 admitted patients, 15 (25%) required intensive care unit (ICU) admission based on the presence of persistent orthostasis despite fluid bolus. The remaining patients were treated in an observation unit or hospital ward. Rebleeding occurred in 4 (7%) of the admitted patients. Although a small single-center study, this study suggests that using orthostatic vital signs and appropriate risk stratification using clinical criteria and esophagogastroduodenoscopy findings can result in accurate patient selection and effective and efficient treatment.

Other studies caution against outpatient management for GIB. A retrospective analysis of Medicare claims data found a 6.3% 30-day mortality rate for patients with non-variceal UGIB treated as an outpatient.[48] These mortality data support a role for the EDOU as an intermediate step between inpatient and outpatient management to provide further care to patients with GIB.

### Observation Unit Management

The provider should consider the appropriateness of placing a patient with GIB on an EDOU protocol based on a number of inclusion and exclusion criteria (**Box 1**).

The EDOU strategy includes frequent patient reassessments with efforts made to identify the source of bleeding. Serial assessments of vital signs, physical examinations, and laboratory testing are required. All patients should have 2 large-bore intravenous catheters and be kept NPO (nothing by mouth) status in case of need for an urgent procedure.

It is recommended that proton pump inhibitor (PPI) treatment is initiated for UGIB or suspected UGIB. In cases of UGIB, the use of PPIs has been shown to reduce endoscopic findings of recent serious bleeding and the need for endoscopic treatments, such as cautery. However, PPIs have not been shown to affect the risk of rebleeding, need for surgery, or risk of death.[49] Performance of EGD for UGIB within 24 hours has been shown to reduce mortality for higher-risk patients.[50] In the EDOU, some patients may become high risk and require urgent endoscopy. Lower-risk patients can be managed with a follow-up endoscopy procedure if one is not readily available.

---

**Box 1**
**EDOU GIB Protocol Suggested Inclusion and Exclusion Criteria**

*Suggested Inclusion Criteria*

Suspected Gastrointestinal Bleed

Low-risk score: Glasgow Blatchford Score = 0 (may permit higher if urgent support available)

Orthostatics: Not orthostatic after 1-L intravenous fluid bolus

*Suggested Exclusion Criteria*

Hemodynamic instability

Persistent orthostasis despite 1-L intravenous fluid bolus

Evidence of active bleeding in the emergency department: frequent episodes of hematemesis, melena, bright red blood per rectum

Coagulopathy

Known esophageal varices

Transfusion requirement

Treatment of a patient with a positive *Helicobacter pylori* test reduces the risk of recurrent bleeding.[51]

Patients with LGIB may require a colonoscopy for accurate diagnosis and to direct treatment. Interventions may include injection, cautery, and band ligation. The gastroenterology service may request a bowel preparation occur in the EDOU before the colonoscopy procedure. Angiography and nuclear scans with technetium Tc 99m–labeled red blood cells are rarely needed by low-risk patients undergoing an EDOU GIB protocol; however, familiarity with these modalities is important in case of clinical deterioration.

The decision to discharge a patient from the EDOU requires evidence of clinical stability. This includes stable hemoglobin/hematocrit level, no evidence of rebleeding, and no concern based on endoscopy for high risk of rebleeding. The patient should receive detailed instructions with regard to the avoidance of NSAIDs, anticoagulants, and alcohol consumption. Timely outpatient follow-up should be arranged.

## ACUTE PANCREATITIS
### Introduction

Acute pancreatitis (AP) is a frequent cause of abdominal pain, with recent data showing approximately 1.2 million ED visits between 2006 and 2009 with approximately 75% of those patients being admitted.[52] The diagnosis of AP requires 2 of the following 3 features: abdominal pain consistent with AP; serum lipase or amylase at least 3 times the upper limit of normal; or characteristic findings on abdominal imaging, generally contrast-enhanced CT.[53] The Atlanta Classification of AP most recently modified its classification of AP into 2 phases: early and late. Further classification is based on severity. Mild AP has no organ failure, or local or systemic complications, and often resolves within the first week, which may be ideal for EDOU management. Moderately severe AP is defined by the presence of transient organ failure, local complications, or exacerbation of comorbid disease. Severe AP is defined by persistent organ failure for more than 48 hours.[54]

### Epidemiology

AP is the most common gastrointestinal reason for hospital admission in the United States, accounting for approximately 275,000 hospitalizations in 2009 and $2.6 billion per year in inpatient costs.[55] The annual incidence of AP worldwide has been described to be in the range of 13 to 45 per 100,000 persons. The incidence of AP is similar among men and women, although alcohol-related pancreatitis is more common in men, whereas in women, pancreatitis is more likely related to gallstones (**Box 2**).[56] The length of stay for patients diagnosed with AP can vary based on severity and etiology. A recent study demonstrated a median length of stay of 8 days, with a range of 1 to 31 days.[57]

### Clinical Presentation

Most patients with AP will present with nausea and vomiting as well as acute upper abdominal pain, which may radiate to the back.[58] Patients may experience restlessness, tachycardia, and low-grade fever. Patients with severe pancreatitis may develop cutaneous manifestations, such as Cullen or Gray Turner sign-ecchymosis in the periumbilical or flank regions, respectively.

### Diagnostic Testing

Standard laboratory testing in a patient with suspected AP would include a complete blood count, a metabolic panel, liver function studies, and pancreatic enzymes.

---

**Box 2**
**Etiologies of acute pancreatitis**

- Gallstones (35%–40%)
- Alcohol (~30%)
- Hypertriglyceridemia
- Mass
- Hypercalcemia
- Genetic mutations
- Infections (viral, bacterial, fungal parasitic)
- Trauma
- Post-ERCP (endoscopic retrograde cholangiopancreatogram)
- Pancreatic divisum
- Iatrogenic
- Pancreatic ischemia
- Medications
- Scorpion envenomation
- Idiopathic

*Data from* Refs.[59–64]

---

Elevated lipase and amylase levels are part of the diagnostic criteria for AP. Pancreatic enzymes increase in parallel at the onset of AP, but amylase returns to normal more quickly.[57] It is also important to note, amylase and lipase also can be elevated in other intra-abdominal diseases. Lipase is the preferred laboratory parameter for testing due to limitations in sensitivity and specificity of the amylase test.[65]

Although not always necessary, abdominal imaging can be useful in the diagnosis of AP. Plain radiographs have limited utility in the diagnosis, but may show findings related to disease severity, such as an ileus, pleural effusions, pulmonary infiltrates, or acute respiratory distress syndrome. Abdominal ultrasound can be helpful in determining if the cause of AP is secondary to gallstones, as this will alter management considerations. Contrast-enhanced CT can be beneficial in equivocal cases, having more than 90% sensitivity and specificity for the diagnosis of AP owing to the ability to detect parenchymal enlargement, inflammation, peri-pancreatic fluid collections, and necrosis.[66] Although not commonly used in the early presentations of AP, MRI is another useful modality in its evaluation.[67]

### Risk Stratification

Clinicians managing patients with AP should determine the severity of disease to make the appropriate treatment and disposition decisions. Select patients may not even require hospitalization. Some may require short observation unit stays, whereas others may require prolonged care in inpatient units or ICUs. The previously mentioned Atlanta Classification is used to provide nomenclature regarding the severity of AP but it does not provide an assessment of risk. Several scoring systems providing an assessment of risk have been published. Some of the most commonly known scores are Ranson criteria, Glasgow score, and the Acute Physiology and Chronic Health Evaluation II (APACHE II) score, which are based on clinical variables.[68–70] Limitations of these scores at the time of ED disposition include that Ranson criteria and the Glasgow score require input of clinical variables at 48 hours, whereas the APACHE II is very complex and not specific to AP.

More recent risk predictors may provide critical information earlier in the course of the presentation of AP. The Harmless Acute Pancreatitis Score (HAPS) is made up of 3 parameters (**Table 3**) and is used to help identify patients with AP who would not require ICU level of care and could potentially not require inpatient treatment at all. In a prospective study, the absence of any of the parameters predicted a mild course of AP in 98% of patients.[71] The HAPS score could provide utility in the evaluation of AP to determine if hospitalization or an observation unit stay is needed or if the patient may be a candidate for discharge home.

Another modern risk score, the Bedside Index of Severity in Acute Pancreatitis (BISAP) score, is currently used to determine AP severity. Calculation of this score depends on 5 parameters that are easily attainable in the ED (see **Table 3**).[72] The BISAP score is simple to use and is an accurate method for identifying patients at increased risk for in-hospital mortality. Several publications have compared the BISAP score with other risk scores in predicting the severity of AP and have noted its usefulness in determining AP severity earlier than other scoring systems.[73–75] The BISAP score may be a useful tool to help divert appropriate patients to an EDOU.

Several CT-based prognostic scoring systems have been described. The CT severity index was published in 1990[76] and later modified to include additional points for extrapancreatic complications.[77] The use of these CT-based scoring systems offers no additional prognostic benefit over the available clinical scoring systems.[78] The 2013 American College of Gastroenterology (ACG) guidelines for the management of AP recommended that contrast-enhanced CT and/or MRI should be reserved for patients in whom the diagnosis is not evident or if the patient does not clinically improve within 48 to 72 hours. They provided a list of clinical findings that are associated with severe pancreatitis (**Table 4**).

**Table 3**
**Risk scores used at initial evaluation for acute pancreatitis**

| Risk Score | Purpose | Clinical Parameters | Scoring | Utility for EDOU |
|---|---|---|---|---|
| BISAP | Predicts mortality from AP | Obtained within first 24 h<br>BUN >25 mg/dL<br>Impaired mental status<br>SIRS<br>Age >60 years<br>Pleural effusion | 1 point for each parameter<br>Maximum score = 5<br>Score = 0: 0.1% mortality<br>Score ≤2: 1.9% mortality | Easily calculated before EDOU disposition<br>Could consider patients with BISAP score ≤2 |
| HAPS | Predicts mild course of AP | Parameters obtained at initial evaluation<br>No rebound tenderness<br>Normal HCT<br>Cr <2 mg/dL | 1 point for each parameter<br>Maximum score = 3<br>Score = 0 may identify patient not requiring hospitalization | Easily calculated before EDOU disposition<br>Patients with score of 0 could be discharged or placed in EDOU |

*Abbreviations:* AP, acute pancreatitis; BISAP, Bedside Index of Severity in Acute Pancreatitis; BUN, blood urea nitrogen; CR, creatinine; EDOU, Emergency Department Observation Unit; HAPS, Harmless Acute Pancreatitis Score; HCT, hematocrit; SIRS, systemic inflammatory response syndrome.

---

**Table 4**
**Findings associated with a severe course of acute pancreatitis**

| Patient characteristics | Laboratory findings |
|---|---|
| • Age >55 years | • BUN >20 mg/dL |
| • Obesity (BMI >30) | • Rising BUN |
| • Altered mental status | • HCT >44% |
| • Comorbid disease | ○ Rising HCT |
| | ○ Elevated creatinine |

| SIRS presence of >2 of the following | Radiology findings |
|---|---|
| • HR >90 beats per min | • Pleural effusions |
| • RR >20/min or Paco₂ >32 mm Hg | • Pulmonary infiltrates |
| • Temp >38°C or <36°C | • Multiple or extensive extrapancreatic |
| • WBC count <4 or >12 × 10⁹/L or >10% Bands | collections |

*Abbreviations:* BMI, body mass index; BUN, blood urea nitrogen; HCT, hematocrit; HR, heart rate; RR, respiratory rate; SIRS, systemic inflammatory response syndrome.

Although risk stratification based on clinical or imaging parameters may help determine which patients are low, moderate, or high risk for mortality, the previously described scoring systems do not predict hospital length of stay, need for ICU care or potential need for surgical intervention. Risk stratifying patients for an observation unit stay should incorporate a risk score that identifies patients at low risk for poor outcomes and uses variables easily obtainable early in the disease course, such as the HAPS or BISAP scores.

### Observation Unit Management

The role of EDOUs in the management of mild AP is emerging. In review of the literature, only 1 article has been published describing management of AP in this setting. In this study, 27 consecutive patients with mild exacerbations of recurrent alcoholic pancreatitis were placed in an EDOU of which 14 (52%) improved enough to be discharged in less than 24 hours.[79] There was no specific method for risk stratification of these patients into the observation unit. Given that there are now several risk scores

---

**Box 3**
**EDOU Pancreatitis Protocol Suggested Inclusion and Exclusion Criteria**

*Suggested Inclusion Criteria*

Mild acute pancreatitis based on risk stratification scores

*Suggested Exclusion Criteria*

Gallstone pancreatitis

Systemic inflammatory response syndrome

Blood urea nitrogen > 20 mg/dL

Hematocrit > 44%

Acute kidney injury

Pleural effusion

Pulmonary infiltrates

Extrapancreatic collections

Altered mental status

available to the emergency provider, there is the potential to select a cohort of patients that would be appropriate for continued care in the observation unit setting. Patients with gallstone pancreatitis or evidence of obstruction are likely to require invasive procedures, and thus would not be suitable for an EDOU (**Box 3**).

The mainstay of treatment of AP is supportive. Early aggressive intravenous fluid hydration is strongly recommended. This helps reduce losses secondary to vomiting, oral intolerance, third spacing, and other factors. Certain groups should be given extra attention when receiving fluids in large volumes, including elderly individuals and those with preexisting renal or cardiac disease. The ACG guidelines recommend aggressive hydration, specifically 250 to 500 mL per hour of isotonic crystalloid solution, noting that this is most beneficial during the first 12 to 24 hours of admission.[64] Lactated Ringer solution is the fluid of choice based on limited but contradictory evidence.[72,80] Clinical volume assessment (eg, vital signs, urine output), and laboratory values should be assessed at regular intervals. The patient should be monitored for complications, such as fluid overload and abdominal compartment syndrome, that may develop as a result of aggressive hydration. Pain control can be achieved with intravenous opioids, as they are known to be safe and effective in AP.[81] In addition, antiemetics, such as ondansetron, metoclopramide, prochlorperazine, or promethazine, can be administered in conjunction with analgesic therapy. Historically, it was recommended that patients with AP be placed on bowel rest. This may be necessary in patients with persistent nausea, vomiting, or severe pain, but possibly not in those with mild AP. Early oral feedings are appropriate and generally preferred, and have been shown to decrease hospital length of stay.[82,83] Diet may be initiated at the time the patient is placed in the observation unit with clear liquids and advanced gradually to a low-fat diet.

The patient can be considered for discharge after demonstrating appropriate clinical improvement. Nausea should be well controlled and the patient should be tolerating oral analgesics and a diet of solid food. Vital signs should be normal and the patient should have an unremarkable abdominal examination. Any complications should have been appropriately addressed. Modifiable risk factors should be addressed, such as provision of alcohol counseling and discontinuation of any medications associated with development of pancreatitis.[84] The patient should be provided with close outpatient follow-up.

## SUMMARY

The EDOU provides a viable alternative to inpatient admission for the management of many acute gastrointestinal conditions with additional opportunities of reducing resource utilization and reducing radiation exposure. Using available evidence-based criteria to determine appropriate patient selection, evaluation, and treatment provides higher-quality medical care and improved patient satisfaction. Descriptions of factors involved in creating an EDOU capable of caring for acute gastrointestinal conditions and clinical protocol examples of acute appendicitis, gastrointestinal hemorrhage, and AP provide a framework from which a successful EDOU can be built.

## REFERENCES

1. Myer PA, Mannalithara A, Singh G, et al. Clinical and economic burden of emergency department visits due to gastrointestinal diseases in the United States. Am J Gastroenterol 2013;108(9):1496–507.
2. Bhuiya FA, Pitts SR, McCaig LF. Emergency department visits for chest pain and abdominal pain: United States, 1999-2008. NCHS Data Brief 2010;(43):1–8.

3. Brenner DJ, Hall EJ. Computed tomography—an increasing source of radiation exposure. N Engl J Med 2007;357(22):2277–84.

4. Zeiger M, Thompson G, Duh Q-Y, et al. American Association of Clinical Endocrinologists and American Association of Endocrine Surgeons medical guidelines for the management of adrenal incidentalomas: executive summary of recommendations. Endocr Pract 2009;15(5):450–3.

5. Available at: http://www.acr.org/~/media/ACR/Documents/PDF/QualitySafety/Radiation%20Safety/Dose%20Reference%20Card.pdf. Accessed September 27, 2016.

6. Brenner DJ, Elliston CD, Hall EJ, et al. Estimated risks of radiation-induced fatal cancer from pediatric CT. AJR Am J Roentgenol 2001;176(2):289–96.

7. Golda T, Kreisler E, Mercader C, et al. Emergency surgery for perforated diverticulitis in the immunosuppressed patient. Colorectal Dis 2014;16(9):723–31.

8. McKean J, Ronan-Bentle S. Abdominal pain in the immunocompromised patient—human immunodeficiency virus, transplant, cancer. Emerg Med Clin North Am 2016;34(2):377–86.

9. Nesher L, Rolston KVI. Neutropenic enterocolitis, a growing concern in the era of widespread use of aggressive chemotherapy. Clin Infect Dis 2012;56(5):711–7.

10. Singh M, Koyfman A, Martinez JP. Abdominal vascular catastrophes. Emerg Med Clin North Am 2016;34(2):327–39.

11. Palmer J, Pontius E. Abdominal pain mimics. Emerg Med Clin North Am 2016; 34(2):409–23.

12. Leuthauser A, McVane B. Abdominal pain in the geriatric patient. Emerg Med Clin North Am 2016;34(2):363–75.

13. Addiss DG, Shaffer N, Fowler BS, et al. The epidemiology of appendicitis and appendecectomy in the United States. Am J Epidemiol 1990;132(5):910–25.

14. Atema JJ, Gans SL, Beenen LF, et al. Accuracy of white blood cell count and C-reactive protein levels related to duration of symptoms in patients suspected of acute Appendicitis. Acad Emerg Med 2015;22(9):1015–24.

15. Alvarado A. A practical score for the early diagnosis of acute appendicitis. Ann Emerg Med 1986;15(5):557–64.

16. Samuel M. Pediatric appendicitis score. J Pediatr Surg 2002;37(6):877–81.

17. Andersson M, Andersson RE. The appendicitis inflammatory response score: a tool for the diagnosis of acute appendicitis that outperforms the Alvarado score. World J Surg 2008;32(8):1843–9.

18. Chong CF, Adi MI, Thien A, et al. Development of the RIPASA score: a new appendicitis scoring system for the diagnosis of acute appendicitis. Singapore Med J 2010;51(3):220–5.

19. Sammalkorpi HE, Mentula P, Leppäniemi A. A new adult appendicitis score improves diagnostic accuracy of acute appendicitis—a prospective study. BMC Gastroenterol 2014;14(1):114.

20. Ohle R, O'Reilly F, O'Brien KK, et al. The Alvarado score for predicting acute appendicitis: a systematic review. BMC Med 2011;9(1):139.

21. Smith MP, Katz DS, Lalani T, et al. ACR appropriateness criteria® right lower quadrant pain—suspected appendicitis. Ultrasound Q 2015;31(2):85–91.

22. Raja AS, Wright C, Sodickson AD, et al. Negative appendectomy rate in the era of CT: an 18-year perspective. Radiology 2010;256(2):460–5.

23. Detmer DE. Regional results of acute appendicitis care. JAMA 1981;246(12): 1318.

24. Cabarrus M, Sun Y-L, Courtier JL, et al. The prevalence and patterns of intraluminal air in acute appendicitis at CT. Emerg Radiol 2012;20(1):51–6.

25. Puylaert JB. Acute appendicitis: US evaluation using graded compression. Radiology 1986;158(2):355–60.

26. Yabunaka K, Katsuda T, Sanada S, et al. Sonographic appearance of the normal appendix in adults. J Ultrasound Med 2007;26(1):37–43.

27. van Randen A, Bipat S, Zwinderman AH, et al. Acute appendicitis: meta-analysis of diagnostic performance of CT and graded compression US related to prevalence of disease. Radiology 2008;249(1):97–106.

28. Lehnert BE, Gross JA, Linnau KF, et al. Utility of ultrasound for evaluating the appendix during the second and third trimester of pregnancy. Emerg Radiol 2012; 19(4):293–9.

29. White J, Santillana M, Haller J. Intensive in-hospital observation: a safe way to decrease unnecessary appendectomy. Am Surg 1975;41(12):793–8.

30. Thomson H, Jones P. Active observation in acute abdominal pain. Am J Surg 1986;152(5):522–5.

31. Brenner DJ. Estimating cancer risks from pediatric CT: going from the qualitative to the quantitative. Pediatr Radiol 2002;32(4):228–31.

32. Wai S, Ma L, Kim E, et al. The utility of the emergency department observation unit for children with abdominal pain. Pediatr Emerg Care 2013;29(5):574–8.

33. Graff L, Radford M, Werne C. Probability of appendicitis before and after observation. Ann Emerg Med 1989;18(4):439.

34. Schultz H, Qvist N, Pedersen BD, et al. Time delay to surgery for appendicitis. Eur J Emerg Med 2015. [Epub ahead of print].

35. Di Saverio S, Sibilio A, Giorgini E, et al. The NOTA study (non operative treatment for acute appendicitis). Ann Surg 2014;260(1):109–17.

36. Salminen P, Paajanen H, Rautio T, et al. Antibiotic therapy vs appendectomy for treatment of uncomplicated acute appendicitis. JAMA 2015;313(23):2340.

37. Rotandano G. Epidemiology and diagnosis of acute nonvariceal upper gastrointestinal bleeding. Gastroenterol Clin North Am 2014;43:643–63.

38. Longstreth GF. Epidemiology and outcome of patients hospitalized with acute lower gastrointestinal hemorrhage: a population-based study. Am J Gastroenterol 1997;92(3):419–24.

39. Strate L, Zyanian J. Risk factors for mortality in lower intestinal bleeding. Clin Gastroenterol Hepatol 2008;6(9):1004–10.

40. Cebollero-Santamaria F. Selective outpatient management of upper gastrointestinal bleeding in the elderly. Am J Gastroenterol 1999;94(5):1242–7.

41. Srygley F, Gerardo C, Tran T, et al. Systematic review of clinical factors to differentiate upper gastrointestinal bleeding from lower gastrointestinal bleeding. Gastroenterology 2011;140(5):S-209.

42. Ko BS, Kim WY, Ryoo SM, et al. Predicting the occurrence of hypotension in stable patients with nonvariceal upper gastrointestinal bleeding. Crit Care Med 2015;43(11):2409–15.

43. Nable JV, Graham AC. Gastrointestinal bleeding. Emerg Med Clin North Am 2016;34(2):309–25.

44. Blatchford O, Murray WR, Blatchford M. A risk score to predict need for treatment for upper gastrointestinal haemorrhage. Lancet 2000;356(9238):1318–21.

45. Stanley A, Ashley D, Dalton H, et al. Outpatient management of patients with low-risk upper-gastrointestinal haemorrhage: multicentre validation and prospective evaluation. Lancet 2009;373(9657):42–7.

46. Meltzer AC, Burnett S, Pinchbeck C, et al. Pre-endoscopic Rockall and Blatchford scores to identify which emergency department patients with suspected

gastrointestinal bleed do not need endoscopic hemostasis. J Emerg Med 2013; 44(6):1083–7.

47. Chandra A, Lewis K, Nouh A, et al. 380: Blatchford clinical risk stratification score may be used in an observation unit setting to risk stratify patients with gastrointestinal bleeding. Ann Emerg Med 2009;54(3):S120.

48. Cooper GS, Kou TD, Wong RCK. Outpatient management of nonvariceal upper gastrointestinal hemorrhage: unexpected mortality in medicare beneficiaries. Gastroenterology 2009;136(1):108–14.

49. Sreedharan A, Martin J, Leontiadis G, et al. Proton pump inhibitor treatment initiated prior to endoscopic diagnosis in upper gastrointestinal bleeding. Cochrane Database Syst Rev 2010;(7):CD005415.

50. Lim L, Ho K, Chan Y, et al. Urgent endoscopy is associated with lower mortality in high-risk but not low-risk nonvariceal upper gastrointestinal bleeding. Endoscopy 2011;43(04):300–6.

51. Ting-Chun H, Chia-Long L. Diagnosis, treatment, and outcome in patients with bleeding peptic ulcers and *Helicobacter pylori* infections. Biomed Res Int 2014;2014:658108.

52. McNabb-Baltar J, Ravi P, Isabwe GA, et al. A population-based assessment of the burden of acute pancreatitis in the United States. Pancreas 2014;43(5): 687–91.

53. Banks PA, Freeman ML. Practice guidelines in acute pancreatitis. Am J Gastroenterol 2006;101(10):2379–400.

54. Banks PA, Bollen TL, Dervenis C, et al. Classification of acute pancreatitis–2012: revision of the Atlanta classification and definitions by international consensus. Gut 2012;62(1):102–11.

55. Peery AF, Dellon ES, Lund J, et al. Burden of gastrointestinal disease in the United States: 2012 update. Gastroenterology 2012;143(5):1179–87.e3.

56. Yadav D, Lowenfels AB. The epidemiology of pancreatitis and pancreatic cancer. Gastroenterology 2013;144(6):1252–61.

57. Francisco M, Valentín F, Cubiella J, et al. Factors related to length of hospital admission in mild interstitial acute pancreatitis. Rev Esp Enferm Dig 2013; 105(2):84–92.

58. Lankisch PG, Apte M, Banks PA. Acute pancreatitis. Lancet 2015;386(9988): 85–96.

59. Gullo L, Migliori M, Oláh A, et al. Acute pancreatitis in five European countries: etiology and mortality. Pancreas 2002;24(3):223–7.

60. Badalov N, Baradarian R, Iswara K, et al. Drug-induced acute pancreatitis: an evidence-based review. Clin Gastroenterol Hepatol 2007;5(6):648–61.e3.

61. Andriulli A, Loperfido S, Napolitano G, et al. Incidence rates of Post-ERCP complications: a systematic survey of prospective studies. Am J Gastroenterol 2007; 102(8):1781–8.

62. Pezzilli R, Morselli-Labate AM, Mantovani V, et al. Mutations of the CFTR gene in pancreatic disease. Pancreas 2003;27(4):332–6.

63. Parenti DM, Steinberg W, Kang P. Infectious causes of acute pancreatitis. Pancreas 1996;13(4):356–71.

64. Bartholomew C. Acute scorpion pancreatitis in Trinidad. BMJ 1970;1(5697): 666–8.

65. Tenner S, Baillie J, DeWitt J, et al. American College of Gastroenterology guideline: management of acute pancreatitis. Am J Gastroenterol 2013;108(9): 1400–15.

66. Balthazar EJ. Acute pancreatitis: assessment of severity with clinical and CT evaluation. Radiology 2002;223(3):603–13.
67. Arvanitakis M, Delhaye M, De Maertelaere V, et al. Computed tomography and magnetic resonance imaging in the assessment of acute pancreatitis. Gastroenterology 2004;126(3):715–23.
68. Ranson JH, Rifkind KM, Roses DF, et al. Objective early identification of severe acute pancreatitis. Am J Gastroenterol 1974;61:443–51.
69. Blamey SL, Imrie CW, O'Neill J, et al. Prognostic factors in acute pancreatitis. Gut 1984;25(12):1340–6.
70. Knaus WA, Draper EA, Wagner DP, et al. APACHE II—A severity of disease classification system. Crit Care Med 1986;14(8):755.
71. Lankisch PG, Weber–Dany B, Hebel K, et al. The harmless acute pancreatitis score: a clinical algorithm for rapid initial stratification of nonsevere disease. Clin Gastroenterol Hepatol 2009;7(6):702–5.
72. Wu BU, Johannes RS, Sun X, et al. The early prediction of mortality in acute pancreatitis: a large population-based study. Gut 2008;57(12):1698–703.
73. Zhang J, Shahbaz M, Fang R, et al. Comparison of the BISAP scores for predicting the severity of acute pancreatitis in Chinese patients according to the latest Atlanta classification. J Hepatobiliary Pancreat Sci 2014;21(9):689–94.
74. Cho Y-S, Kim H-K, Jang E-C, et al. Usefulness of the bedside index for severity in acute pancreatitis in the early prediction of severity and mortality in acute pancreatitis. Pancreas 2013;42(3):483–7.
75. Park JY, Jeon TJ, Ha TH, et al. Bedside index for severity in acute pancreatitis: comparison with other scoring systems in predicting severity and organ failure. Hepatobiliary Pancreat Dis Int 2013;12(6):645–50.
76. Balthazar EJ, Robinson DL, Megibow AJ, et al. Acute pancreatitis: value of CT in establishing prognosis. Radiology 1990;174(2):331–6.
77. Mortele KJ, Zou KH, Banks PA, et al. A modified CT severity index for evaluating acute pancreatitis: improved correlation with patient outcome. Pancreas 2004;29(4):363.
78. Bollen TL, Singh VK, Maurer R, et al. A comparative evaluation of radiologic and clinical scoring systems in the early prediction of severity in acute pancreatitis. Am J Gastroenterol 2011;107(4):612–9.
79. Saunders CE, Gentile DA. Treatment of mild exacerbations of recurrent alcoholic pancreatitis in an emergency department observation unit. South Med J 1988;81(3):317–20.
80. Lipinski M. Fluid resuscitation in acute pancreatitis: normal saline or lactated Ringer's solution? World J Gastroenterol 2015;21(31):9367.
81. Basurto OX, Rigau Comas D, Urrutia G. Opioids for acute pancreatitis pain. Cochrane Database Syst Rev 2013;(7):CD009179.
82. Eckerwall GE, Tingstedt BBÅ, Bergenzaun PE, et al. Immediate oral feeding in patients with mild acute pancreatitis is safe and may accelerate recovery—a randomized clinical study. Clin Nutr 2007;26(6):758–63.
83. Li J, Xue G-J, Liu Y-L, et al. Early oral refeeding wisdom in patients with mild acute pancreatitis. Pancreas 2013;42(1):88–91.
84. Jones MR, Hall OM, Kaye AM, et al. Drug-induced acute pancreatitis: a review. Ochsner J 2015;15(1):45–51.

# Care of Metabolic and Endocrine Conditions in the Observation Unit

Anwar Dayan Osborne, MD, MPM, FACEP

## KEYWORDS

- Metabolic conditions • Observation unit care • Endocrine condition • Hyperglycemia
- Hypokalemia

## KEY POINTS

- Accelerated therapeutic protocols targeting metabolic conditions are ideal for observation unit care.
- Because many conditions, such as hypokalemia and hyperglycemia, have little to no diagnostic uncertainty, the care in unit is often straightforward.
- Some components of care for the endocrine condition may exhaust services, such as phlebotomy.

Accelerated therapeutic protocols targeting metabolic conditions are ideal for observation unit care. Because many conditions, such as hypokalemia and hyperglycemia, have little to no diagnostic uncertainty, the care in unit is often straightforward. To be sure, candidates for this level of care ideally have a more minor manifestation of their chronic condition, thus being sure about the overall severity of the current problem is paramount in the evaluation of these patients. Additionally, some components of care for the endocrine condition may exhaust services, such as phlebotomy. Hence, this discussion focuses on resource utilization and management considerations for the purposes of matching the level of care to the severity of the conditions. When carefully selected candidates are cared for in the observation unit, hospital resources can enable a safe, efficient hospital stay.

Department of Emergency Medicine, Emory University Hospital School of Medicine, Emory University Hospital, 531 Asbury Circle-Annex, Suite N340, Atlanta, GA 30322, USA
*E-mail address:* adosbor@emory.edu

Emerg Med Clin N Am 35 (2017) 589–601
http://dx.doi.org/10.1016/j.emc.2017.03.006
emed.theclinics.com

## HYPERGLYCEMIA

> **Case Study**
>
> Gerald Wilson is a 52-year-old man who lives in transitional housing. He complains of weakness and thirst. He says that it's odd that he's also making multiple trips to the bathroom at night to urinate. He has been rationing his insulin 70/30 mm Hg for it to last until his caseworker provides him with a new identification card. His card was stolen a few weeks ago, along with most of his belongings that he kept in a backpack. In the emergency department (ED) his vital signs are unremarkable. His laboratories are significant for a blood sugar of 469 mg/dL and an anion gap of 13.

Although treatment of hyperglycemia has a wide range of approaches in treatment of the acute phase, the Emergency Department Observation Unit (EDOU) performs well in delivering both rapid and standardized care. Currently, the number of EDOUs using hyperglycemia care pathways is largely unknown; but, in the author's experience, many, if not most units do use some form of standardized approach to patients with hyperglycemia. Most EDOUs should be capable of treating most forms of hyperglycemia, from new-onset diabetes to mild or moderate diabetic ketoacidosis (DKA).

### Patient Evaluation Overview

In the ED setting, patients with hyperglycemia can present in a variety of ways. Classically, patients with hyperglycemia report polyuria, polydipsia, and polyphagia, features that result from increased osmotic burden. Stabilization and evaluation for possible underlying causes of hyperglycemia is the cornerstone of initial management. Hyperglycemia still poses a large mortality burden, particularly in elderly individuals.[1] Laboratory assessment of serum electrolytes will yield several pieces of important information used to direct further care. The typical laboratory findings of DKA and hyperosmolar hyperglycemic state (HHS) are listed in **Table 1**.[2] The presence of hyperglycemia should be the initial finding that prompts further evaluation. The level at which there should be concern for hyperglycemic emergencies is generally accepted as more than 250 mg/dL. However, recent data show that in the setting of known diabetes, the threshold should be closer to 300 mg/dL. When the serum glucose levels exceed this threshold, the anion gap (AG) and serum electrolytes are key to choosing which patients may benefit from the observation unit setting.

**Table 1**
**Electrolyte abnormalities for hyperglycemic crises**

|  | Mild DKA | Moderate DKA | Severe DKA | HHS |
|---|---|---|---|---|
| Arterial pH | 7.25–7.30 | 7.00–7.24 | <7.00 | >7.30 |
| Serum bicarbonate | 15–18 | 10–15 | <10 | >18 |
| Urine ketone | Positive | Positive | Positive | Small |
| Serum ketone | Positive | Positive | Positive | Small |
| Effective serum osmolality | Variable | Variable | Variable | >320 |
| Anion gap | >10 | >12 | >12 | Variable |
| Mental status | Alert | Alert/drowsy | Stupor/coma | Stupor/coma |

Abbreviations: DKA, diabetic ketoacidosis; HHS, hyperosmolar hyperglycemic state.

## Observation Unit Care

A comprehensive discussion of the ED phase of management for hyperglycemia is beyond the scope of this article. There are a wide variety of reasonable approaches in the ED regarding the appropriate care provided and the duration of that care before disposition. There is no clear duration of time that dictates that a patient requires disposition to an inpatient service, an observation unit, or to home. Some conditions are amenable to direct placement in an EDOU from another outpatient setting, such as an office, thus bypassing the ED. The authors do not recommend this practice for patients with hyperglycemia. Even with normal vital signs, the patient may have profound electrolyte abnormalities that could significantly change the disposition and care needs of the patient. Patient selection for EDOU care is dependent on a thorough evaluation in the ED to rule out conditions that warrant a level of care beyond what is available in the EDOU. The following discussion assumes that a thorough ED evaluation has been completed.

### Hyperglycemia without evidence of diabetic ketoacidosis or hyperosmolar hyperglycemic state

Most patients with simple hyperglycemia will have an easily identifiable cause for their elevated glucose. Often, this is due to an inability to access medications. Sometimes, there are more insidious factors responsible for hyperglycemia. These factors should be considered in all patients during the initial ED phase of care. The EDOU provider should still remain vigilant regarding other underlying etiologies, as patient conditions may evolve during their time under observation (**Box 1**).[3] A sample set of patient selection criteria for simple hyperglycemia is provided (**Box 2**).

In these cases of hyperglycemia with an easily identifiable cause without the complications of AG elevation and unremarkable electrolyte abnormalities, there are multiple ways to manage the elevation in blood sugar. Potential EDOU interventions are listed in **Box 3**.

Most patients placed in an EDOU for simple hyperglycemia will be safely discharged home after a relatively short period of care. There is no established safe threshold for serum glucose. Many providers use the 300 mg/dL cutoff. Recently, a retrospective study by Driver and colleagues[4] showed that the incidence of adverse events within 7 days of discharge is very low even with a higher range of glucose levels at discharge. Even so, it would not be common practice to discharge patients with blood glucose levels higher than 400 mg/dL. A basic set of discharge interventions is listed in **Box 4**.

### New-onset diabetes mellitus

Considerations to place a patient with new-onset diabetes in an EDOU include factors related to medication initiation or transition and appropriate education. In the adult population, most patients with new-onset diabetes will have type 2 diabetes, which

---

**Box 1**
**Five I's of hyperglycemia**

1. Infection
2. Infarct
3. Infant
4. Indiscretion (eg, cocaine use)
5. Insulin lack

---

**Box 2**
**Emergency Department Observation Unit acceptance criteria for hyperglycemia**

Inclusion Criteria
  Blood sugar greater than 300 mg/dL and less than 600 mg/dL after emergency department treatment
  Normal to near normal pH and $CO_2$ level
  Readily treatable cause (eg, noncompliance, urinary tract infection, abscess)

Exclusion Criteria
  New-onset hyperglycemia
  Diabetic ketoacidosis
  Obtundation (especially in the setting of hyperosmolar hyperglycemic state)
  Social issues precluding continued outpatient management

---

may or may not require insulin. There are several ways to transition to insulin based on insulin usage in the EDOU setting. A general approach is to obtain an A1c initially and use it to determine if the patient may benefit from insulin at all. If above a threshold of 9%, the patient may benefit from a new insulin start (see the section "Insulin transitioning," later in this article), as these patients are unlikely to ultimately achieve adequate control.[5]

Diabetes education can be provided in a number of ways, depending on the resources of the hospital. Some institutions have a "diabetic educator" who handles much of the dietary and pharmacy-related questions for these patients. Other options include separating the pharmacy and diet education needs to work with a pharmacist and diabetic educator separately.

### Diabetic ketoacidosis

Mild DKA (see **Table 1**) may be appropriate for placement in an EDOU, depending on the resources available and the comfort level of the EDOU providers with managing this condition. Moderate to severe DKA and any patient with significant clinical compromise are not appropriate indications for the observation unit setting because of the necessary intensity of service and low likelihood of discharge in 24 hours. Usually DKA is treated with a regular human insulin infusion until the AG is closed. However, there has been considerable experience with insulin aspart and lispro in successfully closing the gap and resolving DKA without requiring an insulin infusion.[6,7] In mild DKA, the time to resolution is generally between 10 and 11 hours from presentation, making it ideal for an observation unit.[8] Potential EDOU interventions for the treatment of mild DKA is provided in **Box 5**, which lists a sample protocol

---

**Box 3**
**Potential Emergency Department Observation Unit interventions for hyperglycemia**

Intravenous hydration using crystalloids at 150 to 250 mL/h

Bedside glucose checks every 2 hours until level less than 300 mg/dL, then every 4 hours

Sliding-scale insulin

Treat precipitating causes

Diabetic counseling

Repeat serum electrolytes every 4 hours until laboratories stable

---

---

**Box 4**
**Emergency Department Observation Unit disposition criteria for hyperglycemia**

Home
  Blood glucose less than 250 mg/dL (see discussion in text)
  Resolution of symptoms
  Normal vital signs
  Tolerating oral fluids
  Primary care follow-up in 48 hours
  Patient education provided

Admit
  Worsening symptoms
  Development of diabetic keotacidosis or hyperosmolar hyperglycemic state
  Inability to tolerate oral fluids despite appropriate management
  Presence of social conditions that preclude safe home management

---

for insulin administration adapted from these studies including the use of rapid-acting insulin.

An important but sometimes overlooked element in the care of patients with DKA is the administration of subcutaneous long-acting insulin while the patient is still receiving an insulin infusion. The timing of this administration, whether at the time of diagnosis or toward the end of the requirement of insulin infusion, is a matter of debate.[9,10] Current recommendations state that the insulin infusion should continue at least 30 minutes to 2 hours beyond the administration of long-acting insulin.[2,11] Other care considerations include education of staff on feeding patients once blood sugars reach the 200 to 250 mg/dL range. In the experience of this author, patients treated for mild DKA are much more likely to become hypoglycemic as a result of over-zealous treatment rather than to fail to have the AG close.

### Insulin transitioning
Many patients will present to the EDOU on outpatient insulin regimens already and transitioning them back to their home regimen is generally simple. However, some patients with type 2 diabetes placed in an EDOU for a hyperglycemic emergency will only have been on outpatient treatment with oral antihyperglycemic agents. Certain

---

**Box 5**
**Observation unit insulin intervention for hyperglycemia in diabetic ketoacidosis**

During diabetic ketoacidosis
  Hydration at 250 mL/h with NS or ½ NS
  Electrolyte replacement of magnesium and potassium
  Insulin aspart at 0.2 units/kg every 2 hours
  Every 2-hour blood sugar level checks
  Every 4-hour basic metabolic panel, β-hydroxybutyrate levels, and venous blood gas

When blood sugar is less than 250 mg/dL
  Fluids changed to dextrose 5% ½ NS at 125 to 250 mL/h
  Insulin decreased to 0.1 units/kg every 2 hours
  Discontinue nothing by mouth status

As diabetic ketoacidosis resolves (criteria blood sugar <250 mg/dL, pH >7.3, anion gap <14, bicarbonate >18)
  Stop intravenous fluids if tolerating an oral diet and has received home long-acting insulin
  Transition to subcutaneous insulin

*Abbreviation:* NS, normal saline.

---

patients with type 2 diabetes will benefit from outpatient treatment with insulin. There are emerging data that support starting insulin in patients with type 2 diabetes if their hemoglobin A1c level is greater than 9.5%.[12] The EDOU can function to initiate this transition through careful patient selection and appropriate education. Other factors that may complicate patient selection for this indication are patient-level issues, such as their access to various resources.

Patients with appropriate access to outpatient resources who require insulin should be started on an optimal regimen that would be basal dosing of long-acting insulin along with a preprandial bolus dosing of rapid-acting insulin. The overall dosing is individualized, but a dosage of 0.5 to 0.8 units/kg per day having 50% divided between the basal dosing and preprandial dosing.[13] Patients with limited access to outpatient resources can be started on a mixed insulin regimen. An advantage of these 70/30 regimens is the decreased cost and these have evidence showing beneficial safety profiles.[14]

### Special populations

There have been no clinical research trials on the management of DKA in patients with end-stage renal disease. The presence of this comorbidity leads to difficulty in interpretation of electrolyte levels due to the mixed acid picture that exists. This challenge coupled with the propensity for hyperkalemia and difficulty with fluid administration makes this a patient population that should be excluded from EDOU care. Patients with a history of congestive heart failure (CHF), regardless of the presence or absence of an acute exacerbation, also should be avoided for placement in the EDOU. These patients require judicious fluid administration and have a risk of developing acute pulmonary edema due to the fluid administered for the treatment of DKA. Further, there is well-documented increased length of stay for these patients beyond the usual observation stay period.[15]

## HYPOGLYCEMIA

A patient with hypoglycemia who has been evaluated by the ED and determined to have an uncomplicated underlying etiology may be appropriate for further care in an EDOU.

### Patient Evaluation Overview

Generally defined as a blood glucose level less than 60 mg/dL, hypoglycemia remains a very common problem in the United States.[3] In fact, hospitalizations for hypoglycemia have surpassed those of hyperglycemia over the past decades.[16] Patients can present with a variety of symptoms that are divided into either neuroglycopenic or autonomic categories. The neuroglycopenic symptoms would include behavior changes, confusion, agitation, and, at very low blood glucose levels, seizures. Patients often are first aware of the presence of hypoglycemia by the development of these neuroglycopenic symptoms.[17] Autonomic symptoms include tremor, palpitations, and hunger. Patients who present with isolated autonomic symptoms may not have a clinical hypoglycemic disorder and simply require food to eat, whereas patients who present with neuroglycopenic complaints are more likely to have a significant hypoglycemic disorder.[18]

Because there is no asymptomatic specific blood glucose that requires immediate treatment in isolation in a patient without diabetes, expert opinion suggests that the presence of the Whipple triad consisting of hypoglycemia, symptoms that are either autonomic or neuroglycopenic, and resolution with provision of glucose should prompt an evaluation for an underlying cause.[18] **Box 6** lists some of the common causes of hypoglycemia in nondiabetic patients.

---

**Box 6**
**Causes of hypoglycemia in adult patients**

Ill individual
1. Drugs (insulin, alcohol)
2. Critical illnesses
    Hepatic, renal, cardiac failure
    Sepsis
    Starvation
3. Hormone deficiency
    Cortisol
    Glucagon
4. Nonislet cell tumor

Well-appearing patient
1. Endogenous insulin (insulinoma, nesidioblastosis)
2. Surreptitious or accidental hypoglycemia (overdose of oral agents)

*Adapted from* Cryer PE, Axelrod L, Grossman AB, et al. Evaluation and management of adult hypoglycemic disorders: an Endocrine Society clinical practice guideline. J Clin Endocrinol Metab 2009;94(3):709–28.

---

### Observation Unit Care

Known diabetics with episodes of hypoglycemia will be the primary beneficiaries of an EDOU clinical care pathway. The pathway is best described as an accelerated treatment pathway. This author does not recommend using the EDOU to determine the cause for hypoglycemia. This evaluation should occur during the initial ED period. The medical evidence available to support hypoglycemia care pathways is limited to a feasibility study by Goh and colleagues[19] in 2009 for patients in a Singapore hospital. This study of 203 patients used many of the aspects found in observation manuals at other institutions.[20] They found a hospital admission rate of 16% but were not able to identify factors that would be predictive of a need for admission. This study demonstrated benefits in costs and length of stay (LOS). In fact, their historical control had an LOS of more than 100 hours compared with the average LOS for the observation unit of only 23 hours. One limitation to the generalizability of this study is that glucose infusion was not listed as an exclusion to placement in their observation unit.

In selecting patients with hypoglycemia appropriate for the observation unit setting, the ideal scenario would include a patient known to have diabetes with the underlying cause being accidental administration of insulin or administration without carbohydrate consumption. The pharmacokinetics of the longer-acting insulin agents are listed in **Table 2** and criteria for placement in the EDOU are shown in **Box 7**.[21]

### Hypoglycemia secondary to oral antihyperglycemic agents

Classically, biguanides such as metformin (Glucophage) do not cause hypoglycemia, whereas sulfonylurea medications including glipizide and glimepiride do. Contemporary treatment of type 2 diabetes involves combinations of these and other noninsulin oral medications, making the teaching about which agents cause hypoglycemia more complex. The newer agent classes, such as alpha-glucosidase-inhibitors, dipeptidyl peptidase-4 inhibitors, and sodium-glucose cotransporter-2 inhibitors do not have as much data in terms of ability to cause hypoglycemia. In a recent meta-analysis, the meglitinide class including nateglinide as well as the sulfonylurea class are consistently shown to cause more hypoglycemia episodes than the newer agents.[22]

Patients who have taken longer-acting insulins, meglitinides, or sulfonylureas should be considered for 12 to 24 hours of care in the EDOU.

| Table 2 | |
|---|---|
| Pharmacokinetics of longer-acting insulins | |
| **Insulin Type** | **Duration of Action, h** |
| Lispro, aspart, glulisine | 2–4 |
| Regular | 5–8 |
| NPH | 18–24 |
| Insulin glargine | 20–24 |
| Insulin detemir | 6–24 |
| NPL | 15 |
| Insulin degludec | >40 |

*Adapted from* McCulloch DK. Insulin therapy in type 2 diabetes mellitus. In: UpToDate, Post TW (Ed), UpToDate, Waltham, MA. Accessed October 6, 2016.

### Potential Emergency Department Observation Unit interventions

A sample listing of interventions is provided in **Box 8**. Patients not at risk for aspiration should be provided a meal rich in carbohydrates as well as fat and protein for more sustained blood sugar levels. If the hypoglycemia episode was not due to inappropriate diet or overdose of medication, then the patient's home medication regimen will need to be adjusted to prevent further episodes of hypoglycemia. The dose of long-acting sulfonylureas should be adjusted downward if not stopped altogether. Insulin should be reduced to two-thirds the dose of what the patient was previously taking.[19]

### Criteria for discharge

Disposition of patients placed in an EDOU for hypoglycemia is based on a number of factors (**Box 9**). After a reasonable period of observation, patients should have normal vital signs and be free of symptoms. It is important that the patient have stable normoglycemia. The level of glucose that is considered safe for discharge has been suggested to be higher than 80 mg/dL, although this is based on expert opinion only.

---

**Vignette Pearls**

The patient in the vignette likely would benefit from observation care. Patients with a new diagnosis of diabetes are typically started on Glucophage with the addition of a sulfonylurea agent in cases of persistently uncontrolled glucose levels. The patient was taking a sulfonylurea (glipizide), which can classically cause hypoglycemia. Patients taking a sulfonylurea who experience hypoglycemia should be observed for 12 to 24 hours to ensure they do not have recurrent episodes.

---

## ELECTROLYTE ABNORMALITIES OF POTASSIUM, SODIUM, AND CALCIUM

---

**Case Study**

A 56-year-old man presents with muscle cramps for several days. He reports initiation of hydrochlorothiazide 5 weeks before the current visit for the treatment of hypertension. His vital signs today are as follows: temperature 98.1, blood pressure 130/84, heart rate 90, $O_2$ 99% on room air. On examination, there are some occasional visible fasciculations of his quadriceps muscle. Laboratory values are remarkable for a potassium level of 2.6 mmol/L.

---

**Box 7**
**Criteria for Emergency Department Observation Unit placement for hypoglycemia**

Inclusion Criteria
    Blood glucose less than 40 mg/dL at diagnosis and greater than 80 mg/dL after treatment
    History of type 1 or type 2 diabetes
    Underlying serious etiology considered and appropriately evaluated

Exclusion Criteria
    Hypoglycemia secondary to drug ingestion as part of attempt at self-harm
    Dextrose 5% or dextrose 10% infusion required to maintain euglycemia
    Inability to tolerate oral intake

---

Electrolyte disorders are very amenable to EDOU care because of their generally simple treatment plans consisting of merely replacing the missing item. Practitioners can intuit the LOS based on the severity of the deficiency of the electrolyte. **Table 3** shows our guidelines for inclusion of these disorders and several are discussed in more detail in the following sections.

### Hypokalemia

Although hypokalemia remains a common problem among patients with coexisting severe conditions such as DKA, the incidence of hypokalemia in the general ED population may be close to 11%.[23] Most of these cases are the result of diuretic use.[24] This group of patients with less severe concomitant illness would be ideal targets for short-stay care. For patients with hypokalemia, the search for an underlying cause is essential, as is finding additional electrolyte abnormalities. The associated findings of hyponatremia and hypomagnesemia are well documented.[24] In a study by Marti and colleagues[23] in 2013, gastroenteritis and malnutrition were also noted to be significant causes of low potassium. Selected additional causes are listed in **Box 10**.[23]

    There are several key elements of care to note in the placement of patients in an EDOU for correction of low potassium. Electrocardiographic changes are common in both asymptomatic and symptomatic patients with hypokalemia; however, the symptom of muscle cramps is generally seen when potassium levels fall below 2.5 mmol/L. Thus, patients with muscle cramps and near normal potassium should have alternate causes fully evaluated. The major causes of hypokalemia, as discussed previously, can likely be addressed in an EDOU and some hospitals use a potassium repletion protocol that is nurse driven. In fact, in critically ill patients, protocol-driven replacement strategies shorten the time between identification and repletion of the abnormal electrolyte levels.[25] Institutional policies may dictate the manner in which

---

**Box 8**
**Potential interventions of observation unit**

Meal tray

Serial examinations

Intravenous hydration

Point-of-care glucose measurement every 2 hours

Dextrose 50% intravenous bolus for significant hypoglycemia

Diabetic education/teaching

**Box 9**
**Disposition of Emergency Department Observation Unit patients with hypoglycemia**

Discharge
    Resolution of symptoms
    Capable adult supervision
    Bedside glucose more than 80 mg/dL
    Resolution of precipitating factor
    Follow-up with primary care arranged

Admission
    Deterioration of clinical signs
    Persistent deficits in neurologic status
    Bedside glucose consistently less than 80 mg/dL

**Table 3**
**EDOU acceptance criteria for electrolyte abnormalities**

| *Inclusion criteria* | |
| --- | --- |
| Unremarkable vital signs | |
| Underlying cause of electrolyte abnormality does not require hospitalization | |
| No other comorbid condition present requiring more prolonged hospitalization | |
| Mild and rapidly correctable electrolyte abnormality | |
| For hyperkalemia | Level <5.0 mEq/L<br>ECG with clear p waves<br>Some T wave tenting is acceptable<br>No QRS widening after 1 h of treatment during ED stay |
| For hypokalemia | Level >2.5 mEq/L<br>No ventricular ectopy on ED monitoring for >1 h |
| For hyponatremia | Level >120 mEq/L<br>Normal mentation<br>Not due to psychogenic polydipsia or SIADH |
| For hypernatremia | Level <155 mEq/L<br>Normal mentation |
| For hypercalcemia | Level <7.0 mEq/L (ionized) |
| For hypocalcemia | Level >1.0 mEq/L (ionized) |
| For hypomagnesemia | Level >2.0 mEq/L<br>Associated with other minor electrolyte abnormalities |
| *Exclusion criteria* | |
| Unstable vital signs or signs of cardiovascular compromise | |
| Mental status changes | |
| Associated cause not amenable to short-term treatment: bowel obstruction, appendicitis, bowel ischemia, DKA, sepsis, some drug effects, and so forth | |
| Presence of abnormality that will require treatment for longer than usual length of stay in EDOU | |
| More than 2 acute electrolyte disturbances | |

*Abbreviations:* DKA, diabetic ketoacidosis; ECG, electrocardiogram; ED, emergency department; EDOU, Emergency Department Observation Unit; SIADH, syndrome of inappropriate antidiuretic hormone secretion.

---

**Box 10**
**Causes of hypokalemia**

| | |
|---|---|
| Decreased K+ intake/increased cellular entry | Increased gastrointestinal losses |

Elevation of extracellular pH
Increased insulin
Elevated β-adrenergic activity: stress or
administration of beta agonists
Hypokalemic periodic paralysis
Increase in blood cell production
Hypothermia
Chloroquine intoxication
Other

Increased sweat losses
Dialysis
Plasmapheresis

Vomiting
Diarrhea
Enteral tube drainage
Laxative abuse
Increased urinary losses

Diuretics
Primary mineralocorticoid excess
Renal tubular acidosis
Hypomagnesemia
Salt-wasting nephropathies
Polyuria

---

electrolytes are repleted and therefore should be consulted when developing an institutional protocol. The primary advantage of adopting an institutional replacement pathway is that the nurses already may be familiar with its implementation. Obviously, all patients should be monitored by telemetry and the goal level would be >3.0 mmol/L at discharge.

## Hyponatremia/Hypernatremia

Typically, disorders of sodium balance require careful monitoring and are usually associated with other diagnoses. The underlying etiology of most patients with low sodium is the intake of excess fluids and the failure to appropriately excrete the excess.[26] Typically defined as sodium level below 135 mEq/L, the causes of hyponatremia that would lend themselves to EDOU care are hyperglycemia, CHF, gastroenteritis, and volume depletion. These topics are discussed in separate articles in this issue; however, there are a few considerations for each of these conditions.

### Hyperglycemia

Hyperglycemia results in increased serum osmolarity. In hyperglycemic patients, a correction for glucose levels must be calculated to determine the actual sodium concentration. The corrected [Na$^+$] is calculated by adding to measured [Na$^+$] 1.6 mEq/L for every 100 mg/dL increment of serum glucose above normal; a correction factor by 2.4 mEq/L is used when serum glucose concentrations are higher than 400 mg/dL.[27]

### Congestive heart failure

As discussed elsewhere, hyponatremia is generally an exclusion criterion for EDOU management of patients with CHF. This is not without justification, though. A recent retrospective review identified hyponatremia as an independent marker for higher mortality and readmission in patients with decompensated CHF.[28] Hence, placing these patients in the observation unit would be a dubious endeavor.

### Gastroenteritis and volume depletion

Mild hyponatremia is seen in volume-depleted states in which sodium loss has exceeded free water loss. This is frequently encountered in the observation setting. Treatment strategies beyond the repletion of volume are similar, as rapid correction of sodium can result in osmotic demyelination syndrome. Patients with seizures secondary to dysnatremias are critically ill and do not belong in an EDOU. Their risk of developing demyelination is much higher. For all patients, the rate of rise in the serum sodium concentration should be targeted at between 4 and 6 mEq/L over 24 hours. An elevation of more than 9 mEq/L increases the risk of a bad outcome significantly.

The overwhelming majority of cases of hypernatremia encountered in the ED that may be appropriate for an EDOU are due to water loss from either skin or gastric sources. Other causes, such as diabetes insipidus and exogenous salt intake, would not be appropriate for EDOU care. Replacement of this volume is discussed elsewhere.

### Hypercalcemia

Most causes of hypercalcemia would be inappropriate for observation care. However, mild to moderate symptomatic hypercalcemia (12–14 mg/dL) may be encountered in any number of instances, including renal failure, hyperthyroidism, and use of thiazide diuretics. In patients with end-stage renal disease, aggressive volume expansion, the mainstay of therapy of hypercalcemia, would not be appropriate. Most patients with normal renal function can be treated with intravascular volume expansion using isotonic saline at an initial rate of 200 to 300 mL/h. The rate is then adjusted to maintain urine output at 100 to 150 mL/h. Loop diuretics should be avoided because of their potential complications and failure to address the most common underlying cause: bone resorption. Bone resorption can be treated with either calcitonin or a bisphosphonate medication. There is no definitive goal for $[Ca^{++}]$; however, a decrease to near normal levels of 10 to 12 mg/dL often is enough to abate symptoms.

Endocrine care pathways can be simple and patients will benefit from the efficient care in the observation setting. Caution should be exercised in these conditions during the acute phase of care in determining appropriateness of the observation care setting. In addition to being clinically ill, sometimes the burden of laboratory draws and reevaluations precludes the observation unit being the most optimal setting. Ultimately, however, the previously discussed endocrine conditions may prove to be ideal for many types of observation units (see **Box 10**).

### REFERENCES

1. Wang J, Williams DE, Narayan KMV, et al. Declining death rates from hyperglycemic crisis among adults with diabetes, U.S., 1985–2002. Diabetes Care 2006; 29(9):2018–22.
2. Kitabchi AE, Umpierrez GE, Miles JM, et al. Hyperglycemic crises in adult patients with diabetes. Diabetes Care 2009;32(7):1335–43.
3. Ford W, Self WH, Slovis C, et al. Diabetes in the emergency department and hospital: acute care of diabetes patients. Curr Emerg Hosp Med Rep 2013;1(1):1–9.
4. Driver BE, Olives TD, Bischof JE, et al. Discharge glucose is not associated with short-term adverse outcomes in emergency department patients with moderate to severe hyperglycemia. Ann Emerg Med 2016;68(6):697–705.e3.
5. Sherifali D, Nerenberg K, Pullenayegum E, et al. The effect of oral antidiabetic agents on A1C levels. Diabetes Care 2010;33(8):1859–64.
6. Kitabchi AE, Umpierrez GE, Fisher JN, et al. Thirty years of personal experience in hyperglycemic crises: diabetic ketoacidosis and hyperglycemic hyperosmolar state. J Clin Endocrinol Metab 2008;93(5):1541–52.
7. Cohn BG, Keim SM, Watkins JW, et al. Does management of diabetic ketoacidosis with subcutaneous rapid-acting insulin reduce the need for intensive care unit admission? J Emerg Med 2015;49(4):530–8.
8. Umpierrez GE, Cuervo R, Karabell A, et al. Treatment of diabetic ketoacidosis with subcutaneous insulin aspart. Diabetes Care 2004;27(8):1873–8.

9. Doshi P, Potter AJ, De Los Santos D, et al. Prospective randomized trial of insulin glargine in acute management of diabetic ketoacidosis in the emergency department: a pilot study. Acad Emerg Med 2015;22(6):657–62.
10. Houshyar J, Bahrami A, Aliasgarzadeh A. Effectiveness of insulin glargine on recovery of patients with diabetic ketoacidosis: a randomized controlled trial. J Clin Diagn Res 2015;9(5):OC01–5.
11. Savage MW, Dhatariya KK, Kilvert A, et al. Joint British Diabetes Societies guideline for the management of diabetic ketoacidosis. Diabet Med 2011;28(5):508–15.
12. Wallia A, Molitch ME. Insulin therapy for type 2 diabetes mellitus. JAMA 2014; 311(22):2315–25.
13. Gosmanov AR, Gosmanova EO, Dillard-Cannon E. Management of adult diabetic ketoacidosis. Diabetes Metab Syndr Obes 2014;7:255–64.
14. Raja-Khan N, Warehime SS, Gabbay RA. Review of biphasic insulin aspart in the treatment of type 1 and 2 diabetes. Vasc Health Risk Manag 2007;3(6):919–35.
15. Adigopula S, Feng Y, Babu V, et al. Hyperglycemia is associated with increased length of stay and total cost in patients hospitalized for congestive heart failure. World J Cardiovasc Dis 2013;03(02):245–9.
16. Lipska KJ, Ross JS, Wang Y, et al. National trends in US hospital admissions for hyperglycemia and hypoglycemia among medicare beneficiaries, 1999 to 2011. JAMA Intern Med 2014;174(7):1116–24.
17. Hepburn DA, Deary IJ, Frier BM, et al. Symptoms of acute insulin-induced hypoglycemia in humans with and without IDDM. Factor-analysis approach. Diabetes Care 1991;14(11):949–57.
18. Cryer PE, Axelrod L, Grossman AB, et al. Evaluation and management of adult hypoglycemic disorders: an endocrine society clinical practice guideline. J Clin Endocrinol Metab 2009;94(3):709–28.
19. Goh KP. Management of hyponatremia. Am Fam Physician 2004;69(10):2387–94.
20. Observation Medicine Practice Resources. Available at: https://www.acep.org/Physician-Resources/Practice-Resources/Administration/Observation-Medicine/. Accessed November 30, 2016.
21. McCullough D. Insulin therapy in type 2 diabetes. UpToDate. Available at: https://www.uptodate.com/contents/insulin-therapy-in-type-2-diabetes-mellitus?source=search_result&search=insulin%20peak%20times&selectedTitle=4~150. Accessed October 6, 2016.
22. Mearns ES, Sobieraj DM, White CM, et al. Comparative efficacy and safety of antidiabetic drug regimens added to metformin monotherapy in patients with type 2 diabetes: a network meta-analysis. PLoS One 2015;10(4):e0125879.
23. Marti G, Schwarz C, Leichtle AB, et al. Etiology and symptoms of severe hypokalemia in emergency department patients. Eur J Emerg 2014;21(1):46–51.
24. Weiner ID, Wingo CS. Hypokalemia–consequences, causes, and correction. J Am Soc Nephrol 1997;8(7):1179–88.
25. Hijazi M, Al-Ansari M. Protocol-driven vs. physician-driven electrolyte replacement in adult critically ill patients. Ann Saudi Med 2005;25(2):105–10.
26. Sahay M, Sahay R. Hyponatremia: a practical approach. Indian J Endocrinol Metab 2014;18(6):760–71.
27. Hillier TA, Abbott RD, Barrett EJ. Hyponatremia: evaluating the correction factor for hyperglycemia. Am J Med 1999;106(4):399–403.
28. De Vecchis R, Di Maio M, Di Biase G, et al. Effects of hyponatremia normalization on the short-term mortality and rehospitalizations in patients with recent acute decompensated heart failure: a retrospective study. J Clin Med 2016;5(10):92.

# Care of Neurologic Conditions in an Observation Unit

Matthew A. Wheatley, MD*, Michael A. Ross, MD

## KEYWORDS

- Emergency department • Neurologic conditions • Cerebrovascular disease
- Headache • Observation unit

## KEY POINTS

- ED Observation Units are the ideal setting for continued monitoring, and diagnostic testing for patients presenting to the ED with neurologic complaints.
- A transient ischemic attack (TIA) is a sentinel event for stroke. Patients with TIA should be risk stratified and begin risk lowering therapies.
- Similarly, the EDOU can be used for further risk stratification of patients with non-disabling cerebrovascular accidents (CVA).
- The EDOU is appropriate for patients with other neurologic conditions such as headache, seizures and vertigo. Goals can include neuro checks, imaging or specialist consultation.

---

**Case Study**

Carol Brown is a 58-year-old woman who presents to the emergency department with pronounced weakness for 12 minutes that resolved 1 hour before arrival. She has a history of hypertension and hyperlipidemia, but no prior stroke or transient ischemic attack. Her examination is normal, including a National Institutes of Health Stroke Score of zero. In the emergency department her cardiac monitor shows a sinus rhythm, and her noncontrast head computed tomography scan and blood work is normal. Her ABCD$^2$ score is 3. In the observation unit, her serial examinations and cardiac monitoring are normal, her echocardiogram and MRI of the brain are normal; however, her magnetic resonance angiogram of the neck vessels shows greater than 70% carotid stenosis. She was admitted to the hospital and underwent successful endarterectomy 5 days later following preoperative clearance. On 1-month follow-up she was asymptomatic and doing well.

---

Department of Emergency Medicine, Emory University, 49 Jesse Hill Jr Drive, Atlanta, GA 30303, USA
* Corresponding author.
*E-mail address:* mwheatl@emory.edu

Emerg Med Clin N Am 35 (2017) 603–623
http://dx.doi.org/10.1016/j.emc.2017.03.007
0733-8627/17/© 2017 Elsevier Inc. All rights reserved.

## INTRODUCTION

As a group, neurologic conditions represent a substantial portion of emergency department (ED) visits. In 2011, 4.7% of ED visits were for diseases of the nervous system.[1] Cerebrovascular disease was the fifth leading principal hospital discharge diagnosis for admitted ED patients.[1] Between 2001 and 2011 the percentage of patients receiving neuro imaging in the ED increased 39% (from 66% to 92%).[2] Similarly, headache (HA) is the fourth leading principal reason for an ED visit overall, accounting for 4.3 million visits or 3.2% of all visits.

## TRANSIENT ISCHEMIC ATTACK
### Background

In the United States, stroke is the fifth leading cause of death.[3] With roughly 800,000 strokes occurring annually, stroke is also a leading cause of disability, costing the United States roughly $34 billion per year.[4] Eighty-five percent of strokes are ischemic, and between 15% and 30% of ischemic strokes are preceded by a transient ischemic attack (TIA).[5,6] An estimated 240,000 TIAs occur annually. TIA has been redefined by the American Stroke Association (ASA) as a "(t)ransient episode of neurologic dysfunction caused by focal brain, spinal cord, or retinal ischemia without acute infarction."[7] Notable updates in this definition include the addition of "infarction" found on brain imaging and the removal of time elements such as 24 hours or 1 hour. Symptoms lasting more than 1 hour have a less than 1 of 6 chance of not having a stroke.[7] Patients with clinical resolution of stroke symptoms that show brain infarction on computed tomography (CT) imaging have a fourfold higher risk of subsequent stroke, and those with a new infarct on MRI have a fivefold higher incidence of subsequent stroke.[8–10]

Although patients with TIA present with no residual deficits, they are at significant risk of subsequent vascular events. Overall, their approximate 90-day stroke rate is 12%, with half of these strokes occurring within the first 1 to 2 days after a sentinel TIA.[7,11,12] In fact, this 90-day stroke rate is more than twice that of patients who have suffered an actual stroke (4%), suggesting that patients with TIA present in a state of greater vascular vulnerability. Yet this is confounded by the fact that these patients appear clinically normal, and most will not have an adverse event during or shortly after their TIA, making TIA an ideal condition for an ED observation unit (EDOU).

### Emergency Department Management

The initial ED evaluation and subsequent EDOU management of patients with TIA is focused on the early detection and prevention of stroke, the detection of alternate causes of TIA symptoms, and the prevention of future strokes. This includes a history that includes symptom duration, vascular risk factors, and other potential etiologies. Ideally, the examination should include a structured stroke examination, such as the National Institutes of Health Stroke Score (NIHSS), to improve the clinical detection of small or subtle strokes. Obtaining an electrocardiogram and placing the patient on cardiac monitoring is important for the detection of atrial fibrillation. Blood testing should include a complete blood count, serum glucose, and electrolytes. A prothrombin time is often ordered, as well, in the event that the patient subsequently develops stroke requiring reperfusion therapy. Brain imaging, with either CT or MRI, should be obtained if possible. Although the safety of delaying imaging is unknown, there are several benefits to timely imaging.[13]

The transient ischemia that occurs in patients with TIA may be due to a number of different vascular events (**Table 1**). Causes of TIA may be broadly classified as intracranial vascular, extracranial vascular, and cardioembolic. When an etiology is not

**Table 1**
**Causes of transient ischemic attack or ischemic stroke**

| Etiology | Causes |
|---|---|
| Intracranial vascular | Atherosclerotic<br>Branch occlusive disease |
| Extracranial vascular | Carotid plaque with arteriogenic emboli<br>Flow-limiting stenosis |
| Cardioembolic | Paroxysmal atrial fibrillation<br>Paradoxic embolism<br>Valve disease with clot formation<br>Intramural clot formation associated with dyskinesis |
| Cryptogenic | Cardiac etiologies: Paroxysmal atrial fibrillation, subacute bacterial endocarditis (culture negative), papillary fibroelastoma<br>Subtle arterial dissections<br>Central nervous system vasculitis<br>Hypercoagulable state in setting of cancer<br>Metabolic disorders: hyper-homocysteine, Fabry disease<br>Plaque in aortic arch<br>Human immunodeficiency virus, central nervous system infection<br>Drug abuse<br>Genetic etiologies (eg, cerebral autosomal dominant arteriopathy with subcortical infarcts and leukoencephalopathy [CADASIL], mitochondrial encephalomyopathy, lactic acidosis, and stroke-like episodes [MELAS]) |

identified, the etiology is classified as cryptogenic. Although this refers to patients with stroke, the testing for causative etiologies for TIA is similar.

It is important to consider conditions that commonly mimic TIA. These include epilepsy, postictal paralysis, complex migraines, such as hemiplegic or ocular migraines, cervical disc disease, transient global amnesia, intracranial lesions, such as subdural hematomas and mass lesions, inner ear disease with vertigo, and metabolic derangement of the serum glucose, sodium, or calcium.

A unique challenge with the diagnosis of TIA is the lack of a clear gold standard for this diagnosis. When a neurologist is used as the gold standard, false-positive diagnostic rates range from 25% to 38%.[14–16] There is even poor agreement between fellowship-trained stroke neurologists.[17]

To improve diagnostic performance, TIA risk stratification scores have been developed. The most common is the ABCD$^2$ score (**Table 2**).[11] American Heart Association (AHA)/ASA guidelines recommend admission or discharge based on a total score greater or less than 3.[7] Like other clinical prediction tools, the ABCD$^2$ score may be used to estimate the likelihood that a patient is having a TIA mimic. However, many have subsequently found high levels of carotid stenosis, atrial fibrillation, and other cardiac sources of embolism in patients with ABCD$^2$ less than 3.[18] Based on these and other studies, the 2016 American College of Emergency Physicians (ACEP) policy for the evaluation of patients with suspected TIA in the ED recommends that physicians do not rely on current scores, such as the ABCD$^2$ score, to identify patients who may be discharged directly from the ED.[13]

## Observation Unit Care

### Patient selection
Several protocols have been reported (**Box 1**).[13–16,19,20] Patients are selected after being seen in the ED and given the diagnosis of TIA by an attending emergency physician. Patients are excluded from the Accelerated Diagnostic Protocol (ADP) if they

**Table 2**
**ABCD² score**

| Risk Factor | Points |
|---|---|
| Age $\geq$ 60 | 1 |
| Blood pressure (BP) | 1 |
|   Systolic BP $\geq$ 140 mm Hg or diastolic BP $\geq$ 90 mm Hg | |
| Clinical features of transient ischemic attack (TIA) (choose 1) | |
|   Unilateral weakness with or without speech impairment or | 2 |
|   Speech impairment without unilateral weakness | 1 |
| Duration | |
|   TIA duration $\geq$ 60 min | 2 |
|   TIA duration 10–59 min | 1 |
| Diabetes | 1 |
| Total ABCD² score | 0–7 |

*From* Johnson SC, Rothwell PM, Huynh-Huynh MN, et al. Validation and refinement of scores to predict very early stroke risk after transient ischemic attack. Lancet 2007;369:283–92.

have (1) any persistent acute neurologic deficit or crescendo TIAs; (2) a positive head CT; (3) a known cardioembolic source; (4) known carotid stenosis (>50%); (5) nonfocal symptoms; (6) significant other acute or chronic comorbidities necessitating inpatient admission.

### Observation unit interventions

The protocol has 4 key diagnostic components: (1) carotid imaging (2) serial clinical evaluation, which includes serial neuro-assessments every 2 hours by NIHSS-trained nurses, emergency physicians, and associate providers, and a neurologist consultant; (3) cardiac monitoring for at least 12 hours; and (4) echocardiography.[13,16,21] Because brain MRI is more sensitive for tissue injury, and generally takes longer than CT to obtain, it is obtained in the EDOU.[19,22] Additionally, screening for treatable conditions that contribute to stroke occurs, such as uncontrolled diabetes, hypertension, smoking, and substance abuse.[23] EDOU patients are often admitted as inpatients if they develop recurrent neurologic symptoms or a stroke, if significant carotid stenosis or a cardioembolic source of TIA is identified, if it is not possible to complete the workup or safely discharge the patient home within 24 hours, or if admission for other reasons is needed.[13,16,21]

The 2009 ASA/AHA guidelines recommend that noninvasive imaging of the cervicocephalic vessels should be performed routinely as part of the evaluation of patients with suspected TIAs (Class I, Level of Evidence A).[7] There are several options to consider for carotid imaging. Because guidelines recommend that an MRI is obtained in patients with a TIA, a magnetic resonance angiogram (MRA) of the brain and neck vessels also can be performed. If MRI cannot be performed, then CT angiography (CTA) may be obtained. If CTA cannot be obtained, then carotid Doppler imaging may be obtained. Guidelines from ACEP, the National Stroke Association, and ASA do not specify which imaging modality is superior.[7,13,24] Recommendations may be best summarized in the ASA guidelines, which specify that imaging may be selected based on "local availability, expertise, and patient characteristics."[7]

Serial examinations to detect occult stroke are important. In one study, serial examinations were the diagnostic intervention that identified most patients with a positive clinical outcome leading to inpatient admission.[16] Serial examinations may be performed by the EDOU nurses, advanced practice providers, managing emergency

**Box 1**
**Transient ischemic attack accelerated diagnostic protocol**

*Inclusion*

- Transient ischemic attack (TIA): resolved acute deficit, not crescendo TIAs
- Negative head computed tomography (CT) (unless prompt MRI planned; with a normal examination and not high risk for bleed)
- Workup can be completed within ~18 hours

*Exclusion*

- Head CT imaging positive for bleed, mass, or acute infarction
- Known extracranial embolic source: history of atrial fibrillation, cardiomyopathy, artificial heart valve, endocarditis, known mural thrombus, or recent myocardial infarction
- Known carotid stenosis (>50%)
- Any persistent acute (<72 hour) neurologic deficit or crescendo TIAs
- Nonfocal symptoms; for example, confusion, weakness, seizure, transient global amnesia
- Hypertensive encephalopathy
- Unable to pass emergency department dysphagia screen
- Severe headache or evidence of cranial arteritis
- Acute medical or social (poor home support) issues requiring inpatient admission
- Prior large stroke, making serial neurologic examinations problematic
- Pregnancy

*Potential interventions*

- Neuro checks every 2 hours to detect stroke, crescendo TIA, and so forth
- Neurology consult to detect occult stroke
- Fasting lipid panel, HgA1c
- Carotid imaging with MRI/magnetic resonance angiography (MRA) to detect infarct or surgical carotid stenosis (>50%)
  - If contraindications to MRI/MRA and *good* renal function, then *CT angiography* of head and neck vessels
  - If contraindications to MRI/MRA and *poor* renal function, then *Doppler* of neck vessels
- 2-dimensional echocardiography as indicated by neurology to detect a cardioembolic source
- Cardiac monitoring for at least 12 hours for paroxysmal atrial fibrillation
- Antiplatelet therapy (aspirin ⇒ If already on aspirin then clopidogrel OR dipyridamole/aspirin)
- Stroke preventive educational materials (lipids, smoking, diabetes mellitus, hypertension, obesity, alcohol, stroke)

*Disposition*

Home
- No recurrent deficits, negative workup
- Clinically stable for discharge home (ie, on antiplatelet therapy and stroke-prevention medications)

Hospital
- Recurrent symptoms/deficit
- Evidence of treatable vascular disease; for example, greater than 50% stenosis of neck vessels
- Evidence of embolic source requiring treatment (eg, heparin/coumadin); for example, mural thrombus, paroxysmal atrial fibrillation
- Unable to complete workup or safely discharge patient within timeframe
- Physician judgment

physician, and neurology consultants. The examination frequency should allow time to diagnose an interval stroke and initiate reperfusion therapy within 3.0 to 4.5 hours from the time last known normal. For this reason, examinations every 2 hours are often used.[16,21,24] It is ideal for staff to be trained in a structured stroke examination, such as the NIHSS, for better consistency and to focus on the essential stroke features.[25] It is important to focus serial examinations on the specific clinical features for which the patient presented to the ED because this represents the vascular territory that is most at risk; for example, if a patient's presenting TIA symptom was dysarthria and left arm weakness. That specific feature should be reexamined on serial examinations, although other neurologic features may be reexamined as well.

Cardiac monitoring for paroxysmal atrial fibrillation, or other major dysrhythmias, occurs following an initial electrocardiogram (ECG) in the ED to screen for atrial fibrillation.[16] Anticoagulation of patients with atrial fibrillation is associated with a 61% reduction in the annual risk of stroke.[26] Patients with TIA with untreated atrial fibrillation may be admitted as inpatients.[13,16] Although initial ED and observation unit cardiac monitoring for paroxysmal atrial fibrillation is important, studies of patients with TIA or cryptogenic strokes suggest that more prolonged monitoring improves detection rates in selected patients.[27,28] The role of prolonged outpatient monitoring continues to be refined and is generally guided by the neurology consultant or physician who will be following the patient after discharge.

The role of echocardiography in the evaluation of patients with TIA is less clear. The 2009 ASA guidelines suggest that transthoracic echocardiography is reasonable in patients in whom no cause of TIA has been identified to detect conditions, such as patients with patent foramen ovale (PFO) or valvular disease that might benefit from specific treatments (Class IIa, Level of evidence B).[7] However, a recent trial sheds doubt on the efficacy of PFO closure.[29] It is also unclear which patients benefit from echocardiography during their index visit to initiate time-sensitive stroke-prevention treatments, compared with patients who may be discharged for outpatient testing.

Although screening for and initiating treatment of stroke risk factors are not associated with a decrease in the short-term stroke risk, they are associated with considerable benefit.[30] Patients presenting to the ED with TIA are likely to represent a unique teachable moment when these interventions are most effective. For this reason, such interventions are required for hospitals to be accredited as a primary stroke center by the Joint Commission for the Accreditation of Hospital Organizations.[31] The details of these prevention measures are often coordinated with neurology consultants or primary care physicians with whom patients will be following up.

### Beneficial outcomes of transient ischemic attack accelerated diagnostic protocols

Outpatient "TIA clinics" in Europe have been shown to be effective not only in shortening time and reducing overall cost of evaluation, but actually reduce the number of subsequent strokes.[14,15] Similar results have been reported in the United States using EDOUs. In a prospective randomized trial of 149 patients with TIA comparing an EDOU TIA ADP with inpatient admission with standing orders, Ross and colleagues[16] found that ADP patients had a significantly shorter length of stay (25.6 vs 61.2 hours) and lower 90-day costs ($890 vs $1510) with no increase in adverse outcomes. ADP patients were more likely to complete necessary testing, and 85% were discharged from the EDOU. Nahab and colleagues[21] performed a before and after validation of this ADP with 142 patients with TIA at a separate academic medical center. Findings were similar in terms of length of stay and cost differences, with no differences in compliance with stroke quality measures, such as diabetes screening, hyperlipidemia screening, or antithrombotic therapy. Others have reported similar findings as these.[19,20]

These, and other issues, support the use of an ADP for patients with TIA as a best practice for selected patients relative to traditional care. The 2016 ACEP policy "Critical Issues in the Evaluation of Adult Patients with Suspected TIA in the ED," asks the question "In adult patients with suspected TIA, can a rapid ED-based diagnostic protocol safely identify patients at short-term risk for stroke?" The patient management recommendations include that "In adult patients with suspected TIA without high-risk conditions, a rapid ED-based diagnostic protocol may be used to evaluate patients at short-term risk for stroke" (Level B recommendation).[13] The National Stroke Association recommendations for care of patients with a TIA recognize the role of EDOUs as well.[24]

## MINOR STROKE
### Introduction

The efficacy of the EDOU in the management of TIA begs the question: can an EDOU also be used for the management of minor cerebrovascular accidents (mCVA)? This could include patients who present after 24 to 48 hours with persistent symptoms but have been able to perform their activities of daily living (ADLs) at home or patients with acute symptoms who are able to pass a bedside dysphagia screen and ambulate unassisted in the ED.

### What is a "Minor Stroke"?

One of the difficulties in developing an EDOU protocol is that there is no universally accepted definition of minor stroke. Fischer and colleagues[32] evaluated various definitions in 760 consecutive patients with acute ischemic stroke and found best outcomes with a score not greater than 1 on any NIHSS item, a composite NIHSS of no greater than 3 and presence of a normal level of consciousness. Ninety percent of patients defined in this way had a modified Rankin scale score of 2 or less at 3 months, corresponding with slight to no disability (**Table 3**).

### Emergency Department Management

The initial ED workup for patients with mCVA is similar to that of patients with TIA. All patients should have a noncontrast head CT while in the ED. The American College of Cardiology and AHA (ACC/AHA) recommendations for TIA are to obtain a head CT only if MRI is not immediately available. For patients presenting with persistent

| Table 3 Modified Rankin scale | |
|---|---|
| Score | Description |
| 0 | No symptoms at all |
| 1 | No significant disability despite symptoms; able to carry out all usual duties and activities |
| 2 | Slight disability; unable to carry out all previous activities, but able to look after own affairs without assistance |
| 3 | Moderate disability; requiring some help, but able to walk without assistance |
| 4 | Moderately severe disability; unable to walk without assistance and unable to attend to own bodily needs without assistance |
| 5 | Severe disability; bedridden, incontinent and requiring constant nursing care and attention |
| 6 | Dead |

*From* van Swieten J, Koudstaal P, Visser M, et al. Interobserver agreement for the assessment of handicap in stroke patients. Stroke 1988;19(5):604–7.

symptoms, a head CT is necessary during the initial ED evaluation to rule out intracranial hemorrhage or mass lesion. Additionally, an infarct may be visible on CT for patients who present with subacute symptoms. All patients should have basic laboratories and urinalysis sent to screen for comorbid medical conditions. Finally, a neurologist should examine all patients with an mCVA while in the ED.

### Observation Unit Care

To date, there have been no trials examining the use of EDOUs in this patient population. Paul and colleagues[33] published a prospective case series that compared outcomes of 845 patients with TIA or small stroke referred to an outpatient stroke clinic in the United Kingdom versus inpatient admission. In their study, there were 250 patients with minor stroke (NIHSS >3) referred to the outpatient clinic; 237 (95%) of these were discharged the same day. The rehospitalization rate was similar between the inpatient and outpatient groups (6.3% vs 6.8%, $P = .83$), as was the 30-day recurrent stroke rate (3.8% vs 5.3%, $P = .61$). They also reported reduced overall costs for the patients managed as outpatients.

### Patient Selection

The key in selecting appropriate patients for the EDOU is screening for those patients who will benefit from inpatient physical, occupational, or speech therapy as well as subacute rehabilitation. These patients often will require more than 24 hours of care. The Centers for Medicare and Medicaid Services' 3-day rule, also known as the 72-hour rule, requires 3 days of care as an inpatient to have Medicare benefits cover their associated stay in skilled nursing facility. All patients need to pass a bedside dysphagia screen and mobility assessment in the ED. One objective measure of mobility is the "get up and go" test, in which the patient is asked to stand from a seated position, walk a short distance, turn around, walk back and sit down.[34] It is graded on a 5-point scale in which a score of 1 indicates no need for assistance or risk of falling and a score of 5 indicates the patient fell or almost fell during the test (**Table 4**). A score of 3 indicates a risk of falling and should be given if the patient exhibits undue slowness, hesitancy, or stumbling. Although this test has not been validated in this population, the provider needs to perform some functional assessment on patients before EDOU transfer.

### Observation Unit Interventions

EDOU care in patients with mCVA is similar to that for patients with TIAs (**Box 2**). All patients need continuous cardiac monitoring and nurse-performed neurologic checks

| Table 4 Get up and go test | |
| --- | --- |
| Score | Description |
| 1 | Normal: no assistance required; no evidence of falling |
| 2 | Very slightly abnormal |
| 3 | Mildly abnormal: fall risk; patient exhibited undue slowness, hesitancy, abnormal movements of the trunk or upper limbs, staggering or stumbling |
| 4 | Moderately abnormal |
| 5 | Severely abnormal: at risk of falling during the test |

*From* Mathias S, Nayak USL, Isaacs B. Balance in elderly patients: the "get-up and go" test. Arch Phys Med Rehabil 1986;67:387–9.

**Box 2**
**Emergency department observation unit minor stroke protocol**

*Inclusion*

- Nondisabling stroke: will not require nursing home or inpatient rehabilitation on discharge
- Patient is ambulatory
- Independent with activities of daily living (ADLs) (modified Rankin score of <2)
- National Institutes of Health Stroke Score (NIHSS) ≤3; individual component score ≤1
- Passing bedside dysphagia screen
- No high-risk conditions
- Unstable deficit (waxing/waning)
- Evidence of embolic pattern (cortical strokes)
- Acute infarcts >2 cm
- Presence of symptomatic cervical internal carotid artery stenosis (>50%)
- Head CT scan negative for hemorrhage/mass lesion

*Exclusion*

- Disabling stroke (new gait disturbance, unable to perform ADLs, NIHSS >3, fails dysphagia screen)
- Presence of high-risk features
- Altered/depressed mental status
- Known extracranial embolic source (history of atrial fibrillation, cardiomyopathy, artificial heart valve, mural thrombus)
- Active comorbidities
- Poor social support
- Prior large stroke making serial examinations problematic

*Potential interventions*

- Screen for evolving stroke
  - Serial neurology checks
  - Neurology consultation
- Evaluate size of stroke: MRI brain with and without contrast
- Evaluate for embolic sources: MRI head and neck vessels; transthoracic echo, cardiac monitoring
- Evaluate for contributing factors: lipid panel, HgA1c level
- Physical therapy (PT)/occupational therapy (OT) evaluation

*Disposition*

Home
- Improved or nonworsening deficit
- Able to eat, walk, and perform ADLs without assistance
- Reassuring testing

Hospital
- Need for inpatient PT/subacute rehabilitation
- Findings on testing that require further treatment (internal carotid artery stenosis, mural thrombus)
- Recommendation of neurology

every 2 hours. The former will detect dysrhythmias and the latter will detect worsening of their symptoms. Diagnostic workup is aimed at detecting potential sources of the CVA: cardioembolic, large vessel, and small vessel disease. Each patient should have an MRI of the brain to quantify the size of the infarct, as well as an MRA of the head and neck vessels to detect areas of focal stenosis or blockage. In addition, patients should undergo transthoracic echocardiography (TTE) to detect any cardioembolic sources. Patients with known atrial fibrillation need a transesophageal echocardiogram (TEE). Each patient should be screened for hyperlipidemia with a lipid panel and historic glucose control with a hemoglobin A1c level.

The care of a patient undergoing an mCVA protocol in the EDOU should be managed in collaboration with a neurologist. The neurology consultant should examine the patient in the ED or EDOU. The consultant can make recommendations regarding EDOU care and help arrange follow-up on discharge.

### Disposition

Patients may be discharged home if their symptoms have not progressed and testing in the EDOU does not reveal any condition that requires immediate treatment (eg, carotid stenosis, mural thrombus). Patients must be able to ambulate and perform ADLs with minimal assistance.

Education should be provided for patients regarding management of stroke risks, such as smoking cessation, encourage weight loss, exercise, and alcohol consumption in moderation. Patients being discharged should be started on appropriate antiplatelet therapy and have antihypertensive, lipid-lowering, and diabetic therapies maximized.

## BACK PAIN
### Introduction

Back pain is the most common musculoskeletal complaint in the ED.[35] Up to 90% of patients presenting to the ED will have a benign cause for their back pain.[36] Despite this, ED providers must be vigilant in screening patients for life-threatening causes of back pain, as well as cases in which neurologic compromise exists.

### Emergency Department Management

The 2 goals of ED evaluation are to rule in or out life high-risk causes of back pain, such as abdominal aortic aneurysm and spinal cord compression, and to control the patient's symptoms. The former is accomplished through obtaining a thorough history and performing a comprehensive physical examination. For patients with chronic back pain, the presenting complaint should be differentiated based on whether it is different from the usual symptoms. Providers should determine the presence of a subjective or objective neurologic deficit, as well as possible urinary or fecal incontinence. Patients should be assessed for traumatic etiology or intravenous drug use history. A careful examination must be performed to detect weakness and numbness, as well as to determine if the weakness is due to pain or if it is a sensory change in a dermatomal distribution.

Ancillary tests, such as blood work or imaging, are best saved for patients with red flags on history or physical for malignancy, fracture, infection, or epidural compression syndrome.

### Observation Unit Care

The goals of EDOU care for patients with acute back pain are to treat pain for patients with intractable symptoms in the ED and to obtain advanced neuroimaging for patients at mild to moderate risk for lumbar radiculopathy (**Box 3**).

---

**Box 3**
**Emergency department observation unit back pain protocol**

*Inclusion*

- Inability to control pain in the emergency department
- No known malignancy or injection drug use
- No history of trauma
- No fracture seen on imaging (if obtained)

*Exclusion*

- Frequent visits for back pain
- Bowel/bladder incontinence or saddle anesthesia
- Inability to stand or walk due to neurologic deficit
- Fever, concern for discitis or spinal epidural abscess

*Potential interventions*

- Pain control (nonsteroidal anti-inflammatory drugs ± opioids)
- MRI or CT to rule out spinal stenosis, malignancy
- PT assessment
- Neurology or neurosurgery consultation

*Disposition*

Home
- Ability to ambulate and care for self with oral analgesics
- Imaging not concerning for surgical disease

Hospital
- Worsening neurologic examination
- Inability to walk, care for self
- Intractable pain
- Consultant recommendations
- Abnormal imaging

---

### Patient Selection

In terms of pain control, patients in intractable pain, with chronic pain, or with multiple visits to the ED with this complaint are best treated in other settings. Painful conditions are at highest risk for ED recidivism.[37] In terms of disability, the EDOU back pain protocol is designed for patients with mild new subjective or objective neurologic deficits, such as weakness or numbness. Patients at high risk for spinal cord compression due to injection drugs or malignancy or patients with a dense new neurologic deficit will likely need physical therapy or occupational therapy (PT/OT) consultations, possibly surgical correction, and will take more than 15 to 18 hours for their condition to resolve.

Alternatively, EDOU is not an ideal destination for facilitating an outpatient workup on patients with chronic back pain. Obtaining an interval MRI due to patient or physician preference is not the best use of the EDOU and may not meet criteria for observation care, as it is not care rendered to determine the need for admission.

### Potential Interventions

While in the EDOU, the patient will have the symptoms controlled with anti-inflammatory and opioid pain medications as needed. An MRI should be ordered on patients with new subjective or objective neurologic deficits. In addition, neurology, neurosurgery, or PT/OT consultations can be obtained as needed based on amount of disability and findings on imaging.

### Disposition

Patients with resolved symptoms and nonconcerning imaging can be discharged if they are able to ambulate without difficulty. Use of aids, such as walkers or crutches, is appropriate if they can be used at home. Alternatively, patients require admission if their pain or disability does not resolve while in the EDOU. In addition, findings on MRI or recommendations of consultants can influence disposition.

## DIZZINESS/VERTIGO
### Introduction

Dizziness can be a vexing complaint for both the patients who suffer with it and for the providers who are tasked with diagnosing and treating it. It accounts for approximately 4% of ED visits in the United States with a direct cost of approximately $4 billion.[38] As with syncope, it is a symptom, rather than a disease entity. The differential is broad and the underlying etiology may involve many different organ systems as well as pharmacologic and environmental factors. Up to 50% of ED patients with dizziness have peripheral vestibular or brainstem pathology.[39]

### Emergency Department Management

Neurogenic dizziness maps to 2 main anatomic regions: the cerebellum or the peripheral vestibular system. Patients with cerebellar dysfunction may present with ataxia or falls, whereas those with vestibular dysfunction may present with vertigo. A careful neurologic examination, including cerebellar and gait testing, should be performed to detect subtle deficits, especially in patients with waxing and waning symptoms. In patients with vertigo, an attempt should be made to determine if the cause is central or peripheral. This can be difficult, but techniques such as the HINTS examination have been shown to aid in differentiation.[40] Patients with peripheral vertigo should have a Dix-Hallpike maneuver performed to test for nystagmus.

Most patients in the ED will require laboratory tests and many will require imaging. A complete blood count and chemistry panel will screen for anemia, infection, or electrolyte abnormalities, such as hyponatremia, that can contribute to their symptoms. Consider serum vitamin B12 and folic acid levels in those presenting with ataxia of insidious onset, especially if they are at risk for malnutrition. A noncontrast head CT is indicated as the initial test for patients with a suspected central cause of neurogenic dizziness. This will rule out mass lesions, intracranial hemorrhage, subacute ischemic strokes, or cerebellar atrophy. Patients with vertigo that is clearly the result of a peripheral cause do not need imaging.

ED treatment of peripheral causes of vertigo is mainly supportive and can include intravenous (IV) fluids, benzodiazepines, antiemetics, and antihistamines, such as meclizine. The Epley maneuver can resolve benign paroxysmal peripheral vertigo and may be performed by the ED provider or neurology consultant.

### Observation Unit Care

#### Patient selection
The EDOU can be considered for continued diagnostic or therapeutic care of ED patients with vertigo (**Box 4**). Ideal patients for the EDOU are those whose symptoms are likely peripheral. Patients with concern for a central process based on history or physical examination should be admitted for further workup, as they will likely

---

**Box 4**
**Emergency department observation unit vertigo protocol**

*Inclusion*

- Likely peripheral vertigo
- CT negative for mass lesion, hemorrhage, or ischemia
- Normal cerebellar examination (heel to shin, or finger nose finger testing)
- Normal cranial nerve examination (eg, corneal reflex, extraocular movements)

*Exclusion*

- Acute hearing loss, double vision, fixed neurologic deficits
- Severe headache, head trauma associated with vertigo
- Significant vital sign abnormalities
- Fever
- High clinical suspicion for central vertigo or stroke

*Potential interventions*

- Symptomatic control
- Benzodiazepines, anticholinergics (meclizine, diphenhydramine)
- Antiemetics
- Intravenous hydration as needed
- Diagnostic testing
- MRI, neurology consultation

*Disposition criteria*

Home
- Acceptable vital signs
- Able to ambulate and care for self safely in home
- Able to take oral medications/food

Hospital
- Positive finding on testing (MRI or laboratory)
- Consultant recommendation
- Continued symptoms, inability to ambulate/perform ADLs

---

require PT/OT evaluations and take more than 48 hours to improve. If a head CT is performed in the ED, it should be negative for intracranial hemorrhage, ischemia, or mass lesion.

### Potential interventions

While in the EDOU, suppression of the vestibular system with antihistamines, benzodiazepines, and antiemetics can be continued. Neurology consultation can be obtained for patients with refractory or frequently recurring symptoms, as well as those for whom the diagnosis is in doubt.

MRI/MRA can be performed for patients in whom a central cause of vertigo is possible. This will rule out subtle posterior circulation strokes or vertebrobasilar insufficiency. As mentioned previously, patients who are profoundly ataxic, at risk of falls, or thought to need help with ADLs should be admitted rather than go to the EDOU due to intensity of service and complexity of care.

*Disposition*

Patients may be discharged home once their symptoms have resolved. Before discharge, the providers should make sure the patient can ambulate without difficulty and tolerate oral intake food and/or medications. Those with persistent symptoms or are unable to ambulate or tolerate food should be admitted. Patients with positive findings on imaging should be admitted.

## HEADACHE
### Introduction

HA is a common complaint for ED patients, most of whom will have benign conditions and will be released following ED treatment. A select few patients will require additional diagnostic and therapeutic interventions, making them ideal EDOU candidates.

### Emergency Department Management

The 2 primary goals of ED evaluation of patients with HA is to rule out life-threatening causes of HA, such as subarachnoid hemorrhage or meningitis, and to begin appropriate therapy. The differential can be narrowed through a thorough history and examination, and should include characteristics of the current HA as well as an understanding of how this episode compares with previous episodes. Patients thought to have benign causes of HA, such as tension HA or migraine, can be treated with oral analgesia and discharged after satisfactory pain relief is obtained. Patients who are vomiting or appear in distress may require IV fluids, analgesia, and antiemetics. Noncontrast head CT is not recommended for routine evaluation of patients with HA but is a recommended initial step to rule out subarachnoid hemorrhage or mass lesion.

### Observation Unit Care

There are 2 groups of patients with HA who may benefit from care in an EDOU. Each of these conditions requires coordination with ancillary services, specifically neurology, before initiation of an HA protocol to ensure efficient care. The first group is patients with benign HA who need better pain control and the second is patients in whom there is a concern for idiopathic intracranial hypertension (IIH), previously known as pseudotumor cerebri.

### Tension/migraine

**Patient selection** For patients with a migraine HA, it is important to choose patients with either an established diagnosis of migraines or whose current HA is similar to their previous episodes. For new-onset migraines, patients should fit a classic migraine pattern. Patients with fever, neurologic deficits, and other comorbidities should be excluded (**Box 5**).

**Potential interventions** EDOU care for patients with tension/migraine consists of continued supportive care, such as a quiet, dark room where they can rest, routine analgesia, and antiemetics. Usual medications are nonsteroidal anti-inflammatory medications (NSAIDs) or steroids. Neurology consultation may be necessary for HAs that are difficult to abort, as they can recommend other abortifacient medications, such as valproic acid. Some patients may require further imaging, such as MRI/MRA.

**Disposition** Patients whose HAs have aborted and are at their neurologic baseline may be discharged home. Patients should be admitted if they have a change in their neurologic examination, unrelieved pain, or need further workup (eg, electroencephalogram [EEG], lumbar puncture).

---

**Box 5**
**Emergency department observation unit headache and papilledema protocols**

*Headache*

Inclusion
- Persistent pain in tension or migraine headache
- History of migraine with same aura, onset, location, and pattern
- Drug-related headache
- No focal neurologic signs
- Normal CT scan (if done)
- If lumbar puncture is needed, then it must be done and normal (unless failed attempt and interventional radiology consult for lumbar puncture arranged in emergency department (ED) BEFORE transfer to EDOU, and low-risk patient)
- Neurology, neurosurgery, neuro-ophthalmology consult completed in ED for complicated cases

Exclusion
- Focal neurologic signs
- Meningismus or high suspicion of meningitis, encephalitis, or subarachnoid hemorrhage
- Elevated intraocular pressure as cause (ie, glaucoma)
- Abnormal CT scan
- Abnormal lumbar puncture (if performed)
- Hypertensive emergency (diastolic blood pressure >120 mm Hg with symptoms)
- Suspected temporal arteritis
- Blocked ventriculo-peritoneal shunt
- Frequent ED visits: suspected habitual patient, narcotic-seeking behavior

Potential Interventions
- Serial examinations including vital signs
- Neurology checks: level of alertness, speech, motor function
- Analgesics, analgesics appropriate for a headache
- Neurology consult as indicated
- MRI/MR angiogram/MR venogram (MRV) imaging as indicated
- Retina scan if available

Disposition Criteria
  Home
  - Resolution of pain
  - Other to take patient home
  - No deterioration in clinical course
  Hospital
  - No resolution in pain
  - Deterioration in clinical course
  - Rule in of exclusionary causes

*Idiopathic intracranial hypertension (IIH)/Papilledema*

Inclusion
- Patients at moderate risk for IIH or venous thrombosis based on clinical profile (obese, papilledema, headache, and/or visual symptoms)
- Patients with unexplained papilledema
- Hemodynamically and neurologically stable patients

Exclusion
- Febrile patients
- Patients in whom subarachnoid hemorrhage, meningitis, encephalitis is a concern
- Rapidly progressing visual loss
- Patients with an altered mental status or acute neurologic deficits
- Inability to complete protocol within 15 to 24 hours, or if patient declines needed lumbar puncture (LP)/MRI
- Patients whose testing can/should be done electively as an outpatient
- Patients with chronic pain or opioid overuse with low clinical suspicion of an acute process

ED Interventions
- Initial ophthalmologic and neurology examinations
- Complete blood count, platelets, prothrombin time/international normalized ratio if LP under fluoroscopy is planned
- Retina camera pictures using ED equipment if available
- Head CT without contrast
- Neurology consult/notification: clearance for CDU protocol
- LP if indicated emergently

CDU Interventions:
- Pain medications as needed
- Serial neurologic examinations every 4 hours
- Ophthalmology (or neuro-ophthalmology) consult
- Brain venous imaging: MRI/MRV brain, with and without contrast (or CT venogram if unable to tolerate MRI/MRV)
- LP (unless indicated otherwise) to be performed after venous imaging by Neurology or Diagnostic Neuroradiology for opening pressures and cerebrospinal fluid (CSF) analysis (routine CSF plus cryptococcal antigen, tuberculosis/acid-fast bacillus [TB/AFB]/fungal culture, venereal disease research labratory [VDRL])
- Visual fields as indicated by ophthalmology/neuro-ophthalmology
- Completion of neurology consult

Disposition criteria:
Hospital
- Evidence of acute neurologic process: tumor, ischemic infarct, venous thrombosis, infection
- Symptom management that has failed in the CDU
- Visual loss from papilledema (which may require emergent surgical treatment)
- Inability to complete time-sensitive testing within 15 to 24 hours
Home
- Negative diagnostic testing
- Identification of conditions that may be treated as an outpatient
- Adequate symptom control

### Idiopathic intracranial hypertension/papilledema

**Patient selection** These patients can present to the ED in 1 of 3 ways: new HA in which the emergency provider is concerned about IIH, known diagnosis of IIH with pain/vision changes, or referred from outside provider for workup of papilledema. Patients who require a workup for new papilledema require an extensive and coordinated workup that should be attempted only in mature units after meeting with stakeholders from neurology, radiology, and ophthalmology to discuss the timing of diagnostic studies and consults. If this is not possible, patients should be admitted to inpatient services for further workup.

As mentioned previously, patients with fever, neurologic deficits, or active comorbidities should be excluded from the EDOU (see **Box 5**). Also, patients for whom optic neuritis is a diagnostic concern should be admitted, as they often require a few days of IV steroids.

Patients with HA and papilledema require neuroimaging to rule out secondary causes of increased intracranial pressure, such as intracranial mass lesions, venous sinus thrombosis, and obstructive hydrocephalus. Timing of essential studies will vary based on local availability and expertise, but this will dictate what can be done in the ED versus EDOU. Brain MRI is the test of choice, as it is more sensitive in detecting small mass lesions.[41] If this is not rapidly available or there are contraindications for MRI, noncontrast head CT should be obtained in the ED. This will rule out larger mass lesions or hydrocephalus.

**Potential interventions** Workup for papilledema includes the following:

- MRI brain
- MR venogram (MRV) to rule out secondary causes of intracranial hypertension, such as venous sinus thrombosis; CT venogram (CTV) is another option
- Lumbar puncture
- Ophthalmology consultation, including visual field testing
- Neurology consultation

The choice of CTV versus MRV to rule out venous sinus thrombosis should be made in conjunction with local radiology and neurology colleagues. Advantages of CTV are that it is more readily available and could be obtained before EDOU admission and there are no contraindications for metallic devices. MRV is preferred in the setting of renal insufficiency or contrast dye allergy.

**Disposition** Patients may go home if their symptoms are controlled, the workup is unrevealing, and follow-up has been arranged with the appropriate specialists. Patients may require admission for any positive findings on testing, untreated symptoms, or if lumbar puncture is unsuccessful at the bedside.

## SEIZURES
### Introduction

Seizures are a common reason for patients to present to the ED. It can be difficult for the emergency practitioner to determine if a patient's presentation is due to seizure, as there are many things that can mimic seizures, such as syncope or psychiatric conditions.

### Emergency Department Management

Initial ED management in patients presenting with active or recent seizure involves ensuring the seizure has stopped and keeping the patient safe during the postictal period. Patients who receive benzodiazepines from prehospital providers or in the ED need to have their airway and cardiovascular status closely monitored.

In patients with no history of seizures, ED workup is indicated. This should include a complete blood count and basic chemistry to screen for infectious or metabolic precipitants for the seizure. In addition, brain imaging should be obtained to rule out structural brain abnormality.

For patients with epilepsy, there should still be an attempt to isolate the precipitant for the seizure. This can include infectious or metabolic conditions, as well as noncompliance with anticonvulsant medications. Patients whose seizures followed their usual pattern and have returned to their baseline may not need any workup other than determination if drug levels are therapeutic in cases in which levels can be obtained in a timely manner. Patients with evidence of head trauma, fevers, or altered mental status likely need laboratory tests and imaging to ensure another condition does not exist. Neurology consultation may be helpful for establishing the diagnosis of seizures and in deciding whether to start anticonvulsant medications.

### Observation Unit Care

Occasionally patients presenting after a seizure will need further workup or therapeutics beyond their ED visit. The EDOU is an ideal location for patients who need to be loaded with anticonvulsant medications, obtain an MRI or EEG, or have a formal evaluation by neurology.

## Patient Selection

Patients going to the EDOU should be seizure-free and have returned to their baseline before transfer. As with other conditions that involve an alteration in level of consciousness, patients who are still somnolent or confused after their seizure may go to the

---

**Box 6**
**Emergency department observation unit seizure protocol**

*Inclusion*

- Past history of seizures with breakthrough seizure or subtherapeutic anticonvulsant level
- No seizure within past 2 hours
- New-onset seizures with a normal neurology examination, normal head CT, and neurology agreement
- Blood work: electrolytes, blood glucose, anticonvulsant levels (if appropriate), urine drug screen/toxicology laboratories as indicated

*Exclusion*

- Ongoing seizures or postictal state
- Persistent focal neurologic findings (eg, Todd paralysis)
- Clinical suspicion of meningitis or new stroke
- Delirium of any etiology, including alcohol withdrawal syndrome/delirium tremens
- Seizures due to toxic exposure (eg, theophylline or carbon monoxide toxicity) or hypoxemia
- Pregnancy beyond first trimester/eclampsia
- New findings on head CT
- New electrocardiogram changes or significant arrhythmias

*Potential interventions*

- Appropriate anticonvulsant therapy
- Seizure precautions
- Cardiac and oximetry monitoring
- Serial (every 2–4 hours) neurology checks and vital signs
- Toxicologic testing as needed
- Electroencephalogram or neurology consultation as indicated
- Nothing per mouth or liquid diet as indicated
- Neurology consult if new-onset seizures

*Disposition*

Home
- No deterioration in clinical status
- Therapeutic levels of anticonvulsants as needed
- Correction of abnormal laboratories
- Resolution of postictal or benzodiazepine-related sedation
- Appropriate home environment

Hospital
- Deterioration of clinical status, mentation, or neurology examination
- Rule in for exclusionary causes
- Inappropriate home environment
- Recurrent seizures or status epilepticus

EDOU, provided there is enough staff to ensure their safety. Patients with unresolved postictal paresis, concern for meningitis, severe electrolyte abnormalities, or positive findings on head CT should be admitted (**Box 6**).

### Potential Interventions

As mentioned previously, patients being managed for their seizures in the EDOU can get diagnostics and therapeutics at the discretion of the emergency provider or the neurology consultant. Patients needing IV or oral medication loading can have that done with appropriate monitoring. Repeat drug levels can be sent as needed. Diagnostic tests, such as MRI or EEG, can be performed on select patients to assess for precipitants or establish the diagnosis of seizures.

### Disposition

Patients may be discharged home if they are at their neurologic baseline and have received all anticonvulsant medications with therapeutic serum levels (if those are being monitored). Patients with deteriorating neurologic status or continued seizures should be admitted.

### REFERENCES

1. National Hospital Ambulatory Medical care survey: 2011 emergency department summary tables. Center for Disease Control; 2011. p. 3.
2. Talwalkar A, Uddin S. Trends in emergency department visits for ischemic stroke and transient ischemic attack: United States, 2001-2011. NCHS Data Brief 2015;(194):1–8.
3. National Center for Health Statistics. Health, United States, 2015: with special feature on racial and ethnic health disparities. Hyattsville (MD): US Department of Health and Human Services; 2016. Avaialble at: https://www.cdc.gov/nchs/data/hus/hus15.pdf. Accessed April 11, 2017.
4. Mozaffarian D, Benjamin EJ, Go AS, et al. Heart disease and stroke statistics–2015 update: a report from the American Heart Association. Circulation 2015; 131(4):e29–322.
5. Go AS, Mozaffarian D, Roger VL, et al. Heart disease and stroke statistics–2013 update: a report from the American Heart Association. Circulation 2013;127(1):e6–245.
6. Rothwell PM, Warlow CP. Timing of TIAs preceding stroke: time window for prevention is very short. Neurology 2005;64(5):817–20.
7. Easton JD, Saver JL, Albers GW, et al. Definition and evaluation of transient ischemic attack: a scientific statement for healthcare professionals from the American Heart Association/American Stroke Association Stroke Council; Council on Cardiovascular Surgery and Anesthesia; Council on Cardiovascular Radiology and Intervention; Council on Cardiovascular Nursing; and the Interdisciplinary Council on Peripheral Vascular Disease. The American Academy of Neurology affirms the value of this statement as an educational tool for neurologists. Stroke 2009;40(6):2276–93.
8. Ay H, Koroshetz WJ, Benner T, et al. Transient ischemic attack with infarction: a unique syndrome? Ann Neurol 2005;57(5):679–86.
9. Coutts SB, Hill MD, Simon JE, et al. Silent ischemia in minor stroke and TIA patients identified on MR imaging. Neurology 2005;65(4):513–7.
10. Douglas VC, Johnston CM, Elkins J, et al. Head computed tomography findings predict short-term stroke risk after transient ischemic attack. Stroke 2003;34(12): 2894–8.

11. Johnston SC, Rothwell PM, Nguyen-Huynh MN, et al. Validation and refinement of scores to predict very early stroke risk after transient ischaemic attack. Lancet 2007;369(9558):283–92.

12. Giles MF, Rothwell PM. Risk of stroke early after transient ischaemic attack: a systematic review and meta-analysis. Lancet Neurol 2007;6(12):1063–72.

13. American College of Emergency Physicians Clinical Policies Subcommittee on Suspected Transient Ischemic Attack, Lo BM, Carpenter CR, et al. Clinical policy: critical issues in the evaluation of adult patients with suspected transient ischemic attack in the emergency department. Ann Emerg Med 2016;68(3): 354–70.e29.

14. Rothwell PM, Giles MF, Chandratheva A, et al. Effect of urgent treatment of transient ischaemic attack and minor stroke on early recurrent stroke (EXPRESS study): a prospective population-based sequential comparison. Lancet 2007; 370(9596):1432–42.

15. Lavallee PC, Meseguer E, Abboud H, et al. A transient ischaemic attack clinic with round-the-clock access (SOS-TIA): feasibility and effects. Lancet Neurol 2007;6(11):953–60.

16. Ross MA, Compton S, Medado P, et al. An emergency department diagnostic protocol for patients with transient ischemic attack: a randomized controlled trial. Ann Emerg Med 2007;50(2):109–19.

17. Castle J, Mlynash M, Lee K, et al. Agreement regarding diagnosis of transient ischemic attack fairly low among stroke-trained neurologists. Stroke 2010;41(7): 1367–70.

18. Amarenco P, Labreuche J, Lavallée PC, et al. Does ABCD2 score below 4 allow more time to evaluate patients with a transient ischemic attack? Stroke 2009; 40(9):3091–5.

19. Oostema JA, Delano M, Bhatt A, et al. Incorporating diffusion-weighted magnetic resonance imaging into an observation unit transient ischemic attack pathway: a prospective study. Neurohospitalist 2014;4(2):66–73.

20. Stead LG, Suravaram S, Bellolio MF, et al. An assessment of the incremental value of the ABCD2 score in the emergency department evaluation of transient ischemic attack. Ann Emerg Med 2011;57(1):46–51.

21. Nahab F, Leach G, Kingston C, et al. Impact of an emergency department observation unit transient ischemic attack protocol on length of stay and cost. J Stroke Cerebrovasc Dis 2012;21(8):673–8.

22. Oostema JA, Brown MD, DeLano M, et al. Does diffusion-weighted imaging predict short-term risk of stroke in emergency department patients with transient ischemic attack? Ann Emerg Med 2013;61(1):62–71.e1.

23. Furie KL, Kasner SE, Adams RJ, et al. Guidelines for the prevention of stroke in patients with stroke or transient ischemic attack: a guideline for healthcare professionals from the American Heart Association/American Stroke Association. Stroke 2011;42(1):227–76.

24. Johnston SC, Albers GW, Gorelick PB, et al. National Stroke Association recommendations for systems of care for transient ischemic attack. Ann Neurol 2011; 69(5):872–7.

25. Association, N.S. NIH Stroke Scale Certification. NIH Stroke Scale online training and certification site. 2016. Available at: http://www.stroke.org/we-can-help/ healthcare-professionals/improve-your-skills/tools-training-and-resources/training/ nih. Accessed October 31, 2016.

26. Hart RG, Pearce LA, Aguilar MI. Meta-analysis: antithrombotic therapy to prevent stroke in patients who have nonvalvular atrial fibrillation. Ann Intern Med 2007; 146(12):857–67.
27. Dussault C, Toeg H, Nathan M, et al. Electrocardiographic monitoring for detecting atrial fibrillation after ischemic stroke or transient ischemic attack: systematic review and meta-analysis. Circ Arrhythm Electrophysiol 2015;8(2):263–9.
28. Kishore A, Vail A, Majid A, et al. Detection of atrial fibrillation after ischemic stroke or transient ischemic attack: a systematic review and meta-analysis. Stroke 2014; 45(2):520–6.
29. Furlan AJ, Reisman M, Massaro J, et al. Closure or medical therapy for cryptogenic stroke with patent foramen ovale. N Engl J Med 2012;366(11):991–9.
30. Hackam DG, Spence JD. Combining multiple approaches for the secondary prevention of vascular events after stroke: a quantitative modeling study. Stroke 2007;38(6):1881–5.
31. Commission, T.J. The Joint Commission - Core Measure Sets, Topic Library Item, Stroke. [Stroke Certification Core Measures]. 2016. Available at: https://www.jointcommission.org/core_measure_sets.aspx. Accessed October 30, 2016.
32. Fischer U, Baumgartner A, Arnold M. What is a minor stroke? Stroke 2010;41: 661–6.
33. Paul NLM, Koton S, Simoni M, et al. Feasibility, safety and cost of outpatient management of acute minor ischaemic stroke: a population-based study. J Neurol Neurosurg Psychiatry 2013;84:356–61.
34. Mathias S, Nayak US, Isaacs B. Balance in elderly patients: the "get-up and go" test. Arch Phys Med Rehabil 1986;67:387–9.
35. Wipf JE, Deyo RA. Low back pain. Med Clin North Am 1995;79(2):231–46.
36. Chou R, Qaseem A, Snow V, et al. Diagnosis and treatment of low back pain: a joint clinical practice guideline from the American College of Physicians and the American Pain Society. Ann Intern Med 2007;147(7):478–91.
37. Ross MA, Hemphill RR, Abramson J, et al. The recidivism characteristics of an emergency department observation unit. Ann Emerg Med 2010;56(1):34–41.
38. Saber Tehrani AS, Coughlan D, Hsieh Y-H, et al. Rising annual costs of dizziness presentation to US emergency departments. Acad Emerg Med 2013;20(7): 689–96.
39. Herr RD, Zun L, Matthews JJ. A directed approach to the dizzy patient. Ann Emerg Med 1989;18(6):664.
40. Kattah JE, Talkad AV, Wang DZ, et al. HINTS to diagnose stroke in the acute vestibular syndrome: three-step bedside oculomotor examination more sensitive than early MRI diffusion-weighted imaging. Stroke 2009;40(11):3504–10.
41. Friedman DI. Papilledema and pseudotumor cerebri. Ophthalmol Clin North Am 2001;14(1):129.

# Care of Respiratory Conditions in an Observation Unit

Margarita E. Pena, MD[a,b,]*, Viviane M. Kazan, MD[a,b],
Michael N. Helmreich, MD[a], Sharon E. Mace, MD[c]

## KEYWORDS

- Emergency department • Emergency department observation unit • Asthma
- Chronic obstructive pulmonary disease • Community-acquired pneumonia
- Observation

## KEY POINTS

- Asthma, chronic obstructive pulmonary disease, and community-acquired pneumonia are the second most common category of diseases treated in an emergency department observation unit (EDOU).
- EDOU management of respiratory disorders is effective, efficient, safe, and less costly compared with inpatient care.
- Risk stratification ensures appropriate patients are placed in the EDOU.
- Use of condition-specific rapid diagnostic and treatment protocols and clinical pathways allow for standardizing care using evidence-based best practice.

Respiratory conditions are common complaints seen in the emergency department (ED). After initial ED evaluation, stabilization, and treatment, patients may require further testing or treatment. The ED observation unit (EDOU) offers an alternative disposition to inpatient admission for patients who require short-term monitoring, testing, and/or treatment. By using rapid diagnostic and therapeutic protocols, the vast majority of patients can be safely discharged home within 24 hours (or 2 midnights).

This article focuses on 3 respiratory conditions that are frequently managed in an EDOU: exacerbations of asthma and chronic obstructive pulmonary disease (COPD) and treatment of community-acquired pneumonia (CAP). Other authors discuss additional respiratory conditions such as congestive heart failure and pneumothorax elsewhere within this issue.

[a] Department of Emergency Medicine, St. John Hospital and Medical Center, 22101 Moross Road, Detroit, MI 48236, USA; [b] Department of Emergency Medicine, Wayne State University School of Medicine, 540 E. Canfield Street, Detroit, MI, USA; [c] Department of Emergency Medicine, Cleveland Clinic, Cleveland Clinic Lerner College of Medicine, Case Western Reserve University, 9500 Euclid Avenue, Cleveland, OH 44195, USA
* Corresponding author. Department of Emergency Medicine, St. John Hospital and Medical Center, 22101 Moross Road, Detroit, MI 48236.
E-mail address: margarita.pena@ascension.org

Emerg Med Clin N Am 35 (2017) 625–645
http://dx.doi.org/10.1016/j.emc.2017.03.008
0733-8627/17/© 2017 Elsevier Inc. All rights reserved.

---

**Case Study**

Jennifer Andrews, a 35-year-old female asthmatic, complains of shortness of breath and wheezing for 2 days. Despite nebulizer therapy and oral corticosteroids in the ED, her peak flow measurement increases to only 200 L/min (personal best 400 L/min). Auscultation reveals persistent diffuse expiratory wheezing. She is placed in the EDOU, where she receives nebulized bronchodilator therapy. After 15 hours, her peak flow increases to 350 L/min and auscultation reveals only rare expiratory wheezing. Ambulatory pulse oximetry on room air is 98%. She is discharged with prescriptions for oral and inhaled corticosteroids. Follow-up with her primary care physician is arranged.

---

## ASTHMA

The Global Initiative for Asthma defines asthma as "a heterogeneous disease, usually characterized by chronic airway inflammation. It is defined by the history of respiratory symptoms such as wheeze, shortness of breath, chest tightness and cough that vary over time and in intensity, together with variable expiratory airflow limitation."[1] This common disease affects 7.0 million children and 18.7 million adults in the United States.[2] In 2011, asthma accounted for 1.6 million ED visits and 27% (439,000) were hospitalized an average of 3.6 days (1.6 million hospital days).[3–5] Asthma is one of the most common conditions managed in an observation setting for all ages.[6,7]

The cost of asthma care in the United States increased to $56 billion in 2007 with the majority of cost owing to the cost of hospitalization ($50 billion).[8,9] The average annual costs for an asthma-related hospital stay are estimated at $3600 per child and as much as $6600 per adult.[9] Annually, asthma causes adults to miss 14 million days of work and children to miss 10 million days of school.[5,10]

### Evidence for Emergency Department Observation Unit Management of Asthma Exacerbation

The EDOU is ideal for asthma exacerbation care and offers many advantages to traditional admission. Because ED rescue therapy (eg, corticosteroids) may not reach full effect for up to 6 hours, the EDOU allows time for medications to achieve effect and for repeated clinical assessments so that final disposition can be made.[11] This extended period of observation affords time for patient teaching and preventative treatments that may lead to decreased recidivism, admissions, morbidity, and mortality.[11,12]

Numerous studies since the 1980s have demonstrated that treatment of adult and pediatric asthmatics in an EDOU avoids hospitalization, is cost effective, and is clinically beneficial with reduced morbidity and mortality.[13–23] Prospective, randomized, clinical trials found greater patient satisfaction and perceived quality of life.[17,20,24]

Despite evidence favoring EDOU use for asthma exacerbation, reports demonstrate that EDOUs continue to be underused. This is evidenced by large numbers of both pediatric and adult patients treated as inpatients during short-stay admissions.[25–27]

### Patient Selection

Patient assessment should include determination of risk factors, especially those for fatal or near-fatal asthma (**Box 1**). Asthma severity can be classified as mild, moderate, or severe based on vital signs and physical examination findings.[28] Scoring systems assess symptom severity and treatment response but do not assess the need for admission. Commonly used scores include the Pediatric Asthma Severity Score,[29] Pulmonary Index Score,[30] Pediatric Respiratory Assessment Measure,[31] and RAD[32]

---

**Box 1**
**Risk factors for asthma severity**

- Prior intubation
- Prior admission to the intensive care unit
- Frequent emergency department visits (≥3 per year)
- Frequent hospitalizations (≥2 per year)
- Recent steroid use
- Steroid dependence
- Significant comorbidities (eg, cardiovascular disease, other chronic lung disease, chronic psychiatric disease, etc)
- Limited access to health care

---

(respiratory rate, accessory muscle use, decreased breath sounds) score. Unfortunately, there is no one, widely accepted and sufficiently validated scoring system.

## Emergency Department Observation Unit Care of Patients With Asthma Exacerbation

### Protocols

The use of condition-specific protocols are a hallmark of EDOU management that provide an excellent opportunity for standardizing care using evidence-based best practice. Use of asthma protocols in the EDOU for adults and children shows numerous clinical and financial advantages compared with routine nonstandardized care (**Box 2**).[33,34]

Patients suitable for the EDOU include those with low or moderate asthma severity who do not improve adequately with initial ED therapy or who cannot be safely discharged home owing to concerns about treatment adherence or follow-up. Patients at very high risk for poor outcomes may benefit from a period of observation regardless of initial response to therapy.

A study by McCarren and colleagues[35] found patients achieving a peak expiratory flow rate of 40% or greater after 3 β-agonist treatments had high probability of EDOU discharge, peak expiratory flow rate from 32% to 40% had intermediate probability whereas rates of 32% or less had a low probability of discharge and therefore are not appropriate for EDOU placement and require inpatient care.

### Emergency department observation unit interventions

Patients with asthma exacerbations placed in the EDOU require vital sign monitoring, including measurement of oxygen saturation and frequent clinical reassessments to gauge response to therapy. Pulse oximetry measurement during ambulation may provide information regarding response to treatment and aid in disposition decisions. Many patients being placed in an EDOU for an asthma exacerbation will have received a chest radiograph as part of the workup performed in the ED. Clinical judgment should be exercised to determine which patients require imaging. It should be strongly considered in patients with new-onset wheezing, indicators of pneumonia, and risk of other alternative diagnosis, as well as those patients who are either failing to respond to therapy or are worsening clinically despite therapy.

Patient education is important in the management and prevention of recidivism. Patients and caregivers should receive education regarding asthma medications, proper inhaler and peak flow meter use, smoking cessation if applicable, avoidance

---

**Box 2**
**ED observation unit adult asthma protocol example**

*Inclusion criteria*

- Alert and oriented, acceptable vital signs
- Intermediate response to therapy – improving but still wheezing
- PEFR (peak flow) 40% to 70% predicted (or personal best) after $\beta_2$ agonists
- $\beta_2$ agonist nebulizers (2 treatments or 10 mg albuterol) + steroids given in ED
- Minimum ED treatment time greater than 2 hours
- Chest radiography, if done, with no significant acute findings (eg, pneumonia, pneumothorax, congestive heart failure, et.)

*Exclusion criteria*

- Unstable vital signs or clinical condition—severe dyspnea, confusion, drowsiness
- Poor response to initial ED treatment
  - Persistent use of accessory muscles, RR >40, or excessive effort
  - Elevated $Pco_2$ (>50 mm Hg) plus decreased pH (<7.40) if ABG done
  - $O_2$ saturation of less than 92% on room air, unless documented chronic hypoxia
  - PEFR of less than 40% predicted or personal best
- Suspicion of acute coronary syndrome, new-onset congestive heart failure, or pneumonia

*Potential interventions*

- Serial treatments with nebulized $\beta_2$ agonist and ipratropium
- IV magnesium sulfate
- Frequent reassessment (every 2–4 hours)
- Systemic steroids (PO or IV)
- Pulse oximetry and oxygen with cardiac monitoring as needed

*Discharge criteria*

- Home (*Patient to be discharged on steroids, nebulizers, with follow-up and smoking cessation counseling, if relevant*)
  - Acceptable vital signs: HR <100, RR <20 after ambulation (if able)
  - Pulse oximetry ≥95% on room air (or return to baseline)
  - Resolution of bronchospasm or return to baseline status
  - PEFR greater than 70% predicted (or 70% personal best) if reliable reading
- Admit
  - Progressive deterioration in clinical status or vital signs
  - Failure to resolve bronchospasm within 15 hours
  - Persistent PEFR less than 70% of predicted (if reliable)
  - Hypoxic despite therapy, if not chronic state

*Abbreviations:* ABG, arterial blood gases; ED, emergency department; HR, heart rate; PEFR, peak expiratory flow rate; RR, respiratory rate.
*From* Observation Protocols, Asthma. Available at: http://obsprotocols.org/tiki-index.php?page=Asthma. Accessed October 1, 2016.

---

of asthma triggers, and treatment plan after EDOU discharge including close follow-up with a primary care provider.[1]

### Medical Treatments for Asthma Exacerbation

Short-acting $\beta_2$ agonists (SABA) are first-line medications for the treatment of asthma exacerbations. The most commonly used SABA is albuterol sulfate, administered via a nebulizer ('wet' form) or a metered dose inhaler with a holding chamber or spacer ('dry' form). For patients with nonsevere asthma exacerbations, SABA therapy via metered dose inhaler with a spacer is at least as effective as nebulized therapy[36] and is considered by Global Initiative for Asthma as an efficient and cost-effective delivery method.[1] A metered dose inhaler with a spacer is preferred in children with mild to moderate asthma.[1,37] Levalbuterol, the nonracemic enantiomer form of albuterol, has not been shown to offer any significant advantages over albuterol. Its use may be considered in patients at risk for tachyarrhythmias or who have previously shown better tolerance to nonracemic enantiomer form of albuterol.[38]

Short-acting anticholinergics, also known as short-acting muscarinic antagonists, such as ipratropium bromide, reduce bronchoconstriction through blockade of the cholinergic receptors. They are a useful adjunct to SABA, but are not effective as monotherapy. The combination of anticholinergics and SABA improves pulmonary function and reduces admission rates.[39] The effectiveness of anticholinergic therapy has only been demonstrated in the acute setting. Continuation of anticholinergic therapy once a patient is hospitalized has not been shown to improve outcomes.[40]

Systemic corticosteroids (CS), another first-line therapy, should be initiated in the ED and continued in the EDOU. CS reduce $\beta_2$ agonist therapy requirements and hospital admission rates, prevent relapses, and reduces overall mortality.[37] Oral formulations have similar efficacy to intravenous (IV) and intramuscular routes and is the preferred route of administration in patients who can tolerate oral intake. Intramuscular and IV administration should be reserved for patients who do not tolerate oral intake. Patients placed in the EDOU should have CS therapy continued. The use of dexamethasone as the initial CS used in the ED may make additional doses of CS unnecessary. The data are limited, but there seems to be relatively similar rates of relapse for either single-dose or 2-day dosing dexamethasone as compared with a multiday course of prednisolone or prednisone.[41–44] Other benefits of this approach are improved palatability,[45] increased compliance,[46] and parental preference.[47]

Antibiotics are not recommended for routine exacerbations of asthma.[1,37] Even in cases of an infectious cause of asthma exacerbation, viral infections are much more common than bacterial. In cases where there is radiographic evidence of pneumonia or other strong clinical indicators of a bacterial infection, antibiotics would be appropriate.

Patients requiring continued therapy with subcutaneous $\beta_2$-agonists, IV magnesium sulfate, or epinephrine are likely poor candidates for an EDOU protocol and likely require hospital admission **Table 1**.

### Disposition

Patients who fail to improve or worsen significantly require admission to an inpatient service. Patients are likely appropriate for discharge when there has been sufficient clinical improvement such that the patient has at most minimal symptoms and there are objective findings such as normal pulse oximetry and peak flow measurements. Patients should be educated about the plan for outpatient therapy, including systemic CS if required. If the patient is being discharged on prednisone the adult dose is 1 mg/kg/d (maximum dose of 60 mg/d) for 5 to 7 days. The pediatric dose of prednisone is 1 to 2 mg/kg/d (maximum dose of 40–60 mg) for 3 to 5 days.[1] The patient should have a supply of a SABA rescue inhaler. Using a stepwise approach, the National Asthma Education and Prevention Program recommends the addition of controller medications in select patients. These may include inhaled corticosteroids and long-acting $\beta_2$-agonists.[50]

**Table 1**
**Rescue or quick-relief medications for asthma exacerbations in the emergency department observation unit**

| Medication | Pediatric Dose (≤12 y) | Adult Dose |
|---|---|---|
| Inhaled short-acting $\beta_2$-agonists | | |
| Albuterol Nebulizer solution (0.63, 1.25, 2.5 mg/3 mL and 5.0 mg/mL) | 0.15–0.3 mg/kg up to 5 mg every 2–4 h as needed | 2.5–10 mg every 2–4 h as needed |
| Metered-dose inhaler (90 μg/puff) | 4–8 puffs every 2–4 h inhalation maneuver as needed. Use valve holding chamber; add mask in children <4 y | 4–8 puffs every 20 min up to 4 h, then every 2–4 h as needed |
| Levalbuterol (R-albuterol) | | |
| Nebulizer solution (0.63 mg/ 3 mL, 1.25 mg/0.5 mL, 1.25 mg/3 mL) | 0.075–0.15 mg/kg up to 5 mg every 2–4 h as needed | 1.25–5 mg every 2–4 h as needed |
| Metered-dose inhaler (45 μg/puff) | See albuterol metered-dose inhaler dosage | See albuterol metered-dose inhaler dosage |
| Systemic (injected) $\beta_2$-agonists | | |
| Epinephrine 1:1000 (1 mg/mL) | 0.01 mg/kg up to 0.3–0.5 mg every 20 min for 3 doses subcutaneous | 0.3–0.5 mg every 20 min for 3 doses subcutaneous |
| Terbutaline (1 mg/mL) | 0.01 mg/kg every 20 min for 3 doses then every 2–6 h as needed subcutaneous | 0.25 mg every 20 min for 3 doses subcutaneous |
| Anticholinergics | | |
| Ipatropium bromide Nebulizer solution (0.25 mg/mL) | 0.25–0.5 mg every 2–4 h as needed | 0.5 mg every 2–4 h as needed |
| Metered-dose inhaler 18 μg/puff) | 4–8 puffs every 2–4 h as needed | 8 puffs every 2–4 h as needed |
| Systemic corticosteroids (Applies to all 3 corticosteroids) | | |
| Prednisone Methylprednisolone Prednisolone | 1–2 mg/kg given in divided dose BID (maximum 60 mg/d) until peak expiratory flow is 70% of predicted or personal best | 40–80 mg/d given once daily or BID in divided dose (maximum 80 mg/d) until peak expiratory flow reaches 70% of predicted or personal best |
| Dexamethasone[42,48,49] | 0.6 mg/kg (maximum of 16 mg/d), 1 dose at discharge, and/or second dose the following day | 12–16 mg/d, 1 dose at discharge, and/or second dose the following day |

*Abbreviation:* BID, 2 times per day.

*Adapted from* Camargo CA, Rachelefsky G, Schatz M. Managing asthma exacerbations in the emergency department: summary of the National Asthma Education And Prevention Program Expert Panel Report 3 guidelines for the management of asthma exacerbations. Proc Am Thorac Soc 2009;6(4):357–66.

## CHRONIC OBSTRUCTIVE PULMONARY DISEASE

---

**Case Study**

Dan Brown, a 66-year-old smoker with COPD, complains of increasing cough, purulent sputum, and difficulty breathing for 3 days. Despite treatment in the ED, he continues to have dyspnea with persistent wheezing. His room air pulse oximetry is only 90%. He is placed in the EDOU, where he is given nebulizer therapy, azithromycin, oral steroids, and smoking cessation education. Twenty hours later, he feels much better and has only occasional, scattered wheezes. Pulse oximetry has increased to 95%. He is discharged with prescriptions for oral steroids, azithromycin, and an albuterol inhaler; primary care follow-up is arranged for the following day.

---

COPD is a common disease that has been diagnosed in more than 15 million Americans with estimates of more than 10 million that are undiagnosed.[51] It is the third leading cause of death in the United States and annually accounts for almost 1.8 million ED visits and 700,000 hospitalizations.[52] The prevalence of COPD in the United States was stable from 1998 to 2009.[53] Exacerbations of COPD are characterized by a worsening of symptoms from the patient's baseline. The primary symptoms of an exacerbation include increased dyspnea, increased sputum volume, and sputum purulence. Patients with COPD who are admitted to the hospital have a high rate of 30-day readmission: 21% for any diagnosis and 7% for principle diagnosis of COPD or bronchiectasis. The economic burden in the United States attributable to COPD is estimated to be greater than $36 billion annually.[52]

### Evidence for Emergency Department Observation Unit Management of Chronic Obstructive Pulmonary Disease Exacerbation

In contrast with other commonly seen diagnoses such as chest pain, asthma, and heart failure, there is a paucity of research regarding observation care for patients with an COPD exacerbation of COPD.[54] A retrospective Spanish study[55] of patients with COPD exacerbation found a decreased length duration stay (3.4 days vs 12 days) and lower mortality (1.7% vs 8.1%) for those treated in an ED short stay unit compared with inpatient care. The cohorts were not matched according to disease severity or comorbid conditions. There was also a significant increase in the rate of readmission by 10 days (9.9% vs 7.0%). Despite the lack of rigorous research, extrapolation of the beneficial results seen in exacerbations of other chronic disease such as asthma and congestive heart failure leads to the reasonable assumption that there would be similar benefits for a patient with an acute exacerbation of COPD.

### Patient Selection

Patients placed in an EDOU for continued treatment of a COPD exacerbation should be selected carefully to avoid patients at high risk for decompensation. An analysis[56] of the data from the recent ECLIPSE study (Evaluation of COPD Longitudinally to Identify Predictive Surrogate Endpoints) distinguished factors that were associated with need for hospitalization. These included a prior hospitalization for COPD, increased airflow limitation, poorer overall health status, advanced age, presence of radiographic evidence of emphysema, and leukocytosis. Factors associated with high risk for adverse events owing to acute COPD exacerbations include rapid respiratory rate, paradoxic breathing, hypoxia, altered mental status, previous intensive care unit admission, chronic steroid use, previous home oxygen use, and history of intubation.[57,58]

Several risk stratification tools exist to predict outcomes of patients with COPD exacerbations. The Global Initiative for Obstructive Lung Disease (GOLD) grades the severity of airflow restriction based on postbronchodilator predicted $\%FEV_1$, a measurement that is not practical in acutely ill ED patients.[59] A validated risk stratification tool is available known as the BAP-65 criteria,[60] which takes into account 5 measurements easily obtainable in the ED setting: blood urea nitrogen 25 mg/dL or greater, altered mental status, pulse 109 bpm or greater, and age greater than 65 years. Patients with none of the 3 main risk factors are categorized as class I if 65 years of age or younger and class II if older than age 65. Designation to classes III, IV, and V are based on the presence of 1, 2, 3 of the main risk factors, respectively. Use of the BAP-65 has been found to be a valid prognostic score in estimating risk of death and mechanical ventilation with increasing risk associated with high class. Mortality rates and need for intubation associated with each class were as follows: class I (0.5%, 2.1%), class II (1.4%, 2.2%), class III (3.7%, 8.4%), class IV (12.7%, 30.1%), and class V (26.2%, 54.6%).

Patients who are at low risk for significant adverse events based on absence of high-risk features and who have a lower BAP-65 classification may be appropriate EDOU candidates. Available resources and capabilities of a individual receiving EDOU will be the final determining factor of how severe a patient's COPD exacerbation that is acceptable for placement in that EDOU.

### Emergency Department Observation Unit Care of Patients with Chronic Obstructive Pulmonary Disease Exacerbation

#### Protocols
The use of a standardized COPD protocol will aid in patient selection and provides for evidence-based management in an effort to reduce complications, decrease the duration of stay, and reduce readmissions. We provide a sample protocol in **Box 3**.

#### Emergency department observation unit interventions
The nonpharmaceutical interventions that can be implemented in an EDOU mirror those done for asthma exacerbations. The patient should have frequent vital sign assessment with strong consideration for continuous cardiac monitoring with pulse oximetry, because patients with COPD are prone to developing arrhythmias. A walking pulse oximetry evaluation may aid in the eventual disposition of the patient. Supplemental oxygen should be provided with careful consideration of the potential harmful effects of oxygen in this patient population. GOLD recommends that supplemental oxygen should be provided to patients with hypoxemia to a target oxygenation of 88% to 92%.[59] The patient should receive education as applicable regarding smoking cessation, avoidance of other triggers, and medication compliance. Successful management of comorbid conditions can help to manage the impact of COPD. The discharging provider should arrange for appropriate outpatient follow-up.

### Medical Treatments for Exacerbation of Chronic Obstructive Pulmonary Disease

Most of the treatments initiated during the initial ED phase of treatment will be continued in the EDOU. The mainstay of treatment of a COPD exacerbation is with bronchodilators. Although COPD is considered generally to be an irreversible condition owing to permanent structural changes to the lung, there is usually a reversible component that can be acted on to improve symptoms during an exacerbation. As with treatment of acute asthma exacerbations, the mainstay of treatment is with short-acting $\beta_2$-agonists, such as albuterol, and short-acting anticholinergic agents, such as ipratropium bromide.

**Box 3**
**ED observation unit chronic obstructive pulmonary disease protocol example**

*Inclusion criteria*

- Stable or acceptable vital signs (pulse oximetry ≥90% with normal home requirements)
- Intermediate response to therapy in ED; improving but still wheezing/symptomatic and high likelihood of further improvement and subsequent discharge home within 24 hours
- No acute mental status changes
- Plan of care established

*Exclusion criteria*

- Depressed mental status or altered level of consciousness
- Signs/symptoms of impending respiratory fatigue or failure (eg, high respiratory rate, requiring BiPAP, accessory muscle use, $PaO_2$ <60 mm Hg, ± $PaCO_2$ >50 mm Hg)
- Significant dysrhythmia, ischemic ECG changes, or theophylline toxicity
- Findings suggesting an alternative etiology for respiratory symptoms (eg, PE, drug overdose or toxic ingestion) excludes from this protocol
- Presence of serious active comorbidities (eg, congestive heart failure, pneumonia, new arrhythmia)
- Clinical decline despite 24 hours of outpatient steroids
- ED or observation provider concern (ie, similar prior hospitalizations requiring intubation or ICU, requiring continuous nebulized bronchodilator therapy in the ED)

*Potential interventions*

- Serial vital signs and reevaluations including mental status evaluation
- Pulse oximetry monitoring
- Cardiac monitoring
- Oxygen
- CXR
- BNP, ECG, cardiac enzymes, ABG
- Scheduled short-acting nebulized $\beta_2$-agonists and anticholinergics
- Systemic corticosteroids
- Systemic antimicrobial therapy
- IV hydration
- IV magnesium sulfate
- Smoking cessation counseling

*Discharge criteria*

- Home
  - Improved clinical symptoms
  - Acceptable vital signs, pulse oximetry ≥90% on room air or home $O_2$ and/or at baseline
  - No longer needing albuterol at least every 4 hours
  - Adequate follow-up plan established and patient education
- Admit
  - Interval development of any exclusion criteria
  - Subjective worsening and/or failure to improve

*Abbreviations:* ABG, arterial blood gases; BiPAP, biphasic intermittent positive airway pressure; BNP, brain natriuretic peptide; CXR, chest radiograph; ECG, electrocardiograph; ICU, intensive care unit; PE, pulmonary embolism.
*From* the Michigan College of Emergency Physicians Observation Committee. Available at: https://www.mcep.org/imis15/mcepdocs/Newsletters/2016/March16newsletter.pdf. Accessed November 30, 2017.

Treatment with systemic glucocorticoids is indicated in patients with COPD exacerbations. Its use decreases hospital duration of stay, hospital admission rates, and treatment failures (ie, relapse or hospitalization within 30 days).[61–63] The GOLD recommendation is that duration of therapy should be 5 to 7 days.[59]

Antibiotic use is somewhat controversial owing to the fact that many previously cited studies purporting to show beneficial effects of antibiotic treatment were poorly structured or otherwise not generalizable. In select patients, antibiotic treatment decreases sputum purulence, treatment failures, and short-term mortality.[61] The most recent GOLD recommendations[59] are based on the presence of 3 cardinal symptoms, namely, increased dyspnea, sputum purulence, and sputum volume. Antibiotics should be given when there is increased sputum purulence with either increased sputum volume or increased dyspnea. This is a change from previous recommendations that did not require the presence of sputum purulence for the provision of antibiotics. The duration of treatment is for 5 to 7 days.

### Disposition

Disposition of patients with COPD exacerbation is based on response to therapy. Patients who respond to treatment in the EDOU may be discharged home if their symptoms are minimal and vital signs are unremarkable. A walking pulse oximetry evaluation may assist in the disposition decision. Close outpatient follow-up should be arranged. The patient should be discharged with prescriptions for steroids, antibiotics (if indicated), and rescue inhalers.

Patients who have not improved significantly or worsen despite appropriate treatment in the EDOU should be admitted as inpatients. Alternative diagnoses for dyspnea, such as pneumonia and pulmonary embolism, should be considered in patients that fail to improve. Patients with severe hypoxic or hypercapnic respiratory failure requiring noninvasive positive pressure ventilation or endotracheal intubation will require admission and intensive care monitoring.

## COMMUNITY-ACQUIRED PNEUMONIA

---

**Case Study**

Robert Jones, a 54-year-old smoker with a history of diabetes, complains of fever and vomiting. Vital signs are temperature, 103.4°F; blood pressure, 115/85 mm Hg; pulse, 135; respiratory rate, 28; and room air oxygenation 91%. On examination, he is alert and oriented with dry mucous membranes. Right-sided rales are noted on auscultation. His chest radiography reveals an infiltrate in the right middle lobe. He is started on ceftriaxone and placed in the EDOU, where he receives IV fluids, azithromycin, and acetaminophen. The next morning, he is drinking fluids, vital signs are unremarkable, and room air pulse oximetry is 96%. Smoking cessation counseling is provided. After arranging for outpatient follow-up in 2 days, he is discharged with a prescription for antibiotics.

---

Pneumonia, an infection of the lung parenchyma caused by bacteria, viruses, and fungi, is commonly seen in the ED. In 2007, there were an estimated 4.5 million visits for pneumonia in ambulatory settings with almost one-third of those visits occurring in EDs[64] and leading to 1.1 million hospitalizations.[65] In 2014, lower respiratory tract infections, including pneumonia and influenza, comprised the leading cause of infection-related death in the United States with more than 55,000 deaths.[66] The economic burden of pneumonia is high, with direct costs just for hospitalization exceeding $10 billion in 2011.[67]

Pneumonia is frequently classified based on the location where it was presumed to have been acquired. Hospital-acquired (nosocomial) pneumonia is one that is diagnosed after a minimum of 48 hours of hospital admission. Ventilator-associated pneumonia is defined by the development of pneumonia more than 48 hours after endotracheal intubation. CAP is pneumonia that is neither hospital-acquired (nosocomial) pneumonia nor ventilator-associated pneumonia. The term health care-associated pneumonia was first introduced in the 2005 guidelines published by the Infectious Diseases Society of America (IDSA) and American Thoracic Society (ATS).[68] This designation was given to pneumonia that was thought to have been acquired in a health care setting, such as a nursing home, dialysis center, or during a recent hospitalization. It was assumed that health care-associated pneumonia was more likely to be caused by multidrug-resistant organisms, but this was not shown in recent studies.[69] With the 2016 IDSA/ATS guidelines, this class has been removed.[70]

Frequently, CAP develops in otherwise healthy patients with fewer or no significant comorbidities and thus has a lower risk of morbidity and mortality. The EDOU is an appropriate alternative disposition for select ED patients with CAP requiring additional treatment and not yet suitable for discharge.

### Evidence for Emergency Department Observation Unit Management of Community-Acquired Pneumonia

There are few studies focused on the EDOU management of CAP. Chan and colleagues[71] reported the use of a modified risk stratification rule, the Pneumonia Severity Index (PSI), to guide inpatient versus outpatient management. Patients with PSI class II were eligible for care in an EDOU. Of the 38 PSI class II patients, 14 were placed in the EDOU and 4 subsequently required hospital admission. The average duration of stay in the EDOU was 15 hours. Two separate Spanish studies have shown a decreased duration of stay for patients with CAP that are managed in a short-stay unit compared with traditional inpatient units. These retrospective studies did not control for severity of illness in the comparisons of duration of stay.[72,73]

### Patient Selection

The decision to place a patient in an EDOU for continued management of CAP should be based on the need for continued care as well as the likelihood of successful treatment in the time frame that is appropriate for this clinical setting. Patients with severe CAP should be excluded immediately from placement in the EDOU owing to their high likelihood of treatment failure and intense resource needs. The 2007 IDSA/ATS guidelines for the management of CAP[74] included a predictive rule for determination of severe CAP based on the presence of at least 1 of 2 major criteria or at least 3 of 9 minor severity criteria (**Box 4**). The use of this rule was shown to have a sensitivity of 71% and specificity of 88% for admission to the intensive care unit.[75] Other validated instruments include the PSI, CURB-65, and the Severe Community-Acquired Pneumonia (SCAP) score.

The PSI or pneumonia Patient Outcomes Research Team score, a 2-step scoring system, is the most studied and validated prediction rule for risk stratification of pneumonia patients.[76,77] Patients are assigned a risk class (I–V) based on increasing cumulative points given for the presence of various risk factors. Classes I through III are considered low risk. In the validation study done by Fine and colleagues,[76] classes I through III had mortality rates of 0.1, 0.6%, and 0.9%, respectively. Classes IV and V are high risk with mortality rates of 9.3% and 27.0%, respectively. Most low-risk patients had only 1 pertinent coexisting illness, physical examination finding, or laboratory or radiographic abnormality. The authors concluded that low-risk patients could be appropriately treated in an outpatient setting or with a short-term hospital stay.

---

**Box 4**
**Criteria for severe community-acquired pneumonia**

*Minor criteria[a]*

- Respiratory rate[b] of greater than 30 breaths/min
- $Pao_2/Fio_2$ ratio[b] of less than 250
- Multilobar infiltrates
- Confusion/disorientation
- Uremia (blood urea nitrogen level of $\geq$20 mg/dL)
- Leukopenia[c] (white blood cell count of <4000 cells/mm$^3$)
- Thrombocytopenia (platelet count <100,000 cells/mm$^3$)
- Hypothermia (core temperature <36°C)
- Hypotension requiring aggressive fluid resuscitation

*Major criteria*

- Invasive mechanical ventilation
- Septic shock with the need for vasopressors

[a] Other factors to consider include hypoglycemia (in nondiabetic patients), acute alcoholism/ alcohol withdrawal, hyponatremia, unexplained metabolic acidosis or elevated lactate level, cirrhosis, and asplenia.
[b] A need for noninvasive ventilation can substitute for a respiratory rate of greater than 30 breaths/min or a $Pao_2/Fio_2$ ratio of less than 250.
[c] As a result of infection alone.
*Data from* Mandell LA, Wunderink RG, Anzueto A, et al. Infectious Diseases Society of America/American Thoracic Society consensus guidelines on the management of community-acquired pneumonia in adults. Clin Infect Dis 2007;44(Suppl 2):27–72.

---

The British Thoracic Society developed the CURB-65 score, a validated scoring system that assigns one point for the presence of each of the following variables: confusion, uremia (blood urea nitrogen $\geq$19 mg/dL), respiratory rate $\geq$30 breaths per minute, blood pressure (systolic <90 mm Hg or diastolic $\leq$60 mm Hg) and age 65 years or older. Patients with a score of 0 and 1 are low risk and had low mortality rates (0.6% and 2.7%, respectively).[78]

The SCAP score was developed in 2006 in an effort to develop a clinical prediction rule that could be calculated easily using only variables readily available in the ED.[79] This system assigns various points for major (arterial pH <7.3, systolic blood pressure <90 mm Hg) and minor (confusion, uremia [blood urea nitrogen >30], respiratory rate >30 breaths per minute, chest radiography [bilateral or multifocal infiltrates], $Pao_2$ <54 mm Hg or $Pao_2/Fio_2$ <250, age $\geq$80 years) variables, and risk stratifies patients into low, medium, and high risk groups. One drawback to this score is the use of arterial pH, which is not always measured.

In a prospective validation study of the 3 scoring systems—PSI, CURB-65, and SCAP—patients considered low risk by all 3 had similar low risks of mortality.[80] All 3 scoring systems had similar but not insignificant rates of inpatients identified as low risk that required intensive care unit admission: PSI (4.8%), CURB-65 (2.8%), and SCAP (2.7%). Therefore, these scoring systems may underestimate illness severity, which should be taken into consideration when making disposition decisions.

The IDSA/ATS consensus CAP guidelines states that severity of illness scores (eg, CURB-65 or PSI) may be used for risk stratification (level I recommendation), although physician judgment regarding individual patient factors (including the ability to reliably take oral medications and availability of outpatient support services) must always be considered (level II recommendation).[74] The American College of Emergency Physicians CAP clinical policy recommends the use of scoring systems to aid in disposition decisions.[81]

The provider must take into account other patient-specific factors when deciding if a patient is appropriate for discharge versus EDOU management. These factors include the likelihood of treatment adherence, presence of coexisting conditions (eg, dehydration, oral intolerance), and psychosocial factors (eg, unsafe living conditions, substance abuse) that make outpatient therapy undesirable or unsafe.

## EMERGENCY DEPARTMENT OBSERVATION UNIT CARE OF PATIENTS WITH COMMUNITY-ACQUIRED PNEUMONIA
### Protocols

The use of EDOU-specific protocols for the treatment of CAP ensures appropriate and timely administration of antibiotics and timely recognition of potential patient deterioration. CAP protocols have been associated with decreased health care costs and improved overall quality (**Box 5**).[82]

### Emergency department observation unit interventions

Management of CAP patients in the EDOU includes regular monitoring of vital signs with assessment of pulse oximetry, respiratory status, and mentation. The patient should be reassessed serially for the need for parenteral antibiotics, IV fluids, and other potential interventions. Respiratory care may include suctioning of secretions. Smokers should have smoking cessation counseling provided. Isolation measures should follow local protocols.

### Medical Treatments for Community-Acquired Pneumonia

Antibiotic therapy, ideally initiated in the ED, should be reviewed for appropriateness and continued during the time care is provided in the EDOU. Targeted therapy to a specific organism would be ideal, but this rarely occurs. In the absence of pathogen identification, the provider must decide on the most appropriate treatment based on knowledge of specific patient factors as well as local resistance patterns. Current identification techniques using isolates from culture identifies the pathogen in 30% to 40% of cases. The use of comprehensive molecular identification techniques may result in identification in almost 90% of cases.[83] *Streptococcus pneumoniae* is the most frequent bacterial pathogen isolated in both the inpatient and outpatient setting.[84] Other bacteria frequently isolated include *Haemophilus influenzae*, *Staphylococcus aureus*, and atypical bacteria. Atypical bacteria, including *Legionella pneumophila*, *Mycoplasma pneumoniae*, and *Chlamydophila pneumonia*, are so named because they are not easily identified by conventional laboratory techniques such as Gram staining, not because they are uncommon. **Box 6** lists antibiotic choices per the IDSA/ATS CAP guidelines.[74] Briefly, the guidelines recommend an antipneumococcal fluoroquinolone or combination therapy with a β-lactam plus a macrolide.

If influenza is suspected, early treatment, within 48 hours of symptom onset, with appropriate antiviral medications is recommended. Although antivirals are not recommended for patients with uncomplicated influenza with symptoms for greater than 48 hours, these drugs may be used to reduce viral shedding in hospitalized patients or for influenza pneumonia.[74] The neuraminidase inhibitors, oseltamivir and zanamivir, are effective against influenza A and B. The adamantanes, amantadine and rimantidine, are M2 inhibitors that are only effective against influenza A, and not influenza

**Box 5**
**ED observation unit community-acquired pneumonia protocol example**

*Inclusion criteria*

- Pneumonia documented on chest radiograph or other imaging studies, such as CT scan

- If no radiographic evidence of pneumonia, clinical presentation consistent with pneumonia

- Risk stratification by appropriate scoring system (CURB-65 $\geq$2) or (PSI class I, II, or III)

- Stable vital signs

- Pulse oximetry $\geq$90% on room air

- Normal or baseline mentation (no mew alteration of mental status)

- Probability of discharge in less than 24 hours is $\geq$80%

*Exclusion criteria*

- Respiratory failure; such as, intubation, need for acute use of noninvasive positive pressure intubation (eg, BiPAP or CPAP)

- Severe respiratory distress, such as respiratory rate >40, use of accessory muscles in the neck, severe intercostal retractions, cyanosis

- Altered mental status, which is new

- Pulse oximetry <90% on room air

- Unstable vital signs

- Risk stratification by appropriate scoring systems (CURB-65 score of 4 or 5) or (PSI class IV or V)

*Potential interventions*

- Serial vital signs

- Pulse oximetry

- Serial examinations including respiratory assessment checklist: clinical—respiratory rate, use of accessory muscles, retractions; auscultation—rales, wheezing

- Mental status assessment

- Supplemental oxygen administration

- Chest radiograph

- Antimicrobial therapy

- Respiratory treatments, if indicated

- IV hydration (IV fluids), if indicated

- Smoking cessation counseling

- Patient/family education

*Discharge criteria*

- Home
  - Significant clinical improvement
  - Acceptable, stable vital signs
  - Pulse oximetry $\geq$90% on room air or home oxygen and at baseline
  - Able to tolerate oral intake and oral medications

- Admit
  - Deterioration of clinical condition: worsening vital signs, alteration of mental status, respiratory distress or respiratory failure
  - Worsening of or no significant improvement in clinical symptoms
  - Hypoxia, as indicated by inability to maintain oxygen saturation >90% on room air or return to baseline

○ Unstable vital signs
○ Conversion to exclusion criteria
○ Other considerations including poor social situation and/or inadequate follow-up care

*Abbreviations:* BiPAP, biphasic intermittent positive airway pressure; CPAP, continuous positive airway pressure; CT, computed tomography; CURB-65, confusion, urea, respiratory rate, blood pressure, and age; PSI, Pneumonia Severity Index.
*Data from* Mace SE. Clinical protocols. In: Observation medicine principles and protocols. Cambridge (United Kingdom): Cambridge University Press; 2016. p. 512–44.

B. In the United States, the Advisory Committee on Immunization Practices no longer recommends M2 inhibitors for influenza treatment, except in special circumstances owing to an increase in resistant isolates.[85]

There has been increased interest in the use of adjunctive corticosteroid therapy for CAP. Steroid use would be beneficial to reduce the inflammatory process that accompanies infection of the lung parenchyma. Studies seem to show significant benefit in patients with severe CAP, but not in the type of patients that would be selected for placement in an EDOU.[86]

## Disposition

Patients who have improved clinically with normal vital signs, including room air pulse oximetry and can be successfully transitioned to oral therapy for the remainder of antibiotic dosing, are candidates for discharge. Primary care provider follow-up should be arranged. Antibiotic treatment is for a minimum of 5 days, but may be extended based on patient comorbidities, response to treatment, and based on culture and sensitivity of causative organism, if available.[74]

---

**Box 6**
**Antibiotic therapy for community-acquired pneumonia**

*Outpatient treatment*

- Previously healthy + no risk factors for DRSP: macrolide (drug of choice), alternative doxycycline

- Comorbidities are present (eg, chronic lung, heart, liver, or renal disease; diabetes mellitus, alcoholism, malignancies, asplenia, immunosuppressing conditions or the use of immunosuppressive drugs, antimicrobial use within prior 3 months (if yes, chose an alternative antibiotic from a different antimicrobial drug class), any risk for DRSP (respiratory fluoroquinolone or β-lactam plus a macrolide or amoxicillin-clavulanate). Alternatives include ceftriaxone, cefpodoxime, cefuroxime. Doxycycline is an alternative to the macrolide.

- If in a region with a high rate (>25%) of infection with high-level (MIC $\geq$16 μg/mL) macrolide-resistant *S pneumoniae* consider alternatives noted in b.

*Inpatient, non-ICU treatment*

- Respiratory fluoroquinolone

- β-Lactam plus a macrolide

Preferred β-lactam agents include cefotaxime, ceftriaxone, ampicillin. Ertapenem is used in selected patients. Doxycycline is an alternative to macrolides. Respiratory fluoroquinolones may be used in penicillin-allergic patients.
*Abbreviations:* DRSP, drug-resistant *Streptococcus pneumoniae*; ICU, intensive care unit; MIC, minimum inhibitory concentration.
*Data from* Mandell LA, Wunderink RG, Anzueto A, et al. Infectious Diseases Society of America/American Thoracic Society consensus guidelines on the management of community-acquired pneumonia in adults. Clin Infect Dis 2007;44(Suppl 2):27–72.

Patients whose condition worsens owing to the development of hypoxia, respiratory distress or failure, hypotension or septic shock, or those who are unable to take oral medications require inpatient admission. Other considerations for prolonged care in the EDOU or inpatient admission include unreliable social situations or inadequate follow-up care.

## SUMMARY

In adults, respiratory disorders are the second most frequent diagnoses treated in EDOUs in the United States and worldwide. They account for the most frequent indication for placement of a pediatric patient into an EDOU. Evidence demonstrates that with appropriate patient selection, adult and pediatric patients with asthma and COPD exacerbations as well as CAP can be managed effectively in the EDOU. EDOU management of these respiratory disorders results in equivalent or better outcomes than inpatient care with decreased duration of stay, increased patient satisfaction, lower cost, and in some studies decreased mortality. Evidence-based protocols are an important tool to ensure appropriate patients are placed in the EDOU, standardize best practice interventions, and guide disposition decisions.

## REFERENCES

1. Global Initiative for Asthma (GINA). Global strategy for asthma management and prevention (updated 2016). Available at: http://www.ginasthma.org. Accessed January, 27 2017.
2. Akinbami LJ, Moorman JE, Bailey C, et al. Trends in asthma prevalence, health care use, and mortality in the United States, 2001–2010. NCHS Data Brief No. 94. Hyattsville (MD): National Center for Health Statistics; 2012. Available at: https://www.cdc.gov/nchs/data/databriefs/db94.pdf. Accessed January, 27 2017.
3. Centers for Disease Conrol and Prevention. National Hospital Ambulatory Medical Care Survey: 2013 emergency department summary tables. Available at: https://www.cdc.gov/nchs/data/ahcd/nhamcs_emergency/2013_ed_web_tables.pdf. Accessed February 8, 2017.
4. United States Environmental Protection Agency. Asthma facts. 2013. Available at: http://www.epa.gov/asthma/pdfs/asthma_fact_sheet_en.pdf. Accessed February 8, 2017.
5. Centers for Disease Control and Prevention. National surveillance of asthma: United States, 2001-2010. Available at: http://www.cdc.gov/nchs/data/series/sr_03/sr03_035.pdf. Accessed February 6, 2017.
6. Macy ML, Kim CS, Sasson C, et al. Pediatric observation units in the United States: a systematic review. J Hosp Med 2010;5:172–82.
7. Venkatesh AK, Geisler BP, Gibson Chambers JJ, et al. Use of observation care in US emergency departments, 2001 to 2008. PLoS One 2011;6(9):e24326.
8. Barnett S, Numagambetov T. Costs of asthma in the United States: 2002-2007. J Allergy Clin Immunol 2011;127(1):145–52.
9. Barrett ML, Wier LM, Washington R. Trends in Pediatric and Adult Hospital Stays for Asthma, 2000-2010. HCUP Statistical Brief #169. Rockville (MD): Agency for Healthcare Research and Quality; 2014. Available at: https://www.hcup-us.ahrq.gov/reports/statbriefs/sb169-Asthma-Trends-Hospital-Stays.pdf. Accessed January 15, 2017.
10. Centers for Disease Control and Prevention. CDC AsthmaStats: Asthma-related missed school days among children aged 5–17 Years. Available at: www.cdc.gov/asthma/asthma_stats/default.htm.

11. Partridge MR. Patient-centred asthma education in the emergency department: the case in favour. Eur Respir J 2008;31(5):920–1.

12. Gibson PG, Powell H, Coughlan J, et al. Self-management education and regular practitioner review for adults with asthma. Cochrane Database Syst Rev 2003;(1):CD001117.

13. Scribano PV, Wiley JF, Platt K. Use of an observation unit by a pediatric emergency department for common pediatric illnesses. Pediatr Emerg Care 2001; 17(5):321–3.

14. Browne GJ. A short stay or 23-hour ward in a general and academic children's hospital: Are they effective? Pediatr Emerg Care 2000;16(4):223.

15. Gouin S, Macarthur C, Parkin PC, et al. Effect of a pediatric observation unit on the rate of hospitalization for asthma. Ann Emerg Med 1997;29(2):218–22.

16. Marks MK, Lovejoy FH, Rutherford PA, et al. Impact of a short stay unit on asthma patients admitted to a tertiary pediatric hospital. Qual Manag Health Care 1997; 6(1):14–22.

17. McDermott MF, Murphy DG, Zalenski RJ, et al. A comparison between emergency diagnostic and treatment unit and inpatient care in the management of acute asthma. Arch Intern Med 1997;157(18):2055–62.

18. Miescier MJ, Nelson DS, Firth SD, et al. Children with asthma admitted to a pediatric observation unit. Pediatr Emerg Care 2005;21(10):645–9.

19. O'Brien SR, Hein EW, Sly RM. Treatment of acute asthmatic attacks in a holding unit of a pediatric emergency room. Ann Allergy 1980;45(3):159–62.

20. Rydman RJ, Isola ML, Roberts RR, et al. Emergency department observation unit versus hospital inpatient care for a chronic asthmatic population: a randomized trial of health status outcome and cost. Med Care 1998;36(4):599–609.

21. Willert C, Davis AT, Herman JJ, et al. Short-term holding room treatment of asthmatic children. J Pediatr 1985;106(5):707–11.

22. Zebrack M, Kadish H, Nelson D. The pediatric hybrid observation unit: an analysis of 6477 consecutive patient encounters. Pediatrics 2005;115(5):e535–42.

23. Zwicke DL, Donohue JF, Wagner EH. Use of the emergency department observation unit in the treatment of acute asthma. Ann Emerg Med 1982;11(2):77–83.

24. Rydman RJ, Roberts RR, Albrecht GL, et al. Patient satisfaction with an emergency department asthma observation unit. Acad Emerg Med 1999;6(3):178–83.

25. Ross MA, Hockenberry JM, Mutter R, et al. Protocol-driven emergency department observation units offer savings, shorter stays, and reduced admissions. Health Aff 2013;32(12):2149–56.

26. Baugh CW, Venkatesh AK, Hilton JA, et al. Making greater use of dedicated hospital observation units for many short-stay patients could save $3.1 billion a year. Health Aff (Millwood) 2012;31(10):2314–23.

27. Macy ML, Stanley RM, Lozon MM, et al. Trends in high-turnover stays among children hospitalized in the United States, 1993-2003. Pediatrics 2009;123(3): 996–1002.

28. Camargo CA, Rachelefsky G, Schatz M. Managing asthma exacerbations in the emergency department: summary of the National Asthma Education And Prevention Program Expert Panel Report 3 guidelines for the management of asthma exacerbations. Proc Am Thorac Soc 2009;6(4):357–66.

29. Gorelick MH, Stevens MW, Schultz TR, et al. Performance of a novel clinical score, the Pediatric Asthma Severity Score (PASS), in the evaluation of acute asthma. Acad Emerg Med 2004;11:10–8.

30. Hsu P, Lam LT, Browne G. The pulmonary index score as a clinical assessment tool for acute childhood asthma. Ann Allergy Asthma Immunol 2010;105(6): 425–9.
31. Ducharme FM, Chalut D, Plotnick L, et al. The Pediatric Respiratory Assessment Measure: a valid clinical score for assessing acute asthma severity from toddlers to teenagers. J Pediatr 2008;152:476–80.
32. Arnold DH, Gebretsadik T, Abramo TJ, et al. The RAD score: a simple acute asthma severity score compares favorably to more complex scores. Ann Allergy Asthma Immunol 2011;107(1):22–8.
33. McFadden ER, Elsanadi N, Dixon L, et al. Protocol therapy for acute asthma: therapeutic benefits and cost savings. Am J Med 1995;99(6):651–61.
34. Norton SP, Pusic MV, Taha F, et al. Effect of a clinical pathway on the hospitalisation rates of children with asthma: a prospective study. Arch Dis Child 2007;92(1): 60–6.
35. McCarren M, Zalenski RJ, McDermott M, et al. Predicting recovery from acute asthma in an emergency diagnostic and treatment unit. Acad Emerg Med 2000;7(1):28–35.
36. Idris AH, McDermott MF, Raucci JC, et al. Emergency department treatment of severe asthma. Metered-dose inhaler plus holding chamber is equivalent in effectiveness to nebulizer. Chest 1993;103(3):665–72.
37. James DR, Lyttle MD. British guideline on the management of asthma: SIGN Clinical Guideline 141, 2014. Arch Dis Child Educ Pract Ed 2016;101(6):319–22.
38. Jat KR, Khairwa A. Levalbuterol versus albuterol for acute asthma: a systematic review and meta-analysis. Pulm Pharmacol Ther 2013;26(2):239–48.
39. Rodrigo G, Rodrigo C. Ipratropium bromide in acute asthma: small beneficial effects? Chest 1999;115(5):1482.
40. Goggin N, Macarthur C, Parkin PC. Randomized trial of the addition of ipratropium bromide to albuterol and corticosteroid therapy in children hospitalized because of an acute asthma exacerbation. Arch Pediatr Adolesc Med 2001; 155(12):1329–34.
41. Kravitz J, Dominici P, Ufberg J, et al. Two days of dexamethasone versus 5 days of prednisone in the treatment of acute asthma: a randomized controlled trial. Ann Emerg Med 2011;58(2):200–4.
42. Rehrer MW, Liu B, Rodriguez M, et al. A randomized controlled noninferiority trial of single dose of oral dexamethasone versus 5 days of oral prednisone in acute adult asthma. Ann Emerg Med 2016;68(5):608–13.
43. Cronin JJ, McCoy S, Kennedy U, et al. A randomized trial of single-dose oral dexamethasone versus multidose prednisolone for acute exacerbations of asthma in children who attend the emergency department. Ann Emerg Med 2016;67(5):593–601.e3.
44. Watnick CS, Fabbri D, Arnold DH. Single-dose oral dexamethasone is effective in preventing relapse after acute asthma exacerbations. Ann Allergy Asthma Immunol 2016;116(2):171–2.
45. Hames H, Seabrook JA, Matsui D, et al. A palatability study of a flavored dexamethasone preparation versus prednisolone liquid in children. Can J Clin Pharmacol 2008;15(1):e95–8.
46. Qureshi F, Zaritsky A, Poirier MP. Comparative efficacy of oral dexamethasone versus oral prednisone in acute pediatric asthma. J Pediatr 2001;139(1):20–6.
47. Williams KW, Andrews AL, Heine D, et al. Parental preference for short- versus long-course corticosteroid therapy in children with asthma presenting to the pediatric emergency department. Clin Pediatr (Phila) 2013;52(1):30–4.

48. Aboeed AMJ, Riss A, McNamee J, et al. Dexamethasone versus prednisone in the treatment of acute asthma in adults: can an easier regimen provide the same results? Am J Respir Crit Care Med 2014;189:A1360.

49. Keeney GE, Gray MP, Morrison AK, et al. Dexamethasone for acute asthma exacerbations in children: a meta-analysis. Pediatrics 2014;133(3):493–9.

50. US Department of Health and Human Services. Asthma care quick reference: diagnosing and managing asthma. Available at: https://www.nhlbi.nih.gov/files/docs/guidelines/asthma_qrg.pdf. Accessed January 27, 2017.

51. Rosenberg SR, Kalhan R, Mannino DM. Epidemiology of chronic obstructive pulmonary disease: prevalence, morbidity, mortality, and risk factors. Semin Respir Crit Care Med 2015;36(4):457–69.

52. Ford ES. Hospital discharges, readmissions, and ED visits for COPD or bronchiectasis among us adults. Chest 2015;147(4):989–98.

53. Akinbami LJ, Liu X. Chronic obstructive pulmonary disease among adults aged 18 and Over in the United States, 1998–2009. NCHS Data Brief No. 63. 2011. Available at: https://www.cdc.gov/nchs/data/databriefs/db63.pdf.

54. Baugh CWM, Mace SE, Pena ME. The evidence basis for observation care for adults based on diagnosis/clinical condition. In: Mace SE, editor. Observation medicine principles and protocols. Cambridge (United Kingdom): Cambridge University Press; 2016.

55. Salazar A, Juan A, Ballbe R, et al. Emergency short-stay unit as an effective alternative to in-hospital admission for acute chronic obstructive pulmonary disease exacerbation. Am J Emerg Med 2007;25(4):486–7.

56. Müllerova H, Maselli DJ, Locantore N, et al. Hospitalized exacerbations of COPD: risk factors and outcomes in the ECLIPSE cohort. Chest 2015;147(4):999–1007.

57. Wiwatcharagoses K, Lueweeravong K. Factors associated with hospitalization of chronic obstructive pulmonary disease patients with acute exacerbation in the emergency department, Rajavithi Hospital. J Med Assoc Thai 2016;99(Suppl 2):S161–7.

58. Stiell IG, Clement CM, Aaron SD, et al. Clinical characteristics associated with adverse events in patients with exacerbation of chronic obstructive pulmonary disease: a prospective cohort study. CMAJ 2014;186(6):E193–204.

59. Vogelmeier CF, Criner GJ, Martinez FJ, et al. Global Strategy for the Diagnosis, Management, and Prevention of Chronic Obstructive Lung Disease 2017 Report: GOLD executive summary. Am J Respir Crit Care Med 2017;195(5):557–82.

60. Shorr AF, Sun X, Johannes RS, et al. Validation of a novel risk score for severity of illness in acute exacerbations of COPD. Chest 2011;140(5):1177–83.

61. Rowe BH, Bhutani M, Stickland MK, et al. Assessment and management of chronic obstructive pulmonary disease in the emergency department and beyond. Expert Rev Respir Med 2011;5(4):549–59.

62. Niewoehner DE, Erbland ML, Deupree RH, et al. Effect of systemic glucocorticoids on exacerbations of chronic obstructive pulmonary disease. Department of Veterans Affairs Cooperative Study Group. N Engl J Med 1999;340(25):1941–7.

63. Bullard MJ, Liaw SJ, Tsai YH, et al. Early corticosteroid use in acute exacerbations of chronic airflow obstruction. Am J Emerg Med 1996;14(2):139–43.

64. Schappert SM, Rechtsteiner EA. Ambulatory medical care utilization estimates for 2007. Vital Health Stat 13 2011;(169):1–38.

65. Hall MJ, DeFrances CJ, Williams SN, et al. National hospital discharge survey: 2007 summary. National health statistics reports; no 29. Hyattsville (MD): National Center for Health Statistics; 2010.

66. Kochanek KD, Murphy SL, Xu J, et al. Deaths: final data for 2014. Natl Vital Stat Rep 2016;65(4):1–122.

67. Pfuntner A, Wier LM, Steiner C. Costs for hospital stays in the United States, 2011. HCUP statistical brief #168. Rockville (MD): Agency for Healthcare Research and Quality; 2013. Available at: http://www.hcup-us.ahrq.gov/reports/statbriefs/sb168-Hospital-Costs-United-States-2011.pdf.

68. American Thoracic Society, Infectious Diseases Society of America. Guidelines for the management of adults with hospital-acquired, ventilator-associated, and healthcare-associated pneumonia. Am J Respir Crit Care Med 2005;171(4):388–416.

69. Chalmers JD, Rother C, Salih W, et al. Healthcare-associated pneumonia does not accurately identify potentially resistant pathogens: a systematic review and meta-analysis. Clin Infect Dis 2014;58:330.

70. Kalil AC, Metersky ML, Klompas M, et al. Management of adults with hospital-acquired and ventilator-associated pneumonia: 2016 clinical practice guidelines by the Infectious Diseases Society of America and the American Thoracic Society. Clin Infect Dis 2016;63:e61–111.

71. Chan SS, Yuen EH, Kew J, et al. Community-acquired pneumonia–implementation of a prediction rule to guide selection of patients for outpatient treatment. Eur J Emerg Med 2001;8(4):279–86.

72. Juan J, Jacob F, Llopis C, et al. Análisis de la seguridad y la eficacia de la unidad de corta estancia en el tratamiento de la neumonía adquirida en la comunidad. [Community-acquired pneumonia management in a short stay unit: analysis of safety and efficacy]. Emergencias 2011;23:175–82.

73. Llorens P, Murcia-Zaragoza J, Sánchez-Payá J, et al. Evaluación de un modelo de atención coordinada entre alternativas a la hospitalización convencional en la neumonía adquirida en la comunidad. [Evaluation of a multidisciplinary alternative hospitalization model in comparison with conventional hospitalization for patients with community acquired pneumonia]. Emergencias 2011;23:167–74.

74. Mandell LA, Wunderink RG, Anzueto A, et al. Infectious Diseases Society of America/American Thoracic Society consensus guidelines on the management of community-acquired pneumonia in adults. Clin Infect Dis 2007;44(Suppl 2):27–72.

75. Liapikou A, Ferrer M, Polverino E, et al. Severe community-acquired pneumonia: validation of the Infectious Diseases Society of America/American Thoracic Society guidelines to predict an intensive care unit admission. Clin Infect Dis 2009;48(4):377–85.

76. Fine MJ, Auble TE, Yealy DM, et al. A prediction rule to identify low-risk patients with community-acquired pneumonia. N Engl J Med 1997;336(4):243–50.

77. Renaud B, Coma E, Labarere J, et al. Routine use of the Pneumonia Severity Index for guiding the site-of-treatment decision of patients with pneumonia in the emergency department: a multicenter, prospective, observational, Controlled Cohort Study. Clin Infect Dis 2007;44(1):41–9.

78. Lim WS, Baudouin A, George R, et al. The British Thoracic Society Guidelines for the management of community acquired pneumonia in adults update 2009. Thorax 2009;64(Suppl 3):iii1–55.

79. España PP, Capelastegui A, Gorordo I, et al. Development and validation of a clinical prediction rule for severe community-acquired pneumonia. Am J Respir Crit Care Med 2006;174(11):1249–56.

80. Espana PP, Capelastegui A, Quintana JM, et al. Validation and comparison of SCAP as a predictive score for identifying low-risk patients in community-acquired pneumonia. J Infect 2010;60:106–13.
81. Decker WW, Jagoda AS, Diercks DB, et al. Clinical policy: critical issues in the management of adult patients presenting to the emergency department with community-acquired pneumonia. Ann Emerg Med 2009;54(5):704–31.
82. Al-Eidan FA, McElnay JC, Scott MG, et al. Use of a treatment protocol in the management of community-acquired lower respiratory tract infection. J Antimicrob Chemother 2000;45(3):387–94.
83. Gadsby NJ, Russell CD, McHugh MP, et al. Comprehensive molecular testing for respiratory pathogens in community-acquired pneumonia. Clin Infect Dis 2016; 62(7):817–23.
84. Capelastegui A, España PP, Bilbao A, et al. Etiology of community-acquired pneumonia in a population-based study: link between etiology and patients characteristics, process-of-care, clinical evolution and outcomes. BMC Infect Dis 2012;12(1):134.
85. Fiore AE, Fry A, Shay D, et al. Antiviral agents for the treatment and chemoprophylaxis of influenza - recommendations of the Advisory Committee on Immunization Practices (ACIP). MMWR Recomm Rep 2011;60(1):1–24.
86. Bi J, Yang J, Wang Y, et al. Efficacy and safety of adjunctive corticosteroids therapy for severe community-acquired pneumonia in adults: an updated systematic review and meta-analysis. PLoS One 2016;11(11):e0165942.

# Care of Infectious Conditions in an Observation Unit

Pawan Suri, MD*, Taruna K. Aurora, MD

## KEYWORDS

- Infectious conditions • Emergency department • Soft tissue infections

## KEY POINTS

- Urinalysis and urine culture are indicated for all patients with acute pyelonephritis, preferably before starting antibiotics.
- Blood cultures rarely impact patient management and should not be routinely ordered.
- Radiographic imaging with a computed tomography scan or renal ultrasound provides a useful adjunct in the evaluation and management of complicated urinary tract infection.
- Indications for radiographic imaging include immunosuppression, persistent symptoms despite antibiotic therapy, recurrent infections, sepsis, diabetes, and prior urologic surgery.

---

**Case Study**

A 38-year-old man presented with a 3-day history of redness, swelling, and pain on his right thigh. He reported subjective fever and chills. Examination revealed oral temperature of 38.0°C, pulse 88, blood pressure 120/70 mm Hg, and respiratory rate 12. Right thigh had a 3 × 3-cm tender, indurated, and fluctuant area consistent with an abscess, which was drained in the Emergency Department (ED). Patient was given IV antibiotics and placed in the Emergency Department Observation Unit (EDOU). There was marked improvement of his cellulitis with extremity elevation and continued antibiotics, and the patient was discharged the next day on oral clindamycin.

---

## INTRODUCTION

Infectious conditions are commonly encountered in the ED. With the emergence and spread of drug-resistant organisms, especially community-acquired methicillin-resistant *Staphylococcus aureus* (CA-MRSA), management of infections poses new challenges.[1–3] These infections have a higher incidence of complications and

---

Department of Emergency Medicine, Virginia Commonwealth University Health System, 1200 E Marshall Street, Richmond, VA 23298, USA
* Corresponding author.
*E-mail address:* psuri@vcu.edu

Emerg Med Clin N Am 35 (2017) 647–671
http://dx.doi.org/10.1016/j.emc.2017.03.009
0733-8627/17/© 2017 Elsevier Inc. All rights reserved.

hospitalization. Choice of initial antibiotic medication and predicting response to therapy may not be straightforward. Sometimes the decision to admit versus discharge home can be a difficult one. The emergency physician may need more time to evaluate response to therapy before making a final disposition. An EDOU provides a convenient and safe option for carefully selected patients with infectious conditions (**Fig. 1**).

## SKIN AND SOFT TISSUE INFECTIONS

Between 1993 and 2005, annual ED visits in the United States for skin and soft tissue infections (SSTIs) increased from 1.2 to 3.4 million[4] and continues to increase.

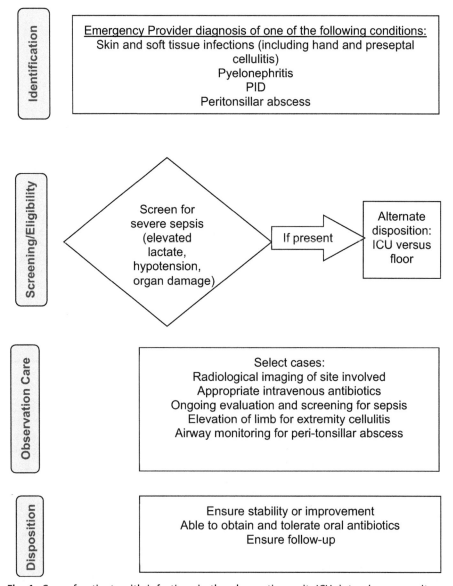

**Fig. 1.** Care of patients with infections in the observation unit. ICU, intensive care unit.

These infections include cellulitis, erysipelas, impetigo, ecthyma, cutaneous abscesses and infected wounds, ulcers, and burns. Although cellulitis can occur at any age, erysipelas occurs most frequently in children and older adults.[5] The lower extremities are the most common anatomic sites of SSTI, where the infection is usually unilateral. Factors that predispose an individual to an SSTI include edema from chronic venous insufficiency, lymphatic obstruction following surgical procedures, disruption of skin barrier from trauma or insect bites, or eczema with secondary bacterial infection. Erysipelas is predominantly caused by β-hemolytic streptococci,[6] whereas cellulitis is usually caused by β-hemolytic streptococci or *S aureus* (including MRSA). Other organisms may include *Haemophilus influenzae*, *Streptococcus pneumoniae*, *Pseudomonas aeruginosa*, *Clostridium perfringens*, *Pasteurella multocida* (animal bites), *Aeromonas hydrophila*, and *Vibrio vulnificus* (water exposure).

Preseptal or periorbital cellulitis is an infection of the soft tissues anterior to the orbital septum, whereas orbital cellulitis is infection of the ocular muscles and fat posterior to the orbital septum. Both conditions are more common in children than in adults. The most common organisms causing preseptal cellulitis are *S aureus* (including MRSA), *S pneumoniae*, other streptococci, and anaerobes.[7,8]

### Patient Evaluation Overview

Clinically, SSTIs manifest as skin erythema, warmth, and edema. Erysipelas typically has an acute onset with fever, chills, and a clear line of demarcation between involved and uninvolved tissue. Cellulitis tends to develop over a few days. Other clinical features may include lymphangitic streaking with regional lymph node enlargement. On occasion, there may be associated bullae, vesicles, or petechiae.

Patients with preseptal cellulitis will invariably have eyelid swelling, ocular pain, and erythema. It is important to distinguish it from orbital cellulitis, which also presents with similar symptoms but in addition can manifest pain with eye movements, proptosis, and ophthalmoplegia with diplopia. Fever is more common in orbital cellulitis. Orbital cellulitis is a much more serious condition and can lead to visual impairment. If there is doubt whether the infection is preseptal or orbital, a computed tomography (CT) scan of the sinus and orbits is indicated.

Pain out of proportion to examination may be an early sign of life-threatening necrotizing fasciitis. Pain that precedes physical findings and delayed development of ecchymosis or sloughing of skin may be a manifestation of toxic shock syndrome. Gas gangrene should be suspected in the presence of severe pain with crepitus. Although evaluating a patient with cellulitis in the EDOU, it is important to determine whether the cellulitis is nonpurulent or purulent with drainage or exudates. This determination will guide the choice of initial antibiotic therapy. Often there will be an obvious abscess, but, when in doubt, bedside ultrasound can be a useful adjunct. For noncomplicated SSTIs, blood cultures are positive in less than 5% of cases and therefore not indicated.[9] Similarly, for mild infections, a skin biopsy or needle aspiration is not necessary.[10] Circumstances that prompt blood cultures include extensive skin involvement, systemic symptoms, or presence of comorbidities like neutropenia, conditions that usually require inpatient admission and would exclude the patient from EDOU management. If the SSTI is not responding to antibiotics, it is worthwhile to consider mimics like acute gout, insect bite with local inflammation, contact or stasis dermatitis, drug reaction, vasculitis, or panniculitis. Gram stain and culture of pus or exudates from cutaneous abscesses are recommended to help identify the causative organism, especially in the case of treatment failure.[11] One exception is an inflamed epidermoid cyst, wherein Gram stain and culture are not recommended. Inflammation and purulence in an epidermoid cyst are a reaction to the rupture of cyst wall and extrusion of its contents into the dermis and not a result of an infectious process.[12]

Factors associated with decision to hospitalize ED patients with SSTIs include patients with fever, larger lesions (erythema >10 cm), and comorbidities. Often the only reason for admission is to administer intravenous (IV) antibiotics.[13] Such patients can be safely and effectively managed in an EDOU. Patients with cellulitis admitted to an EDOU are more likely to be obese, have chronic obstructive pulmonary disease or asthma, and meet at least one systemic inflammatory response syndrome (SIRS) criteria.[14] Patients who meet sepsis criteria, have suspected necrotizing fasciitis, or have an expected length of stay greater than 48 hours should be excluded from the EDOU. The goal of EDOU care is to administer antibiotics, provide analgesics, elevate the involved extremity, and obtain consultation, imaging, and home care coordination if indicated. In a study of 192 children admitted to the EDOU for an SSTI, fever on ED presentation was associated with EDOU treatment failure,[15] although the presence or magnitude of fever does not preclude EDOU or outpatient management.[16,17]

### Treatment Options

Avoiding unnecessary, broad-spectrum antibiotics should be the guiding principle in managing cellulitis in the EDOU. A recent study looking into the treatment of bacterial skin infections in EDOUs found less than half the patients were treated according to Infectious Diseases Society of America (IDSA) guidelines (**Fig. 2**), 42% were over-treated, and 15% were undertreated. Patients greater than 50 years old were at

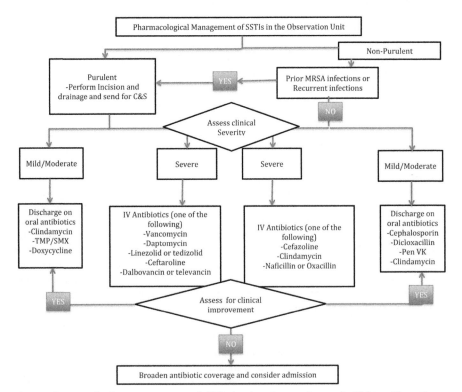

**Fig. 2.** Pharmacologic management of SSTIs in the observation unit. SMX, sulfamethoxazole; TMP, trimethoprim.

risk for overtreatment, whereas women were likely to be undertreated.[18] Patients with mild cellulitis can be treated with oral antibiotics. Patients with nonpurulent cellulitis are empirically treated with antibiotics to cover β-hemolytic streptococci and methicillin-sensitive *S aureus*.[19] Dicloxacillin or cephalexin is an appropriate initial choice. Cure rates were comparable when compared with a combination of cephalexin and trimethoprim-sulfamethoxazole or cephalexin alone in a randomized trial of patients with cellulitis without abscess.[20] It is reasonable to add MRSA coverage in communities where the prevalence of MRSA is greater than 30% and for patients with prior MRSA infection, recurrent infection, or lack of response to initial therapy.[21]

Patients with erysipelas and systemic manifestations are started with parenteral agents like cefazolin or ceftriaxone that have activity against β-hemolytic streptococci. Most of these patients will rapidly respond to initial therapy within 24 hours and can be transitioned to oral therapy with amoxicillin or oral penicillin. Cephalexin or clindamycin can be used if the patient is allergic to penicillin.[21]

Purulent cellulitis is much more likely to be caused by CA-MRSA. MRSA was isolated from 59% of cases in a study of 422 patients with purulent soft tissue infections.[1] Compared with hospital-associated MRSA, CA-MRSA tends to be more virulent, causing tissue necrosis and severe disease.[22] The addition of systemic antibiotics to incision and drainage (I&D) of cutaneous abscesses does not improve cure rates, even in those due to MRSA, but have a modest effect on the time to recurrence of other abscesses.[23–27] The decision to add antibiotic therapy should be based on presence or absence of SIRS, which is temperature greater than 38°C or less than 36°C, respiratory rate greater than 24, heart rate greater than 90 bpm, or white blood cell count greater than 12,000 or less than 400 cells/dL. Empiric therapy should include MRSA coverage pending results from culture and sensitivity of the pus. For moderate infection, oral therapy with trimethoprim-sulfamethoxazole or doxycycline is appropriate. For severe infections, parenteral therapy with IV vancomycin, daptomycin, linezolid, telavancin, or ceftaroline is indicated.

Infected animal bite–related wounds should be irrigated with copious fluid and approximated but not closed (with the exception of those on the face). The patient should be treated with antimicrobial agents active against both aerobic and anaerobic bacteria, such as amoxicillin-clavulanate. Other alternatives include second- or third-generation cephalosporins plus anaerobic coverage with clindamycin or metronidazole. Single-agent therapy with a carbapenem, moxifloxacin, or doxycycline is also appropriate. Tetanus status should be assessed and appropriate prophylaxis administered, if indicated.

Mild cases of preseptal cellulitis can be treated with clindamycin monotherapy or combination therapy with trimethoprim-sulfamethoxazole plus either amoxicillin, amoxicillin-clavulanic acid, cefpodoxime, or cefdinir for 7 to 10 days.

Often overlooked in the treatment of SSTIs is elevation of the affected area. It facilitates gravity drainage of edema and inflammatory substances. The skin should be hydrated with emollients to avoid dryness. It is important to treat underlying predisposing conditions like chronic venous insufficiency, tinea pedis, and lymphedema.

### Evaluation of Outcome and Long-Term Recommendations

Patients with SSTIs managed in the EDOU should have the area of erythema marked with a pen. Lack of response or development of systemic symptoms in the first 24 hours should prompt consideration for imaging, expanding antibiotic coverage, and inpatient admission.

*Summary*

- SSTIs are a growing problem, partly due to emergence of strains of MRSA.
- Preseptal cellulitis is an infection of the soft tissues anterior to the orbital septum and should be differentiated from orbital cellulitis, which is infection of the ocular muscles and fat posterior to the orbital septum
- Antibiotic choice is guided by the presence of purulence. Purulent cellulitis is much more likely to be associated with MRSA.
- For nonpurulent cellulitis, it is not necessary to perform blood cultures or needle aspiration, whereas the drainage from purulent cellulitis should be sent for culture and sensitivity.
- Management of cellulitis should include nonpharmacologic interventions like I&D of an abscess if present and elevation of the affected area.

## HAND INFECTIONS

Hand infections may be surgical emergencies, and misdiagnosis or delayed treatment can lead to hand stiffness, contractures, and even amputations. An EDOU is ideal for the management of hand infections because it allows frequent reevaluation to assess response to therapy while avoiding inpatient admission. The most common hand infections encountered in the ED are superficial infections involving skin and subcutaneous tissue, including cellulitis, paronychia, pulp space infections, herpetic whitlow, web space infections, and felons. Deep infections are deep to the tendon sheath and include tenosynovitis, septic arthritis, and deep fascial space infections. Steroid use, diabetes, immunocompromised state, and IV drug use predispose to infections.[28] Infected animal and human bites can result in both superficial and deep space infections. Although dogs cause most animal bites, it is cat bites that are responsible for most infections.[29] Cats have sharp teeth that cause deep puncture wounds that inoculate bacteria deep into the tissue. *Pasteurella* species are isolated in 50% of dog bites and 75% of cat bites.[30] Human bites to the hand can initially appear benign but almost always require surgical exploration and irrigation. A "fight-bite" is the most common type of human bite caused by a clenched fist injury striking another person's mouth. A human tooth contacting a clenched fist usually violates the extensor tendon and joint capsule and may injure the metacarpal head, inoculating the metacarpophalangeal joint.[31] Human bites have a greater chance of getting infected if there is delay in initial treatment, inadequate debridement, or initial wound closure.[32] Patients with bite infections more than 8 days after the initial injury have an 18% chance of requiring amputation.[33] Most deep infections will require operative management and inpatient admission. A significant proportion of patients with hand infections are young and healthy individuals who may have ignored seemingly minor trauma.[34]

The most common bacteria implicated in hand infections are *S aureus* and β-hemolytic streptococci. The incidence of MRSA ranges from 34% to 73% of all hand infections.[34] Human bite wounds tend to be infected by mixed bacterial flora and have the highest complication rates.[35]

### Patient Evaluation Overview

A good history and physical examination are important to narrow the diagnosis of the type of hand infection and to exclude mimics like inflammatory arthropathies, tendinitis, or pyoderma gangrenosum. Among other things, the history should include hand dominance and immune and tetanus immunization status. Physical examination should note if there is swelling, deformity, tenderness, erythema, fluctuance, crepitus, adenopathy, skin necrosis, or limited range of motion. Neurovascular status and alignment should be documented. Laboratory evaluation is tailored to the presentation and underlying patient condition. Blood cultures can be obtained if the patient is febrile or has the presence of one or more SIRS criteria. Complete blood count and renal or liver function can be ordered if the patient is immunocompromised or has known renal or hepatic impairment. If the patient has an open wound or if an I&D is performed, a sample should be sent for Gram stain as well as aerobic and anaerobic cultures. A plain radiograph should be obtained to look for a fracture, foreign body, osteomyelitis, or gas in the soft tissues. Imaging studies may be used to confirm osteomyelitis, fluid collection along tendon sheaths, or a soft tissue abscess. The area of erythema is outlined with an indelible marker to monitor progress. Acute paronychia is evidenced by erythema, swelling, and tenderness along the dorsolateral nail fold. Trauma from hangnails, manicures, or nail biting introduces bacteria into the area. An abscess can form along the nail fold and sometimes extend into the pulp space. Patients with pulp space infection or felon present with severe, throbbing pain, most commonly in the thumb and index fingers,[36] often with a history of penetrating trauma. Pulp space infections account for 15% to 20% of all hand infections. A felon can sometimes be confused with a herpetic whitlow, a viral infection of the hand caused by inoculation of herpes simplex virus (HSV) into broken skin. HSV type 1 is the primary cause of herpetic whitlow in patients less than 10 year old, whereas adults can be infected with either HSV-1 or HSV-2.[37] Patients present with a prodrome of influenza-like symptoms and fever, followed by tingling, burning, erythema, swelling, and 1- to 2-mm vesicles containing clear fluid in the involved digit.[38] In contrast to a felon, the pulp space in herpetic whitlow is soft, not tense.

### Treatment Options

Superficial infections, with the exception of necrotizing fasciitis, can be treated with antibiotics alone. On the other hand, deep infections usually need surgical debridement and irrigation in conjunction with antibiotic treatment. Oral antibiotics are appropriate for skin and other soft tissue infections. Initial choice of antibiotic should cover CA-MRSA. Trimethoprim-sulfamethoxazole and clindamycin are good first-line agents. IV antibiotics are recommended for bone or flexor sheath infections. Vancomycin and piperacillin/tazobactam are the most commonly used IV antibiotics. Animal bite wounds should be treated with irrigation and oral amoxicillin-clavulanate or IV ampicillin-sulbactam. If patients are allergic to penicillin, they can be treated with doxycycline, sulfamethoxazole-trimethoprim, or a fluoroquinolone plus clindamycin.

Splinting, elevation, and heat are important in the treatment of hand infections. Splinting protects the affected area, limits opening of tissue planes restricting the spread of infection, and decreases pain. Splinting in a position of function can help protect against flexion contractures, reduce stiffness, and hasten rehabilitation. The principle of elevation is to keep the hand above the level of the heart. Elevation helps to reduce edema by improving venous and lymphatic drainage. Short, frequent, warm soaks improve patient comfort, enhance antibiotic delivery to the tissue, and increase the delivery of inflammatory cells to the affected area by local vasodilation. Herpetic whitlow is self-limiting and resolves within 3 weeks without treatment. The vesicles drain and ulcerate before resolution and are contagious during the first 2 weeks. A dry dressing should be worn over the involved digit at all times during this period to prevent spreading the infection.

### Evaluation of Outcome and Long-Term Recommendation

Patients who respond to therapy with either IV or oral antibiotics can be safely discharged from the EDOU. If a hand surgery service was consulted from the ED, they will follow the patient in the EDOU. If hand surgery was not consulted or is not available in the hospital, there should be an attempt to arrange a follow-up appointment with a hand surgeon upon discharge.

### Summary

- Superficial hand infections can be treated with antibiotics alone and can be safely managed in an EDOU. Delayed treatment or misdiagnosis of hand infections can lead to hand stiffness, contractures, or even amputations.
- Dogs cause most animal bites, but cats are responsible for most infections.
- The most common bacteria implicated in hand infections are S aureus and β-hemolytic streptococci. Human bites tend to be infected by mixed bacterial flora and have the highest complication rates.
- Splinting, elevation, and heat are important in the treatment of hand infections.

## PERITONSILLAR ABSCESS

Peritonsillar abscess (PTA) is the most common deep infection of the head and neck in young adults with the highest incidence between the ages of 10 and 40.[38,39] Although tonsillitis is a disease of childhood, only a third of PTA cases are found in this age group. A retrospective study found that PTA is affecting an older population more often than in the past. Its course in adults is longer and worse than in children, and smoking may be a predisposing factor.[40] Prompt diagnosis and treatment are essential to prevent complications, which are rare but can be fatal. The EDOU provides a buffer zone for those patients that are not stable for immediate discharge from ED. There are no published studies from the EDOU looking at this specific condition.

### Patient Evaluation Overview

The typical clinical presentation of PTA is a severe sore throat (usually unilateral), fever, and a "hot potato" or muffled voice. Pooling of saliva or drooling may be present. Trismus, related to irritation and reflex spasm of the internal pterygoid muscle, occurs in nearly two-thirds of patients; it helps to distinguish PTA from severe pharyngitis or tonsillitis.[41,42] Patients often have neck swelling and pain and may have ipsilateral ear pain.[43] Weakness, fatigue, and decreased oral intake may occur as a result of discomfort.

The presence of trismus may limit the ability to perform an adequate examination. If there is doubt about whether the patient has a PTA, epiglottitis, or other deep neck space infection, imaging or examination in the operating room may be necessary.

Examination findings consistent with PTA include an extremely swollen and fluctuant tonsil with deviation of the uvula to the opposite side. Alternatively, there may be fullness or bulging of the posterior soft palate near the tonsil with palpable fluctuance. Cervical and submandibular lymphadenopathy may be present. Bilateral PTAs are rare, but have been reported.[44,45]

Laboratory evaluation is not necessary to make a diagnosis of PTA, but may help gauge the level of illness and direct therapy. Throat culture for group A β-hemolytic streptococcus should be sent to the laboratory. Other studies include Gram stain, culture (aerobic and anaerobic), and susceptibility testing of abscess fluid if a drainage procedure is performed. Although these results rarely affect management of uncomplicated patients,[39] cultures may help guide antimicrobial therapy in immuno-compromised patients, those with complications, treatment failures, or extension of infection.

Imaging is usually not necessary to make the diagnosis of PTA. Indications for imaging may include the following:

- Distinguishing cellulitis from abscess
- Looking for spread of infection to the parapharyngeal space
- Inadequate examination secondary to trismus
- Exclusion of other conditions that present with sore throat and signs of respiratory obstruction, such as epiglottitis and retropharyngeal abscess (**Box 1**).

CT and intraoral ultrasound are similar in regard to PTA diagnosis.[46,47] CT with IV contrast can distinguish PTA from cellulitis and also demonstrate the spread of infection to contiguous deep neck spaces. CT should be omitted in patients with moderate to severe respiratory distress, particularly when sedation is necessary; such patients generally undergo evaluation in the operating room, where, if necessary, an artificial airway can be established. Intraoral ultrasound is becoming the imaging of choice to distinguish PTA from cellulitis and to guide needle aspiration.[46,48–53] However, intraoral ultrasonography may be limited by trismus.[46] PTA appears as an echo-free cavity with an irregular border, and peritonsillar cellulitis appears as a homogeneous or striated area without a distinct fluid collection.[48,49]

Clinical features and imaging cannot always distinguish PTA from cellulitis.[54,55] A 24-hour trial of antimicrobial therapy (with or without antecedent imaging) may be helpful in this regard.[54,56] Failure to respond to a trial of appropriate antibiotic therapy suggests PTA, whereas response to therapy suggests cellulitis. Response is defined by improvement in at least one clinical parameter: sore throat, fever, trismus, or tonsillar bulge.

### Treatment Options

Antibiotic therapy should be directed to cover group A β-hemolytic streptococci, S aureus, and oral anaerobes.[57–59] Although PTAs are polymicrobial infections, several studies have shown IV penicillin alone to be as clinically effective as broader-spectrum antibiotics, provided the abscess has been adequately drained.[39,57] Some physicians choose to use broader spectrum antibiotics based on studies demonstrating more than 50% of aspirates show β-lactamase producing bacteria.[57,58,60] Decision to add MRSA coverage depends on patient's clinical condition and prevalence of MRSA in the community. **Table 1** shows the most common organisms associated with peritonsillar infections, and **Table 2** illustrates the proposed antimicrobial regimens for treatment.[61]

Evidence regarding the benefits of glucocorticoids in the management of PTA is inconsistent.[55] In one trial of 62 patients, glucocorticoids appeared to hasten

---

**Box 1**
**Major considerations in the differential diagnosis of peritonsillar abscess**

Epiglottitis

Retropharyngeal abscess or cellulitis

Abscess of the parapharyngeal space

Severe tonsillopharyngitis

| Table 1 | |
|---|---|
| **Bacteriology of peritonsillar abscess** | |
| Aerobic | Anaerobic |
| Group A streptococcus | Fusobacterium |
| S aureus | Peptostreptococcus |
| H influenzae | Pigmented prevotella |

symptomatic improvement in adolescent (>16 years) and adult patients treated with needle aspiration and IV antimicrobial therapy.[62] In another small trial of 41 adult patients undergoing needle aspiration for PTA, IV dexamethasone was associated with less pain at 24 hours than placebo but no other benefits.[63] In a retrospective case series of 249 episodes of PTA in children less than 18 years, glucocorticoids were used in 37% but without clear benefit or adverse outcomes.[55]

Drainage, antimicrobial therapy, and supportive care are the cornerstones of management for PTA; peritonsillar cellulitis responds to antimicrobial therapy and supportive care alone.[39,41,54,64–67] Supportive care includes provision of adequate hydration and analgesia and monitoring for complications.

Surgical intervention (eg, tonsillectomy or I&D) is reserved for those who do not respond to medical therapy.[54] This strategy was evaluated in a retrospective series of 102 children (8 months to 19 years).[56] Approximately 50% of patients responded to medical therapy and 50% underwent tonsillectomy, 80% of which had abscesses at the time of surgery. Children younger than 6 years were more likely to respond to medical therapy.

PTA usually requires surgical drainage through needle aspiration.[64] Ultrasound may be used to guide the procedure.[48,53] A meta-analysis found needle aspiration to be 94% (range 85%–100%) successful in acute resolution.[39] Repeat aspiration may be necessary in 4% to 10% of patients.[67,68]

Patients must be observed after the procedure to make sure they can tolerate oral antimicrobial therapy, pain medications, and liquids. **Fig. 3** describes a proposed algorithm for patients presenting to the ED with PTA.

### Evaluation of Outcome and Long-Term Recommendations

Early diagnosis and prompt, appropriate management of peritonsillar infection is critical to avoiding complications. Complications of PTA occur rarely, but are potentially fatal (**Box 2**). Infection can spread from the peritonsillar space to other deep neck spaces, to adjacent structures, and to the bloodstream.[69–75] Treatment failure may occur in patients who have developed complications, are infected with unusual organisms, or have underlying problems. Reevaluation of such patients may include repeat imaging (CT with contrast to look for extension of infection) or surgical intervention. Broadening antimicrobial coverage may also be indicated.

| Table 2 | |
|---|---|
| **Proposed antimicrobial regimes for peritonsillar abscess** | |
| IV therapy | Oral therapy |
| Ampicillin/sulbactam 3 g every 6 h | Amoxicillin/clavulanic acid 875 mg |
| Penicillin G 10 million units every 6 h plus | twice daily |
| metronidazole 500 mg every 6 h | Penicillin VK 500 mg 4 times a day plus |
| Clindamycin 900 mg every 8 h | metronidazole 500 mg 4 times a day |
| | Clindamycin 300 mg 4 times a day |

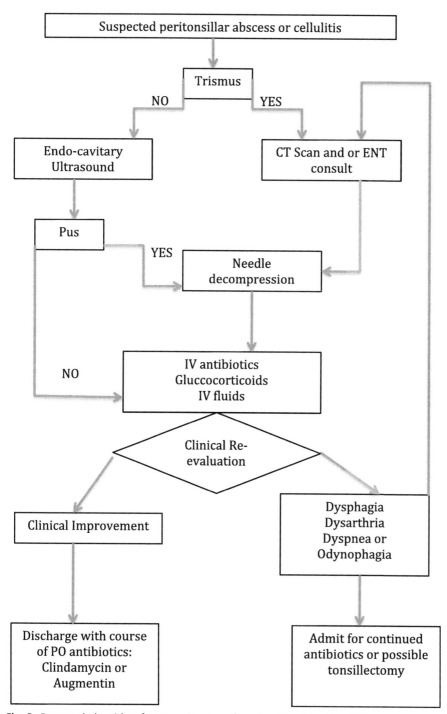

**Fig. 3.** Proposed algorithm for management of peritonsillar infection. ENT, ear, nose, and throat.

---

**Box 2**
**Complications of peritonsillar abscess**

Airway obstruction

Aspiration pneumonia if the abscess ruptures into the airway

Septicemia

Internal jugular vein thrombosis

Jugular vein suppurative thrombophlebitis (Lemierre syndrome)

Carotid artery rupture

Pseudoaneurysm of the carotid artery

Mediastinitis

Necrotizing fasciitis

---

After therapy for peritonsillar infection, patients should be instructed that prompt reevaluation is necessary for the following:

- Dyspnea
- Worsening throat pain, neck pain, or trismus
- Enlarging mass
- Fever
- Neck stiffness
- Bleeding

With early and appropriate treatment, most peritonsillar infections resolve without sequelae. Recurrence is estimated to occur in 10% to 15%.[39,76,77] The risk of recurrence is increased in patients with a history of recurrent tonsillitis before development of the abscess (40 vs 9.6%).[78]

*Summary*

- PTA is the most common deep infection of head and neck in young adults. It is difficult to distinguish from cellulitis in the early stages.
- Imaging may be helpful for distinguishing cellulitis from abscess, when examination is inadequate due to presence of trismus and to exclude life-threatening conditions like epiglottitis and parapharyngeal abscess.
- Intraoral ultrasonography is becoming the imaging of choice to distinguish PTA from cellulitis and to guide needle aspiration of the abscess.
- Adequate drainage, supportive care with analgesics, and antibiotic therapy to cover group A β-hemolytic streptococci, S aureus, and oral anaerobes is the recommended therapy for PTA.
- Evidence regarding the benefit of concomitant steroid use in PTA is inconsistent.

## PELVIC INFLAMMATORY DISEASE

Pelvic inflammatory disease (PID) is a spectrum of disorders of the upper female genital tract that occurs among women who are sexually active. Based on a nationally representative sample from 2006 to 2010, 5% of US women have reported being treated for PID in their lifetime.[79] EDOU care specifically for treatment of PID has not been reported in the literature. In a recent review of PID by Das and colleagues,[80] it has been suggested that the EDOU would be an effective model for treating such patients.

## Patient Evaluation Overview

The diagnosis of PID is challenging, because the symptoms and signs vary widely, ranging from mild vaginal discomfort to severe abdominal pain requiring surgical intervention.[81–83] Fever and other systemic manifestations like nausea and vomiting can occur but are not a prominent feature of PID. Rarely, PID can be complicated by perihepatitis, which is inflammation and adhesion formation in the liver capsule, and presents with right upper quadrant pain (Fitz-Hugh–Curtis syndrome).[84,85]

The Centers for Disease Control and Prevention (CDC) diagnostic criteria for PID using minimum clinical criteria are based on the finding of pelvic organ tenderness, as indicated by cervical motion tenderness, adnexal tenderness, or uterine compression tenderness on bimanual examination, in conjunction with signs of lower genital tract inflammation (**Table 3**).

All patients with suspected PID should undergo cervical or vaginal nucleic acid amplification tests (NAATs) for *Neisseria gonorrhoeae* and *Chlamydia trachomatis* infection because these are implicated in many cases, and a positive test increases the likelihood that PID is present.[86] Recent studies suggest that the proportion of PID attributable to *N gonorrhoeae* and *C trachomatis* is declining.[87,88] Newer data suggest that *Mycoplasma genitalium* may play a role in PID[89]; however, molecular tests for *M genitalium* are not yet commercially available.[90] Vaginal fluid should be evaluated for signs of bacterial vaginosis and white blood cells. Normally, bacterial vaginosis is a noninflammatory condition, and if white cells accompany clue cells, this suggests PID.[87,91]

A pregnancy test should be performed in all patients being evaluated for PID.[84] Serologic testing for human immunodeficiency virus (HIV) should be strongly considered because HIV increases the risk of a tuboovarian abscess (TOA).[92] Erythrocyte sedimentation rate and C-reactive protein level can be used as adjuncts for diagnosing PID; however, these tests are not routinely needed.[86]

| Table 3<br>Pelvic inflammatory disease diagnostic criteria per 2015 Centers for Disease Control and Prevention guidelines | |
|---|---|
| Minimal clinical criteria[a] | Cervical motion tenderness<br>Uterine tenderness<br>Adnexal tenderness |
| Additional criteria[b] | Oral temperature >101°F (38.3°C)<br>Abnormal cervical mucopurulent discharge or cervical friability<br>Abundant white blood cells on microscopic evaluation of vaginal fluid<br>Elevated erythrocyte sedimentation rate<br>Elevated C-reactive protein<br>Laboratory documentation of cervical infection with *N gonorrhoeae* or *C trachomatis* |
| Specific criteria[c] | Endometrial biopsy with histopathologic evidence of endometritis<br>Transvaginal US or MRI showing thickened, fluid-filled tubes with or without free pelvic fluid or tubo-ovarian complex, or Doppler studies suggesting pelvic infection<br>Laparoscopic findings consistent with PID |

[a] Initiate treatment if one or more of these criteria are met.
[b] In addition to one or more minimal criteria, one or more of the additional criteria increases specificity of the diagnosis of PID.
[c] One or more of these criteria provides the most specific diagnosis of PID.
*Reproduced from* CDC. 2015 sexually transmitted diseases treatment guidelines. Atlanta (GA): Department of Health and Human Services; 2015.

Imaging is not required to diagnose PID but can rule out complications such as TOA or make an alternative diagnosis, such as ovarian cyst, endometriosis, ectopic pregnancy, or acute appendicitis. These conditions can be found in 10% to 25% of women who are thought to have acute PID.[84] TOAs occur in up to a third of women hospitalized with PID.[93,94] It is challenging to distinguish PID from PID complicated by TOA based on clinical presentation alone.[94–97]

### Treatment Options

The CDC has developed guidelines for the treatment of PID (**Table 4**).[98] Most patients are successfully treated as outpatients with single-dose intramuscular ceftriaxone, cefoxitin plus probenicid, or another third-generation cephalosporin (cefotaxime or ceftizoxime), followed by oral doxycycline with or without metronidazole for 2 weeks.

The reasons for hospitalization for PID currently include pregnancy, an inability to rule out competing diagnoses, severe illness combined with an inability to take oral medications, or presence of tubal abscess.

The Pelvic Inflammatory Disease Evaluation and Clinical Health study showed that among women with mild to moderate PID, the efficacy of cefoxitin-doxycycline therapy, with respect to both short-term and long-term complications, was similar in inpatient and outpatient settings.[87]

The EDOU offers a unique interface between inpatient and outpatient management. The CDC recommends that patients be transitioned from parental to oral antibiotic treatment in 24 to 48 hours, which is well within scope of EDOU practice. **Fig. 4** describes a proposed algorithm for patients diagnosed with PID.

### Evaluation of Outcome and Long-Term Recommendations

Patients who respond well to treatment may be transitioned to oral antibiotics and discharged home. Empiric therapy for gonorrhea and chlamydia is recommended for all male sexual partners within the past 60 days, or the most recent sexual partner if >60 days ago regardless of symptoms or the result of gonorrhea and chlamydia testing in the female partner with PID. Repeat testing for gonorrhea or chlamydia in

| Table 4 | |
|---|---|
| **PID antibiotic regimens per 2015 Centers for Disease Control and Prevention pelvic inflammatory disease treatment guidelines** | |
| Parenteral treatment | |
| Regimen A | Cefotetan 2 g IV every 12 h + doxycycline 100 mg orally (PO) or IV every 12 h |
| Regimen B | Cefoxitin 2 g IV every 6 h + doxycycline 100 mg PO or IV every 12 h |
| Regimen C | Clindamycin 900 mg every 8 h + gentamicin 2 mg/kg loading dose IV or intramuscularly (IM) followed by 1.5 mg/kg every 8 h (can substitute single daily dosage of 3–5 mg/kg) |
| Alternate regimen | Ampicillin/sulbactam 3 g IV every 6 h + doxycycline 100 mg PO or IV every 12 h |
| Oral treatment | |
| Regimen A | Ceftriaxone 250 mg IM in a single dose + doxycycline 100 mg PO twice a day (BID) for 14 d ± metronidazole 500 mg PO BID for 14 d |
| Regimen B | Cefoxitin 2 g IM and probenicid 1 g PO in a single dose + doxycycline 100 mg PO BID for 14 d ± metronidazole 500 mg PO BID for 14 d |
| Regimen C | Other parenteral third-generation cephalosporin + doxycycline 100 mg PO BID for 14 d ± metronidazole 500 mg PO BID for 14 d |

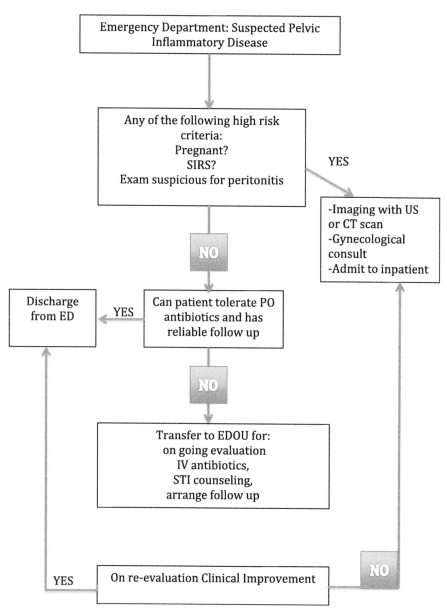

**Fig. 4.** Algorithm for ED: suspected pelvic inflammatory disease. STI, sexually transmitted infection.

3 to 6 months is recommended if initial testing was positive for either infection. Patients who fail to respond to initial EDOU management should get a gynecology consult and require inpatient admission. Repeat imaging may be indicated to look for developing complications.

### *Summary*

- All patients with suspected PID should have NAATs for *N gonorrhoeae* and *C trachomatis* infection.

- Imaging is not required to diagnose PID but can rule out complications such as TOA or make an alternative diagnosis, such as ovarian cyst, endometriosis, ectopic pregnancy, or acute appendicitis.
- Most patients are successfully treated as outpatients with single-dose intramuscular ceftriaxone, cefoxitin plus probenicid, or another third-generation cephalosporin (cefotaxime or ceftizoxime), followed by oral doxycycline with or without metronidazole for 2 weeks.

## ACUTE PYELONEPHRITIS

Urinary tract infections (UTI) can range from uncomplicated cystitis to acute pyelonephritis and septic shock. It is the most common infection seen in ambulatory and emergency settings, accounting for 8.6 million visits a year.[99] Although most patients presenting to the ED with a UTI can be safely discharged home, 16.7% will need an admission for further management.[100] Cystitis is limited to the bladder and manifests with symptoms such as dysuria, urgency, and frequency. Acute pyelonephritis is more serious and involves the upper urinary tract, including the kidneys. It presents with fever, flank pain, and costovertebral angle tenderness with or without lower urinary tract symptoms. The annual incidence of acute pyelonephritis is about 12 to 13 cases per 10,000 women and 2 to 3 cases per 10,000 men.[101] An estimated 10% to 30% of all patients with acute pyelonephritis are hospitalized for treatment in the United States.[102] Emergency physicians need to differentiate complicated from uncomplicated UTIs, choose appropriate antimicrobial treatment based on likely bacterial cause as well as local bacterial resistance patterns, and make a disposition decision. The EDOU can provide a safe and cost-effective alternative to inpatient admission for patients needing further management. Patients who receive IV antibiotics in the EDOU over the first 12 hours usually have a good response and can be discharged home.[103,104]

### Patient Evaluation Overview

In most cases, the diagnosis of acute pyelonephritis is straightforward with typical symptoms.[105] Rarely, elderly or immunocompromised patients may present with a history of malaise, fatigue, nausea, or nonspecific abdominal pain. In patients with diabetes, urinary tract obstruction or infection with antibiotic-resistant bacterial strains, pyelonephritis can progress to renal corticomedullary abscess, perinephric abscess, emphysematous pyelonephritis, or papillary necrosis. Patients with acute complicated pyelonephritis may present with sepsis, multiple organ system dysfunction, shock, and/or acute renal failure. In some cases, the presentation may mimic PID and a pelvic examination is warranted if the history suggests vaginitis or urethritis. A pregnancy test should be performed in women of childbearing age.

Urinalysis and urine culture are indicated for all patients with acute pyelonephritis.[106] Ideally urine sample should be collected before starting antibiotic therapy. Most patients with complicated UTI will have pyuria with rare exceptions where the infection does not communicate with collecting system or if the collecting system is obstructed.

Bacteremia is present in 18% to 42% of patients with pyelonephritis.[107–110] Although some guidelines recommend blood cultures,[106,111] this rarely alters management.[107,108,112,113] Blood cultures may be of benefit in patients with severe sepsis or septic shock resulting from complicated pyelonephritis.[110]

Radiographic imaging with a CT scan or renal ultrasound provides a useful adjunct in the evaluation and management of complicated UTI. Indications for radiographic imaging include immunosuppression, persistent symptoms despite antibiotic therapy,

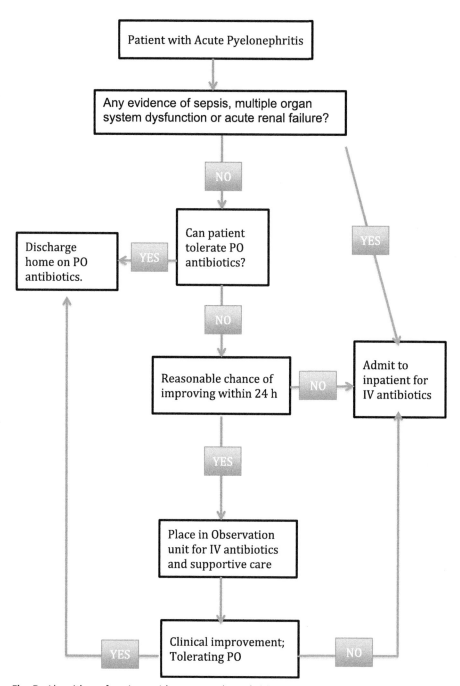

**Fig. 5.** Algorithm of patient with acute pyelonephritis.

recurrent infections, sepsis, diabetes, and prior urologic surgery.[114] A non-contrast-enhanced renal CT is sufficient in most cases and can detect renal calculi, obstruction, hemorrhage, or abscess.[115] Renal ultrasound, although not as sensitive as a CT scan, offers the advantage of avoiding radiation and/or contrast exposure and is now easily available in most EDs.[116]

### Treatment Options

Patients with pyelonephritis who are not ready to be discharged from ED can be admitted to the EDOU if they meet certain criteria (**Fig. 5**). Moderately ill patients with acute complicated pyelonephritis are usually given monotherapy with a fluoroquinolone or third-generation cephalosporin. Previous urine cultures, if available, may help tailor therapy. Severe infections require parenteral antibiotics such as a carbapenem or a combination β-lactam/β-lactamase inhibitor. Proposed antibiotic regimens (**Box 3**) are based on IDSA and Association of Medical Microbiology and Infectious disease Canadian guidelines committee.[106,117]

Patients with recurrent infections or failure to respond to antibiotic therapy may have a genitourinary anomaly, obstruction, or neurogenic bladder. These individuals should have a urologic consultation to correct the underlying problem.

### Evaluation of Outcome and Long-Term Recommendations

Patients who fail to respond to initial therapy in the EDOU, have persistent fever, nausea, and vomiting, or develop sepsis need inpatient admission. Patients who have resolution of symptoms in the EDOU and do not have significant comorbidities can be treated with a 5-day course of oral antibiotics upon discharge. A 2-week course of antibiotics may be more appropriate in patients with severe infection upon presentation, known resistant organisms, or abnormal anatomy. Repeat cultures

---

**Box 3**
**Acute pyelonephritis antibiotic regimens**

*Parenteral therapy*

Fluoroquinolones
    Ciprofloxacin 400 mg IV every 12 hours
    Levofloxacin 750 mg IV every 24 hours

Beta-Lactams
    Ampicillin-sulbactam 3 g every 6 hours
    Piperacillin-tazobactam 3.375 g every 6 hours
    Ceftriaxone 1 g every 24 hours
    Cefepime 2 g every 12 hours

Suspected extended spectrum beta-lactamases
    Meropenem 500 mg every 8 hours
    Imepenem 500 mg every 6 hours

*Oral regimens*

Fluoroquinolones
    Ciprofloxacin 500 mg PO twice daily for 7 d or 1000 mg extended release once daily for 7 days
    Levofloxacin 750 mg once daily for 7 d

Bactrim (trimethoprim-sulfamethoxazole)
    160/800 mg (one double-strength tablet) twice daily for 14 d

Oral beta-lactam if susceptibility is known
    Duration 10 to 14 d

or radiographic imaging are warranted in patients with recurrent symptoms or failure to respond to antibiotics. Patients with a renal transplant may require up to 3 weeks of antibiotics.[118]

**Fig. 5** describes a proposed algorithm for patients diagnosed with acute pyelonephritis.

*Summary*

- Urinalysis and urine culture are indicated for all patients with acute pyelonephritis, preferably before starting antibiotics. Blood cultures rarely impact patient management and should not be routinely ordered.
- Radiographic imaging with a CT scan or renal ultrasound provides a useful adjunct in the evaluation and management of complicated UTI. Indications for radiographic imaging include immunosuppression, persistent symptoms despite antibiotic therapy, recurrent infections, sepsis, diabetes, and prior urologic surgery

## REFERENCES

1. Moran GJ, Krishnadasan A, Gorwitz RJ, et al. Methicillin-resistant S. aureus infections among patients in the emergency department. N Engl J Med 2006; 355(7):666-74.
2. Edelsberg J, Taneja C, Zervos M, et al. Trends in US hospital admissions for skin and soft tissue infections. Emerg Infect Dis 2009;15(9):1516-8.
3. Yarbrough PM, Kukhareva PV, Spivak ES, et al. Evidence-based care pathway for cellulitis improves process, clinical, and cost outcomes. J Hosp Med 2015; 10(12):780-6.
4. Pallin DJ, Egan DJ, Pelletier AJ, et al. Increased US emergency department visits for skin and soft tissue infections, and changes in antibiotic choices, during the emergence of community-associated methicillin-resistant Staphylococcus aureus. Ann Emerg Med 2008;51(3):291-8.
5. Ellis Simonsen SM, van Orman ER, Hatch BE, et al. Cellulitis incidence in a defined population. Epidemiol Infect 2006;134(2):293-9.
6. Bernard P, Bedane C, Mounier M, et al. Streptococcal cause of erysipelas and cellulitis in adults. A microbiologic study using a direct immunofluorescence technique. Arch Dermatol 1989;125(6):779-82.
7. Chaudhry IA, Shamsi FA, Elzaridi E, et al. Inpatient preseptal cellulitis: experience from a tertiary eye care centre. Br J Ophthalmol 2008;92(10):1337-41.
8. Charalampidou S, Connell P, Fennell J, et al. Preseptal cellulitis caused by community acquired methicillin resistant staphylococcus aureus (CAMRSA). Br J Ophthalmol 2007;91(12):1723-4.
9. Perl B, Gottehrer NP, Raveh D, et al. Cost-effectiveness of blood cultures for adult patients with cellulitis. Clin Infect Dis 1999;29(6):1483-8.
10. Kielhofner MA, Brown B, Dall L. Influence of underlying disease process on the utility of cellulitis needle aspirates. Arch Intern Med 1988;148(11):2451-2.
11. Hirschmann JV. Impetigo: etiology and therapy. Curr Clin Top Infect Dis 2002;22: 42-51.
12. Diven DG, Dozier SE, Meyer DJ, et al. Bacteriology of inflamed and uninflamed epidermal inclusion cysts. Arch Dermatol 1998;134(1):49-51.
13. Talan DA, Salhi BA, Moran GJ, et al. Factors associated with decision to hospitalize emergency department patients with skin and soft tissue infection. West J Emerg Med 2015;16(1):89-97.

14. Claeys KC, Lagnf AM, Patel TB, et al. Acute bacterial skin and skin structure infections treated with intravenous antibiotics in the emergency department or observational unit: experience at the detroit medical center. Infect Dis Ther 2015;4(2):173–86.

15. Mistry RD, Hirsch AW, Woodford AL, et al. Failure of emergency department observation unit treatment for skin and soft tissue infections. J Emerg Med 2015;49(6):855–63.

16. Nguyen HH. Hospitalist to home: outpatient parenteral antimicrobial therapy at an academic center. Clin Infect Dis 2010;51(Suppl 2):S220–3.

17. Jauregui LE, Babazadeh S, Seltzer E, et al. Randomized, double-blind comparison of once-weekly dalbavancin versus twice-daily linezolid therapy for the treatment of complicated skin and skin structure infections. Clin Infect Dis 2005;41(10):1407–15.

18. Haran JP, Wu G, Bucci V, et al. Treatment of bacterial skin infections in ED observation units: factors influencing prescribing practice. Am J Emerg Med 2015; 33(12):1780–5.

19. Liu C, Bayer A, Cosgrove SE, et al. Clinical practice guidelines by the Infectious Diseases Society of America for the treatment of methicillin-resistant Staphylococcus aureus infections in adults and children: executive summary. Clin Infect Dis 2011;52(3):285–92.

20. Pallin DJ, Binder WD, Allen MB, et al. Clinical trial: comparative effectiveness of cephalexin plus trimethoprim-sulfamethoxazole versus cephalexin alone for treatment of uncomplicated cellulitis: a randomized controlled trial. Clin Infect Dis 2013;56(12):1754–62.

21. Stevens DL, Bisno AL, Chambers HF, et al. Practice guidelines for the diagnosis and management of skin and soft tissue infections: 2014 update by the Infectious Diseases Society of America. Clin Infect Dis 2014;59(2):147–59.

22. Naimi TS, LeDell KH, Como-Sabetti K, et al. Comparison of community- and health care-associated methicillin-resistant Staphylococcus aureus infection. JAMA 2003;290(22):2976–84.

23. Duong M, Markwell S, Peter J, et al. Randomized, controlled trial of antibiotics in the management of community-acquired skin abscesses in the pediatric patient. Ann Emerg Med 2010;55(5):401–7.

24. Schmitz GR, Bruner D, Pitotti R, et al. Randomized controlled trial of trimethoprim-sulfamethoxazole for uncomplicated skin abscesses in patients at risk for community-associated methicillin-resistant Staphylococcus aureus infection. Ann Emerg Med 2010;56(3):283–7.

25. Klempner MS, Styrt B. Prevention of recurrent staphylococcal skin infections with low-dose oral clindamycin therapy. JAMA 1988;260(18):2682–5.

26. Sjoblom AC, Eriksson B, Jorup-Ronstrom C, et al. Antibiotic prophylaxis in recurrent erysipelas. Infection 1993;21(6):390–3.

27. Whitman TJ, Herlihy RK, Schlett CD, et al. Chlorhexidine-impregnated cloths to prevent skin and soft-tissue infection in marine recruits: a cluster-randomized, double-blind, controlled effectiveness trial. Infect Control Hosp Epidemiol 2010;31(12):1207–15.

28. Houshian S, Seyedipour S, Wedderkopp N. Epidemiology of bacterial hand infections. Int J Infect Dis 2006;10(4):315–9.

29. Aghababian RV, Conte JE Jr. Mammalian bite wounds. Ann Emerg Med 1980; 9(2):79–83.

30. Stevens DL, Bisno AL, Chambers HF, et al. Practice guidelines for the diagnosis and management of skin and soft-tissue infections. Clin Infect Dis 2005;41(10): 1373–406.
31. Osterman M, Draeger R, Stern P. Acute hand infections. J Hand Surg Am 2014; 39(8):1628–35 [quiz: 1635].
32. Gonzalez MH, Papierski P, Hall RF Jr. Osteomyelitis of the hand after a human bite. J Hand Surg Am 1993;18(3):520–2.
33. Shoji K, Cavanaugh Z, Rodner CM. Acute fight bite. J Hand Surg Am 2013; 38(8):1612–4.
34. Tosti R, Ilyas AM. Empiric antibiotics for acute infections of the hand. J Hand Surg Am 2010;35(1):125–8.
35. Stern PJ, Staneck JL, McDonough JJ, et al. Established hand infections: a controlled, prospective study. J Hand Surg Am 1983;8(5 Pt 1):553–9.
36. Stern PJ. Selected acute infections. Instr Course Lect 1990;39:539–46.
37. Rubright JH, Shafritz AB. The herpetic whitlow. J Hand Surg Am 2011;36(2): 340–2.
38. Franko OI, Abrams RA. Hand infections. Orthop Clin North Am 2013;44(4): 625–34.
39. Herzon FS. Harris P. Mosher Award Thesis. Peritonsillar abscess: incidence, current management practices, and a proposal for treatment guidelines. Laryngoscope 1995;105(8 Pt 3, Suppl 74):1–17.
40. Marom T, Cinamon U, Itskoviz D, et al. Changing trends of peritonsillar abscess. Am J Otolaryngol 2010;31(3):162–7.
41. Ungkanont K, Yellon RF, Weissman JL, et al. Head and neck space infections in infants and children. Otolaryngol Head Neck Surg 1995;112(3):375–82.
42. Szuhay G, Tewfik TL. Peritonsillar abscess or cellulitis? A clinical comparative paediatric study. J Otolaryngol 1998;27(4):206–12.
43. Nwe TT, Singh B. Management of pain in peritonsillar abscess. J Laryngol Otol 2000;114(10):765–7.
44. Fasano CJ, Chudnofsky C, Vanderbeek P. Bilateral peritonsillar abscesses: not your usual sore throat. J Emerg Med 2005;29(1):45–7.
45. Mobley SR. Bilateral peritonsillar abscess: case report and presentation of its clinical appearance. Ear Nose Throat J 2001;80(6):381–2.
46. Scott PM, Loftus WK, Kew J, et al. Diagnosis of peritonsillar infections: a prospective study of ultrasound, computerized tomography and clinical diagnosis. J Laryngol Otol 1999;113(3):229–32.
47. Patel KS, Ahmad S, O'Leary G, et al. The role of computed tomography in the management of peritonsillar abscess. Otolaryngol Head Neck Surg 1992; 107(6 Pt 1):727–32.
48. Lyon M, Blaivas M. Intraoral ultrasound in the diagnosis and treatment of suspected peritonsillar abscess in the emergency department. Acad Emerg Med 2005;12(1):85–8.
49. Boesen T, Jensen F. Preoperative ultrasonographic verification of peritonsillar abscesses in patients with severe tonsillitis. Eur Arch Otorhinolaryngol 1992; 249(3):131–3.
50. Buckley AR, Moss EH, Blokmanis A. Diagnosis of peritonsillar abscess: value of intraoral sonography. AJR Am J Roentgenol 1994;162(4):961–4.
51. Strong EB, Woodward PJ, Johnson LP. Intraoral ultrasound evaluation of peritonsillar abscess. Laryngoscope 1995;105(8 Pt 1):779–82.

52. Costantino TG, Satz WA, Dehnkamp W, et al. Randomized trial comparing intraoral ultrasound to landmark-based needle aspiration in patients with suspected peritonsillar abscess. Acad Emerg Med 2012;19(6):626–31.
53. Blaivas M, Theodoro D, Duggal S. Ultrasound-guided drainage of peritonsillar abscess by the emergency physician. Am J Emerg Med 2003;21(2):155–8.
54. Brodsky L, Sobie SR, Korwin D, et al. A clinical prospective study of peritonsillar abscess in children. Laryngoscope 1988;98(7):780–3.
55. Millar KR, Johnson DW, Drummond D, et al. Suspected peritonsillar abscess in children. Pediatr Emerg Care 2007;23(7):431–8.
56. Blotter JW, Yin L, Glynn M, et al. Otolaryngology consultation for peritonsillar abscess in the pediatric population. Laryngoscope 2000;110(10 Pt 1):1698–701.
57. Kieff DA, Bhattacharyya N, Siegel NS, et al. Selection of antibiotics after incision and drainage of peritonsillar abscesses. Otolaryngol Head Neck Surg 1999; 120(1):57–61.
58. Brook I. Microbiology and management of peritonsillar, retropharyngeal, and parapharyngeal abscesses. J Oral Maxillofac Surg 2004;62(12):1545–50.
59. Brook I. Failure of penicillin to eradicate group A beta-hemolytic streptococci tonsillitis: causes and management. J Otolaryngol 2001;30(6):324–9.
60. Ozbek C, Aygenc E, Unsal E, et al. Peritonsillar abscess: a comparison of outpatient i.m. clindamycin and inpatient i.v. ampicillin/sulbactam following needle aspiration. Ear Nose Throat J 2005;84(6):366–8.
61. Galioto NJ. Peritonsillar abscess. Am Fam Physician 2008;77(2):199–202.
62. Ozbek C, Aygenc E, Tuna EU, et al. Use of steroids in the treatment of peritonsillar abscess. J Laryngol Otol 2004;118(6):439–42.
63. Chau JK, Seikaly HR, Harris JR, et al. Corticosteroids in peritonsillar abscess treatment: a blinded placebo-controlled clinical trial. Laryngoscope 2014; 124(1):97–103.
64. Herzon FS, Martin AD. Medical and surgical treatment of peritonsillar, retropharyngeal, and parapharyngeal abscesses. Curr Infect Dis Rep 2006;8(3): 196–202.
65. Ophir D, Bawnik J, Poria Y, et al. Peritonsillar abscess. A prospective evaluation of outpatient management by needle aspiration. Arch Otolaryngol Head Neck Surg 1988;114(6):661–3.
66. Savolainen S, Jousimies-Somer HR, Makitie AA, et al. Peritonsillar abscess. Clinical and microbiologic aspects and treatment regimens. Arch Otolaryngol Head Neck Surg 1993;119(5):521–4.
67. Weinberg E, Brodsky L, Stanievich J, et al. Needle aspiration of peritonsillar abscess in children. Arch Otolaryngol Head Neck Surg 1993;119(2):169–72.
68. Stringer SP, Schaefer SD, Close LG. A randomized trial for outpatient management of peritonsillar abscess. Arch Otolaryngol Head Neck Surg 1988;114(3): 296–8.
69. Thapar A, Tassone P, Bhat N, et al. Parapharyngeal abscess: a life-threatening complication of quinsy. Clin Anat 2008;21(1):23–6.
70. da Silva PS, Waisberg DR. Internal carotid artery pseudoaneurysm with life-threatening epistaxis as a complication of deep neck space infection. Pediatr Emerg Care 2011;27(5):422–4.
71. Roccia F, Pecorari GC, Oliaro A, et al. Ten years of descending necrotizing mediastinitis: management of 23 cases. J Oral Maxillofac Surg 2007;65(9): 1716–24.
72. Wenig BL, Shikowitz MJ, Abramson AL. Necrotizing fasciitis as a lethal complication of peritonsillar abscess. Laryngoscope 1984;94(12 Pt 1):1576–9.

73. Stevens HE. Vascular complication of neck space infection: case report and literature review. J Otolaryngol 1990;19(3):206–10.
74. Greinwald JH Jr, Wilson JF, Haggerty PG. Peritonsillar abscess: an unlikely cause of necrotizing fasciitis. Ann Otol Rhinol Laryngol 1995;104(2):133–7.
75. Goldenberg NA, Knapp-Clevenger R, Hays T, et al. Lemierre's and Lemierre's-like syndromes in children: survival and thromboembolic outcomes. Pediatrics 2005;116(4):e543–8.
76. Johnson RF, Stewart MG, Wright CC. An evidence-based review of the treatment of peritonsillar abscess. Otolaryngol Head Neck Surg 2003;128(3):332–43.
77. Apostolopoulos NJ, Nikolopoulos TP, Bairamis TN. Peritonsillar abscess in children. Is incision and drainage an effective management? Int J Pediatr Otorhinolaryngol 1995;31(2–3):129–35.
78. Kronenberg J, Wolf M, Leventon G. Peritonsillar abscess: recurrence rate and the indication for tonsillectomy. Am J Otolaryngol 1987;8(2):82–4.
79. CDC. Sexullay transmitted disease surveillance, 2013. Atlanta (GA): Department of Health and Human Services; 2014.
80. Das BB, Ronda J, Trent M. Pelvic inflammatory disease: improving awareness, prevention, and treatment. Infect Drug Resist 2016;9:191–7.
81. Eschenbach DA, Wolner-Hanssen P, Hawes SE, et al. Acute pelvic inflammatory disease: associations of clinical and laboratory findings with laparoscopic findings. Obstet Gynecol 1997;89(2):184–92.
82. Wiesenfeld HC, Hillier SL, Meyn LA, et al. Subclinical pelvic inflammatory disease and infertility. Obstet Gynecol 2012;120(1):37–43.
83. Peipert JF, Ness RB, Blume J, et al. Clinical predictors of endometritis in women with symptoms and signs of pelvic inflammatory disease. Am J Obstet Gynecol 2001;184(5):856–63 [discussion: 863–4].
84. Brunham RC, Gottlieb SL, Paavonen J. Pelvic inflammatory disease. N Engl J Med 2015;372(21):2039–48.
85. CDC. 2015 sexually transmitted diseases treatment guidelines. Atlanta (GA): Department of Health and Human Services; 2015.
86. Peipert JF, Boardman L, Hogan JW, et al. Laboratory evaluation of acute upper genital tract infection. Obstet Gynecol 1996;87(5 Pt 1):730–6.
87. Ness RB, Soper DE, Holley RL, et al. Effectiveness of inpatient and outpatient treatment strategies for women with pelvic inflammatory disease: results from the pelvic inflammatory disease evaluation and clinical health (PEACH) randomized trial. Am J Obstet Gynecol 2002;186(5):929–37.
88. Burnett AM, Anderson CP, Zwank MD. Laboratory-confirmed gonorrhea and/or chlamydia rates in clinically diagnosed pelvic inflammatory disease and cervicitis. Am J Emerg Med 2012;30(7):1114–7.
89. Bjartling C, Osser S, Persson K. Mycoplasma genitalium in cervicitis and pelvic inflammatory disease among women at a gynecologic outpatient service. Am J Obstet Gynecol 2012;206(6):476.e1-8.
90. Manhart LE, Broad JM, Golden MR. Mycoplasma genitalium: should we treat and how? Clin Infect Dis 2011;53(Suppl 3):S129–42.
91. Haggerty CL, Hillier SL, Bass DC, et al, PID Evaluation and Clinical Health Study Investigators. Bacterial vaginosis and anaerobic bacteria are associated with endometritis. Clin Infect Dis 2004;39(7):990–5.
92. Cohen CR, Sinei S, Reilly M, et al. Effect of human immunodeficiency virus type 1 infection upon acute salpingitis: a laparoscopic study. J Infect Dis 1998;178(5):1352–8.

93. Zeger W, Holt K. Gynecologic infections. Emerg Med Clin North Am 2003;21(3): 631–48.

94. Slap GB, Forke CM, Cnaan A, et al. Recognition of tubo-ovarian abscess in adolescents with pelvic inflammatory disease. J Adolesc Health 1996;18(6): 397–403.

95. Boardman LA, Peipert JF, Brody JM, et al. Endovaginal sonography for the diagnosis of upper genital tract infection. Obstet Gynecol 1997;90(1):54–7.

96. Romosan G, Valentin L. The sensitivity and specificity of transvaginal ultrasound with regard to acute pelvic inflammatory disease: a review of the literature. Arch Gynecol Obstet 2014;289(4):705–14.

97. Hiller N, Sella T, Lev-Sagi A, et al. Computed tomographic features of tuboovarian abscess. J Reprod Med 2005;50(3):203–8.

98. Workowski KA. Centers for Disease Control and Prevention sexually transmitted diseases treatment guidelines. Clin Infect Dis 2015;61(Suppl 8):S759–62.

99. Schappert SM, Rechtsteiner EA. Ambulatory medical care utilization estimates for 2007. Vital Health Stat 13 2011;169:1–38.

100. Sammon JD, Sharma P, Rahbar H, et al. Predictors of admission in patients presenting to the emergency department with urinary tract infection. World J Urol 2014;32(3):813–9.

101. Czaja CA, Scholes D, Hooton TM, et al. Population-based epidemiologic analysis of acute pyelonephritis. Clin Infect Dis 2007;45(3):273–80.

102. Foxman B, Klemstine KL, Brown PD. Acute pyelonephritis in US hospitals in 1997: hospitalization and in-hospital mortality. Ann Epidemiol 2003;13(2): 144–50.

103. Ward G, Jorden RC, Severance HW. Treatment of pyelonephritis in an observation unit. Ann Emerg Med 1991;20(3):258–61.

104. Israel RS, Lowenstein SR, Marx JA, et al. Management of acute pyelonephritis in an emergency department observation unit. Ann Emerg Med 1991;20(3):253–7.

105. Fairley KF, Carson NE, Gutch RC, et al. Site of infection in acute urinary-tract infection in general practice. Lancet 1971;2(7725):615–8.

106. Gupta K, Hooton TM, Naber KG, et al. International clinical practice guidelines for the treatment of acute uncomplicated cystitis and pyelonephritis in women: a 2010 update by the Infectious Diseases Society of America and the European Society for Microbiology and Infectious Diseases. Clin Infect Dis 2011;52(5): e103–20.

107. Thanassi M. Utility of urine and blood cultures in pyelonephritis. Acad Emerg Med 1997;4(8):797–800.

108. McMurray BR, Wrenn KD, Wright SW. Usefulness of blood cultures in pyelonephritis. Am J Emerg Med 1997;15(2):137–40.

109. Finkelstein R, Kassis E, Reinhertz G, et al. Community-acquired urinary tract infection in adults: a hospital viewpoint. J Hosp Infect 1998;38(3):193–202.

110. Hsu CY, Fang HC, Chou KJ, et al. The clinical impact of bacteremia in complicated acute pyelonephritis. Am J Med Sci 2006;332(4):175–80.

111. Coburn B, Morris AM, Tomlinson G, et al. Does this adult patient with suspected bacteremia require blood cultures? JAMA 2012;308(5):502–11.

112. Velasco M, Martinez JA, Moreno-Martinez A, et al. Blood cultures for women with uncomplicated acute pyelonephritis: are they necessary? Clin Infect Dis 2003; 37(8):1127–30.

113. Smith WR, McClish DK, Poses RM, et al. Bacteremia in young urban women admitted with pyelonephritis. Am J Med Sci 1997;313(1):50–7.

114. Nikolaidis P, Casalino D, Remer E, et al, Expert Panel on Urologic Imaging. ACR appropriateness criteria® acute pyelonephritis. Reston (VA): American College of Radiology (ACR); 2012. p. 6.
115. Kawashima A, LeRoy AJ. Radiologic evaluation of patients with renal infections. Infect Dis Clin North Am 2003;17(2):433–56.
116. Browne RF, Zwirewich C, Torreggiani WC. Imaging of urinary tract infection in the adult. Eur Radiol 2004;14(Suppl 3):E168–83.
117. Nicolle LE, AMMI Canada Guidelines Committee. Complicated urinary tract infection in adults. Can J Infect Dis Med Microbiol 2005;16(6):349–60.
118. Parasuraman R, Julian K, AST Infectious Diseases Community of Practice. Urinary tract infections in solid organ transplantation. Am J Transplant 2013; 13(Suppl 4):327–36.

# Care of Traumatic Conditions in an Observation Unit

Christopher G. Caspers, MD

## KEYWORDS

• Observation • Trauma • Unit • Emergency • Value • Medicine

## KEY POINTS

- Observation units can be used to care for patients in need of short-term management of acute traumatic injuries.
- Some injured patients with an unrevealing initial clinical evaluation are at risk for delayed deterioration that can be detected during a period of observation.
- Emergency physicians have the necessary skills to provide observation services to a variety of conditions that may be present in injured patients.

*Even in trauma, signs and symptoms take time to develop and the diagnosis of "no injury" is more difficult to make than the positive.[1]*

---

**Case Study**

A 29-year-old woman who was a restrained passenger in a motor vehicle collision arrives to the emergency department (ED) at 11 PM on a Saturday night. Emergency Medical Service reports moderate front-end damage to the vehicle. The patient is 26 weeks pregnant and reports mild abdominal pain. Her vitals are stable. She has a Glasgow Coma Scale (GCS) of 15, and her physical examination demonstrates no evidence of traumatic injury. The trauma service responds to the ED and assists with management. Her focused assessment with sonography for trauma (FAST) examination is normal. A computed tomography (CT) of her chest, abdomen, and pelvis are performed and are also normal. The obstetrics and gynecology (ob/gyn) service is consulted, who initiates cardiotocographic monitoring (CTM) and notes that the initial tracings appear reassuring. They recommend observation with further CTM overnight. The patient is placed in the observation unit (OU) where she receives serial physical examinations, CTM, and a repeat FAST examination. The following day, her pain is resolved, and she is asymptomatic with no maternal obstetric signs. The trauma and ob/gyn services clear the mother for discharge, provide follow-up information, and counsel the patient on warning signs to return to the ED. The OU team arranges for transportation, and the patient returns home uneventfully.

---

Disclosure Statement: The author has nothing to disclose.
Ronald O. Perelman Department of Emergency Medicine, New York University Langone Medical Center, 560 First Avenue, New York, NY 10016, USA
*E-mail address:* Christopher.Caspers@nyumc.org

Emerg Med Clin N Am 35 (2017) 673–683
http://dx.doi.org/10.1016/j.emc.2017.03.010
0733-8627/17/© 2017 Elsevier Inc. All rights reserved.

emed.theclinics.com

## INTRODUCTION

Emergency department observation units (EDOUs) have been used to manage patients with injuries over the past several decades in an effort to reduce hospital overcrowding and improve throughput.[1–3] In 2012, the first prospective study evaluating the use of EDOUs for all types of trauma was performed.[4] Ten percent required inpatient conversion from the EDOU, and there were no deaths, intubations, loss of vital signs, or other adverse outcomes for patients placed in the EDOU under the trauma protocol. Overall, the EDOU was shown to be a safe, cost-effective alternative to routine inpatient admission for the short-term management of injured patients.[4]

## MILD TRAUMATIC BRAIN INJURY

Head injury is one of the most commonly encountered types of trauma in the ED, comprising 20% to 30% of all traumas. In 2010, 2.2 million ED visits in the United States were due to a traumatic brain injury (TBI).[5] However, only 10% to 15% of these patients have severe head injuries that require hospitalization.[6]

The severity of TBI is categorized according to the GCS. Approximately 80% of brain injuries are considered mild traumatic brain injury (mTBI) (GCS 13–15).[7,8] The optimal evaluation and treatment strategy of mTBIs remains controversial.[9–13] Some patients with an initially normal GCS will have an abnormal CT scan.[14] Furthermore, some patients with normal neurologic examinations and CT scans will subsequently deteriorate.[15,16] Mendelow and colleagues[17] reported that mTBI patients occupied 1959 of 5288 total bed days and incurred 37% of total cost for all TBI patients, although the incidence of subsequent deterioration was low. In a separate retrospective analysis by Jones and colleagues,[18] if observation was not performed, 35 additional beds would be made available for inpatients each year, but 30 patients with neurologic deterioration after mTBI would be erroneously discharged.

The ability to predict which alert, responsive ED patients with mTBI require monitoring for subsequent deterioration is limited. In one study, observation of patients with loss of consciousness or amnesia who had no evidence of impaired consciousness, focal neurologic deficit, seizure, vomiting, severe headache, or skull fracture led to no negative outcomes and no missed injuries.[19] The incidence of significant neurologic deterioration after minor head injury is less well known and estimated at 0.59% to 3.9%.[17,18] Unpredictable neurologic deterioration may occur regardless of GCS score, so focused and frequent reassessments in observation are necessary to detect any change that suggests the development or expansion of an intracranial hematoma or edema.[20–22]

The predictive value of head CT in identifying patients at risk for neurologic deterioration has been unclear. A retrospective review concluded that in patients who presented with a GCS of 15, if the patient had a normal mental status and a normal neurologic examination in the ED, the chance of the patient developing a serious complication from mTBI was exceedingly small.[23] However, in the presence of an abnormal mental status or focal neurologic deficit, even if no operative lesion is present on CT, the patient should be observed in the hospital. This recommendation was based on the finding that 3 of the 137 patients developed operative hematomas and an additional 3 had significant deterioration while in the hospital under observation.

It has also been noted that relying on neurologic signs at the time of arrival at the ED and observation may not be adequate in all settings. Stein and Ross[24] reported 18% of patients with mTBI and a nonfocal neurologic examination had abnormalities on CT scan, which increased 3-fold as GCS decreased from 15 to 13. Five percent of the total study population eventually needed surgery as the result of their mTBI. Similar to other investigators, they were unable to determine who would experience delayed deterioration from intracranial lesions not yet clinically evident.[25]

Two large investigations attempted to derive criteria to predict the need for CT in ED patients with mTBI.[12,13] The investigators of the New Orleans Criteria (NOC) study attempted to develop and validate a set of 100% sensitive clinical criteria for identifying patients with mTBI presenting with a GCS of 15 who should undergo CT scanning.[12] The primary endpoint of the NOC was the detection of any acutely positive finding on CT scan.

The following year, a second clinical decision tool, the Canadian CT Head Rule (CCHR), was derived to guide decision making regarding the use of CT in patients with mTBI.[13] Patients were enrolled if they experienced mTBI and presented with a GCS of 13 to 15. The primary goal of the CCHR was predicting the need for neurosurgical intervention, whereas the secondary outcome was predicting clinically important brain injury on CT. The CCHR was not calibrated to detect any of the following in a neurologically intact patient: solitary contusion less than 5 mm diameter, localized subarachnoid hemorrhage less than 1 mm thick, isolated pneumocephaly or closed depressed skull fracture not extending through the inner table. The investigators concluded they had developed a highly sensitive tool for the use of CT in patients with mTBI who were at high risk for the primary or secondary outcomes. However, TBI that does not require immediate neurosurgical intervention may still lead to significant clinical problems, and patients with these injuries may benefit from being observed for the development of these conditions.

Subsequent validation studies of the CCHR and NOC have been attempted. Sensitivities ranged from 79% to 100% for the CCHR and 86% to 100% for NOC, although confidence intervals were wide when perfect sensitivity was reported and specificity was low.[10,11,26,27] In addition, there is a reported risk of subsequent deterioration in those with initially normal CTs, or those with positive CTs with normal neurologic examinations that these instruments are unable to address. Missing any acute intracranial injuries may not be acceptable to some practitioners, regardless of their clinical significance. The benefits of using observation in such patients include the opportunity to provide symptomatic support as well as monitoring neurologic status and coordinating care with specialists for expedited evaluation and follow-up.

Anticoagulated patients with mTBI and normal initial CT scan are at an increased risk for delayed intracranial hemorrhage (ICH).[28–32] The rate of delayed traumatic ICH in anticoagulated patients with mTBI and a normal CT scan was 0.6% in one prospective evaluation.[27] In a separate review of 77 anticoagulated patients with mTBI, neurologic deterioration was most likely to occur at 8 to 18 hours after injury, whereas other small series demonstrated most patients deteriorated within 24 hours of injury.[29–32]

Observation can also be used to manage patients with acute intracranial findings on CT that do not require immediate neurosurgical intervention.[33] In a series of 1078 patients with mTBI, 110 patients with small intracranial bleeds were managed in an OU. No patients experienced delayed deterioration or needed neurosurgical intervention, and there were no readmissions. This concept was supported in a subsequent evaluation comparing observation to routine admission to manage patients with mTBI and acute intracranial hematoma on head CT.[9] The hospital length of stay (LOS) was shortened by 2 days when patients were managed in an OU instead of routine admission. In a separate study of 1185 patients with mTBI, all patients with isolated traumatic subarachnoid hemorrhage managed in an OU did well.[34] Some traumatic ICHs are at low risk for decompensating and should be considered safe for EDOU management to decrease resource utilization. More work is needed to identify these types of conditions.

## SMALL TRAUMATIC PNEUMOTHORACES

A pneumothorax (PTX) is one of the most common complications of chest trauma.[35] With more widespread use of CT in the evaluation of trauma patients, small PTXs not seen on the supine anteroposterior chest radiograph are being diagnosed with CT at an increasing rate, most of which would otherwise have gone unnoticed and presumably untreated. This type of PTX is called an occult pneumothorax (OPTX). Management of the OPTX is controversial, and it is not clear if this condition should be managed with tube thoracostomy, or if it can be managed with observation alone. Proponents of tube thoracostomy argue for the definitive procedure over the risk of progression of the PTX or development of a tension pneumothorax (TPTX). However, tube thoracostomy carries its own risks, such as lung injury, vascular damage, malpositioning, or infection in up to 20% of those receiving the procedure.[36]

Several prospective, randomized evaluations have been conducted to address the management of this condition. Enderson and colleagues[37] compared the risks and benefits of tube thoracostomy versus observation for 40 patients diagnosed with OPTX and included some patients receiving positive-pressure ventilation (PPV). The overall incidence of OPTX in their study population was 5.6%. LOS was shorter in the tube thoracostomy cohort, although not by a statistically significant duration. Eight patients in the observation group developed a need for tube thoracostomy while on PPV, with 3 of these developing a TPTX. The investigators concluded that patients with OPTX who require PPV are at risk for progression of their OPTX and development of TPTX.

These initial studies were followed by a separate investigation of 39 patients with OPTX to compare management with tube thoracostomy versus observation alone in patients with OPTX, regardless of the size of OPTX or requirement for PPV.[38] The overall incidence of OPTX in this study was 5.9%. The median LOS was shorter for the observation cohort than the routine thoracostomy group (5 days vs 8 days). There was no statistically significant difference in rate of OPTX progression or OPTX size between the groups. Similarly, the overall likelihood of progression of OPTX for those patients on PPV was not statistically significant. There was no difference between the groups in overall complication rate, and most patients treated by observation that received PPV did not have progression of their OPTX or require tube thoracostomy placement.

These 2 prior trials yielded differing results, with Enderson and colleagues reporting that 53% of observed patients had progression of their OPTX, including 3 with TPTX, while Brasel and colleagues found that only 22% experienced progression of OPTX, both including patients with OPTX requiring PPV. A third prospective, randomized study of 24 patients with OPTX was performed in an effort to evaluate the management of patients with OPTX requiring PPV with tube thoracostomy or observation alone. Four of 13 patients in the observation cohort required tube thoracostomy; however, no patient required an emergent chest tube. The investigators concluded that observation may be at least as safe and effective as tube thoracostomy for managing OPTX with respect to mortality, progression of PTX, and complication.[39,40]

Recently, Moore and colleagues[41] conducted a prospective study over 2 years at 16 US trauma centers to determine which factors were associated with failed observation (defined as the need for tube thoracostomy while being observed) in patients with OPTX. Five hundred sixty-nine patients with OPTX were enrolled. Six percent of patients who were observed failed observation. No patients in the failed observation group developed a TPTX or an adverse event related to delayed thoracostomy. LOS was reduced by almost half in those who were successfully observed versus those who failed observation (7.6 vs 15 days), resembling findings from a separate study by Wilson and colleagues[42] when OPTX were managed with observation alone versus tube thoracostomy.

Recently, an interim analysis of the American Association for the Surgery of Trauma workgroup was conducted to report the outcomes in an ongoing multicenter randomized controlled trial comparing tube thoracostomy with observation alone for the management of OPTX.[43] There was no difference in the primary outcome noted between the 2 groups. Only one (2%) observed patient developed a TPTX, which occurred during sustained PPV and resolved with tube thoracostomy. There were no differences in mortality or LOS between the 2 groups.

Currently, the Eastern Association for the Surgery of Trauma (EAST) Practice Management Guidelines supports the position that OPTXs in a stable patient can be managed with observation alone.[44] Most patients with OPTX will not have progression of the OPTX. However, the guidelines concluded that more information was needed in determining with accuracy which OPTXs are at risk of progression. Other nonclinical factors may impact decision making, including the level of monitoring while being observed, the availability of a clinician to perform an invasive intervention without delay should OPTX progress or TPTX develop, and patient preference regarding risks and benefits of tube thoracostomy versus observation alone for OPTX.

## TRAUMATIC ORTHOPEDIC CONDITIONS

Data are limited regarding the use of EDOUs for isolated orthopedics trauma. Injuries well suited for EDOUs include nonoperative fractures requiring pain control and coordination of postdischarge services, injuries requiring bracing, and extremity fractures requiring monitoring for compartment syndrome (CS).[45] The vast majority of patients placed in the EDOU with nonoperative orthopedic trauma can be discharged home on the index visit without a need for inpatient admission.

It has been demonstrated that older adults in the ED with orthopedic trauma can be managed with pathways incorporating resources available to most EDOUs.[46,47] The EDOU provides an ideal setting for care coordination and discharge planning and an opportunity for assessment by a geriatrician, pharmacist, physical therapist, social worker, and care manager. These patients receive focused interventions in mobility, gait training, and functional status improvements. Therapists in the EDOU setting are skilled in managing patients with acute pain with the focus of safe disposition planning and also serve as an educational resource to patients and families in preventing future injuries.

## FRACTURES NEEDING SERIAL COMPARTMENT EXAMINATIONS

CS is a syndrome in which increased pressure within a limited anatomic space compromises the circulation and function of tissues within that space. In most cases, a combination of factors is responsible. Complications of CS include infection, contracture, and amputation. CS may be clinically obvious on initial evaluation, or the onset may be more insidious with some cases occurring 12 to 24 hours after injury.[48] The most important determinant of a poor outcome from acute CS after injury is delay to diagnosis, resulting from incomplete appreciation of risk factors and lack of a standard definition of the disease.[49] An OU provides an ideal setting for the ongoing monitoring and frequent reassessments required to make this clinical diagnosis.

The most common fractures causing an extremity CS are the tibial shaft and forearm.[48–51] A greater incidence of CS is also seen with comminuted fractures, a result of higher-energy mechanism of injury resulting in higher damage to the tissues. Vascular tone, systemic blood pressure, duration of compartment pressure elevation, and the metabolic demand of the tissue also impact the development of CS and can be assessed in an OU.[52]

If the diagnosis of CS is clinically apparent, it is not necessary to measure compartment pressures.[48] However, if the clinical scenario is equivocal, compartment pressures can be used as an adjunct to assist the decision to perform a fasciotomy or continue observation. A compartment pressure value must be interpreted in clinical context and there is no universally agreed upon definition of compartment pressure that should automatically trigger a fasciotomy.[47,50,51,53–57]

CS is a clinical diagnosis that can be observed for and diagnosed in an EDOU when the appropriate resources are available. Observation for the development of CS should be considered in those patients wherein there is increased risk for CS, especially in young men with fractures of the tibial diaphysis, and those with high-energy injuries to the forearm diaphysis or distal radius. Accurate measurement of compartment pressure varies based on technique, device, and distance from the fracture site and is not a sole determinant of CS.[58] Emergent fasciotomy should be considered in any patient who is suspected to have CS.

## PREGNANT PATIENTS NEEDING FETAL MONITORING

Trauma is common in pregnancy, affecting approximately 1 in 14 pregnant patients.[59] The most common causes of blunt maternal injury during pregnancy are motor vehicle collisions, falls, and assaults.[60] Trauma results in the death of the fetus much more often than the death of the mother.[61] Pregnant patients with non-catastrophic trauma benefit from observation for monitoring of the patient as well as fetal monitoring. Such observation requires availability of a multidisciplinary team able to care for the mother as well as the fetus. Most obstetric findings will be present within 2 hours of trauma, although some may not be detected until many hours after the trauma, presenting a need for observation.[62]

The initial evaluation should focus on the detection of obstetric finding (ie, vaginal bleeding, uterine tenderness, or contractions). In patients without these findings, the pregnancy is rarely affected (19.3% vs 0.9%). Conversely, when those findings are present, there is a strong association of adverse effect on the pregnancy. The most common cause of fetal death after trauma is placental abruption.[63] Fetal deaths due to direct injury or uterine rupture are much less common that deaths due to placental abruption, which complicates about 1% to 5% of minor injuries and 20% to 50% of major injuries. Uterine rupture due to blunt trauma is a rare injury unique to pregnancy and complicates about 0.6% of trauma, tending to occur only in serious accidents involving direct abdominal trauma.

Cardiotocographic monitoring (CTM) is used to identify a change in fetal physiology and should begin as soon after the trauma as possible.[63–65] There is controversy regarding the optimal duration of monitoring. American College of Obstetricians and Gynecologists and EAST guidelines recommend all pregnant women greater than 20-weeks gestation who suffer trauma have CTM for a minimum of 6 hours. Monitoring should be continued with further evaluation and management if uterine contractions, a nonreassuring fetal heart rate (FHR), vaginal bleeding, uterine tenderness, significant maternal injury, or rupture of the amniotic membranes is present.[66,67] Even after minor injuries to the mother, CTM should be initiated as soon as possible.[58,63] After 4 to 6 hours of CTM, if no maternal obstetric symptoms have developed and CTM is reassuring, traumatic complications to the fetus can be ruled out with high sensitivity.[68] Otherwise, CTM should be continued for 24 hours (**Box 1**).[58,69] Although a normal FHR tracing is associated with a favorable outcome, an abnormal recording does

---

**Box 1**
**Trauma in pregnancy risk factors**

Fetal heart rate and uterine activity monitoring by electronic fetal monitoring for 24 hours for trauma patients with:

Uterine tenderness

Significant abdominal pain

Vaginal bleeding

Contraction frequency greater than once per 10 minutes during a monitoring period of 4 hours

Rupture of the membranes

Atypical or abnormal fetal heart rate pattern (fetal tachycardia, bradycardia, or decelerations)

High-risk mechanism of injury (motorcycle, pedestrian, high-speed crash)

Serum fibrinogen less than 200 mg/dL

---

not always indicate fetal injury.[70] Therefore, FHR monitoring is largely a screening tool to indicate when more definitive instigations are required, such as nonstress test or biophysical profile.

Ultrasound can assist in the diagnosis of abruption and evaluate fetal well-being if CTM is equivocal, although a normal ultrasound does not rule out placental abruption. Fetal ultrasound allows direct visualization of the heartbeat, gestational age, presentation, amniotic fluid volume, placental integrity, biparietal diameter, abdominal circumference, and femur length, allowing gestational age and weight to be estimated, essential for planning if delivery is considered.[58,63]

The mother should be observed for specific clues to complications following trauma such as leakage of fluid, vaginal bleeding, abdominal pain or cramping, increased intensity and frequency of contractions, and decreased maternal perception of fetal movements.[61] Factors that should be taken into consideration when deciding to observe an injured pregnant patient are the severity of the injuries, gestational age, and viability of the fetus. Maternal health should always take priority over interventions for the fetus.[61,71,72]

## SUMMARY

An OU is an effective setting to provide short-term care and monitoring for patients presenting to the ED with trauma. Examples of other traumatic conditions that can be considered for OU management included rhabdomyolysis, rib fractures, abdominal contusions, minor burns, and soft tissue injuries requiring pain management, among others. Clinical protocols should be developed with consideration to the availability of surgeons, proximity to the nearest trauma center should a patient suddenly become more acute, and in collaboration with trauma surgeons.

## REFERENCES

1. Conrad L, Markovchick V, Mitchiner J, et al. The role of an emergency department observation unit in the management of trauma patients. J Emerg Med 1985;2: 325–33.
2. Madsen TE, Bledsoe JR, Bossart PJ. Observation unit admission as an alternative to inpatient admission for trauma activation patients. Emerg Med J 2009;26: 421–3.

3. Dinh MM, Bein KJ, Byrne CM, et al. Deriving a prediction rule for short stay admission in trauma patients admitted at a major trauma centre in Australia. J Emerg Med 2014;31:263–7.

4. Holly J, Bledsoe J, Black K, et al. Prospective evaluation of an ED observation unit protocol for trauma activation patients. Am J Emerg Med 2012;30:1402–6.

5. Injury Prevention & Control: Traumatic Brain Injury & Concussion. Centers for Disease Control and Prevention. 2016. Available at: http://www.cdc.gov/traumaticbraininjury/get_the_facts.html. Accessed November 18, 2016.

6. Fischer RP, Carlson J, Perry JF. Postconcussive hospital observation of alert patients in a primary trauma center. J Trauma 1981;21(11):920–5.

7. Jager TE, Weiss HB, Coben JH, et al. Traumatic brain injuries evaluated in U.S. emergency departments, 1992-1994. Acad Emerg Med 2000;7:134–40.

8. Jennett B. Epidemiology of head injury. J Neurol Neurosurg Psychiatry 1996;60: 362–9.

9. Halbert CA, Cipolle MD, Fulda GJ, et al. Admission to an observational unit improves length of stay for patients with mild traumatic brain injuries. Am Surg 2015;81(2):176–9.

10. Papa L, Stiell IG, Clement CM, et al. Performance of the Canadian CT head rule and the New Orleans criteria for predicting any traumatic intracranial injury on computed tomography in a United States level I trauma center. Acad Emerg Med 2012;19:2–10.

11. Kavalci C. Comparison of the Canadian CT head rule and the New Orleans criteria in patients with minor head injury. World J Emerg Surg 2014;9:31.

12. Haydel MJ, Preston CA, Mills TJ, et al. Indications for computed tomography in patients with minor head injury. N Engl J Med 2000;343(2):100–5.

13. Stiell IG, Wells GA, Vandemheen K, et al. The Canadian CT Head Rule for patients with minor head injury. Lancet 2001;357:1391–6.

14. Mikhail MG, Levitt MA, Christopher TA, et al. Intracranial injury following minor head injury. Am J Emerg Med 1992;10:24.

15. Marshall LF, Toole BM, Bowers SA. The national traumatic coma data bank: II. Patients who talk and deteriorate: implications for treatment. J Neurosurg 1983; 59:285.

16. Snoey ER, Levitt MA. Delayed diagnosis of subdural hematoma following normal computed tomography scan. Ann Emerg Med 1994;23:1127.

17. Mendelow AD, Campbell DA, Jeffrey RR, et al. Admission after mild head injury: benefits and costs. BMJ 1982;285:1530–2.

18. Jones J, Jeffreys R. Relative risk of alternative admission policies for patients with head injuries. Lancet 1981;2(8251):850–3.

19. Weston PA. Admission policy for patients following head injury. Br J Surg 1981; 68(9):663–4.

20. Dacey RG, Alves WM, Rimel RW, et al. Neurosurgical complications after apparently minor head injury. J Neurosurg 1986;65:203–10.

21. Ransohoff J, Fleischer A. Head injuries. JAMA 1975;234(8):861–4.

22. Klauber MR, Marshall LF, Luerssen TG, et al. Determinants of head injury mortality: importance of the low risk patient. Neurosurgery 1989;24(1):31–6.

23. Feuerman T, Wackym PA, Gade GF, et al. Value of skull radiography, head computed tomographic scanning, and admission for observation in cases of minor head injury. Neurosurgery 1988;22(3):449–53.

24. Stein SC, Ross SE. The value of computed tomographic scans in patients with low-risk head injuries. Neurosurgery 1990;26(4):638–40.

25. Saunders CE, Cota R, Barton CA. Reliability of home observation for victims of mild closed-head injury. Ann Emerg Med 1986;15(2):160–3.

26. Smits M. External validation of the Canadian CT head rule and the New Orleans criteria for CT scanning in patients with minor head injury. JAMA 2005;294(12): 1519–25.

27. Stiell IG, Clement CM, Rowe BH, et al. Implementation of the Canadian C-Spine Rule: prospective 12 centre cluster randomised trial. BMJ 2009;339:b4146.

28. Nishijima DK, Offerman SR, Ballard DW, et al. Immediate and delayed traumatic intracranial hemorrhage in patients with head trauma and preinjury warfarin or clopidogrel use. Ann Emerg Med 2012;59(6):460–8.e1-7.

29. Cohen DB, Rinker C, Wilberger JE. Traumatic brain injury in anticoagulated patients. J Trauma Inj Infect Crit Care 2006;60(3):553–7.

30. Itshayek E, Rosenthal G, Fraifeld S, et al. Delayed posttraumatic acute subdural hematoma in elderly patients on anticoagulation. Neurosurgery 2006;58(5): E851–6 [discussion: E851–6].

31. Reynolds FD, Dietz PA, Higgins D, et al. Time to deterioration of the elderly, anti-coagulated, minor head injury patient who presents without evidence of neuro-logic abnormality. J Trauma Inj Infect Crit Care 2003;54(3):492–6.

32. Vos PE, Battistin L, Birbamer G, et al. EFNS guideline on mild traumatic brain injury: report of an EFNS task force. Eur J Neurol 2002;9(3):207–19.

33. Schaller B, Evangelopoulos DS, Muller C, et al. Do we really need 24-h observa-tion for patients with minimal brain injury and small intracranial bleeding? The Bernese Trauma Unit Protocol. Emerg Med J 2010;27:537–9.

34. Pruitt PB, Borczuk P. 74: an observational study to evaluate subarachnoid hem-orrhage discharge from observation. Acad Emerg Med 2015;22(Suppl S1):S38.

35. Yadav K, Jalili M, Zehtabchi S. Management of traumatic occult pneumothorax. Resuscitation 2010;81:1063–8.

36. Etoch SW, Bar-Natan MF, Miller FB, et al. Tube thoracostomy factors related to complications. Arch Surg 1995;130(5):521–6.

37. Enderson BL, Abdalla R, Frame SB, et al. Tube thoracostomy for occult pneumothorax-a prospective, randomized study of its use. J Trauma Inj Infect Crit Care 1993;35(5):726–30.

38. Brasel KJ, Stafford RE, Tenquist JE, et al. Treatment of occult pneumothoraces from blunt trauma. J Trauma Inj Infect Crit Care 1999;46(6):987–91.

39. Ouellet JF, Trottier V, Kmet L, et al. The OPTICC trial: a multi-institutional study of occult pneumothoraces in critical care. Am J Surg 2009;197(5):581–6.

40. Kulshrestha P, Munshi I, Wait R. Profile of chest trauma in a level I trauma center. J Trauma Inj Infect Crit Care 2004;57(3):576–81.

41. Moore FO, Goslar PW, Coimbra R, et al. Blunt traumatic occult pneumothorax: is observation safe?—results of a prospective, AAST multicenter study. J Trauma Inj Infect Crit Care 2011;70(5):1019–25.

42. Wilson H, Ellsmere J, Tallon J, et al. Occult pneumothorax in the blunt trauma pa-tient: tube thoracostomy or observation? Injury 2009;40:928–31.

43. Kirkpatrick AW, Rizoli S, Ouellet JF, et al. Occult pneumothoraces in critical care: a prospective multicenter randomized controlled trial of pleural drainage for me-chanically ventilated trauma patients with occult pneumothoraces. J Trauma Acute Care Surg 2013;74(3):747–55.

44. Mowery NT, Gunter OL, Collier BR, et al. Practice management guidelines for management of hemothorax and occult pneumothorax. J Trauma Inj Infect Crit Care 2011;70(2):510–8.

45. Ernst AA, Jones J, Weiss SJ, et al. Emergency department orthopedics observation unit as an alternative to admission. South Med J 2014;107(10):648–53.
46. Southerland LT, Gure TR, Caterino JM, et al. 232: geriatric observation unit protocols. Acad Emerg Med 2016;23(Suppl S1):S106.
47. Plummer L, Sridhar S, Beninato M, et al. Physical therapist practice in the emergency department observation unit: descriptive study. Phys Ther 2014;95(2):249–56.
48. McQueen M, Court-Brown C. Compartment monitoring in tibial fractures: the pressure threshold for decompression. J Bone Joint Surg Br 1996;78-B:99–104.
49. Köstler W, Strohm P, Südkamp N. Acute compartment syndrome of the limb. Injury 2005;36(8):992–8.
50. Park S, Ahn J, Gee A. Compartment syndrome in tibial fractures. J Orthop Trauma 2009;23(7):514–8.
51. Olson SA, Glasgow RR. Acute compartment syndrome in lower extremity musculoskeletal trauma. J Am Acad Orthop Surg 2005;13(7):436–44.
52. Heckman MM, Whitesides TE, Grewe SR, et al. Compartment pressure in association with closed tibial fractures. The relationship between tissue pressure, compartment, and the distance from the site of the fracture. J Bone Joint Surg Am 1994;76(9):1285–92.
53. Whitesides TE, Haney TC, Morimoto K, et al. Tissue pressure measurements as a determinant for the need of fasciotomy. Clin Orthop Relat Res 1975;(113):43–51.
54. Collinge C, Kuper M. Comparison of three methods for measuring intracompartmental pressure in injured limbs of trauma patients. J Orthop Trauma 2010;24(6):364–8.
55. Hammerberg EM, Whitesides TE, Seiler JG. The reliability of measurement of tissue pressure in compartment syndrome. J Orthopaedic Trauma 2012;26(1):24–31.
56. Whitney A, O'Toole RV, Hui E, et al. Do one-time intracompartmental pressure measurements have a high false-positive rate in diagnosing compartment syndrome? J Trauma Acute Care Surg 2014;76(2):479–83.
57. Nelson JA. Compartment pressure measurements have poor specificity for compartment syndrome in the traumatized limb. J Emerg Med 2013;44(5):1039–44.
58. McQueen M, Gaston P, Court-Brown C. Acute compartment syndrome. Who is at risk? J Bone Joint Surg Br 2000;82(2):200–3.
59. Kuhlmann RS, Cruikshank DP. Maternal trauma during pregnancy. Clin Obstet Gynecol 1994;37(2):274–93.
60. Barraco RD, Chiu WC, Clancy TV, et al. Practice management guidelines for the diagnosis and management of injury in the pregnant patient: the EAST practice management guidelines Work Group. J Trauma Inj Infect Crit Care 2010;69(1):211–4.
61. ACOG educational bulletin. Obstetric aspects of trauma management. Number 251, September 1998 (replaces number 151, January 1991, and Number 161, November 1991). American College of Obstetricians and Gynecologists. Int J Gynaecol Obstet 1999;64(1):87–94.
62. Jain V, Chari R, Maslovitz S, et al. Guidelines for the management of a pregnant trauma patient. J Obstet Gynaecol Can 2015;37(6):553–74.
63. Goodwin TM, Breen MT. Pregnancy outcome and fetomaternal hemorrhage after noncatastrophic trauma. Am J Obstet Gynecol 1990;162(3):665–71.
64. Pearlman MD, Tintinalli JE, Lorenz RP. Blunt trauma during pregnancy. New Engl J Med 1990;323(23):1609–13.

65. Williams JK, McClain L, Rosemurgy AS, et al. Evaluation of blunt abdominal trauma in the third trimester of pregnancy: maternal and fetal considerations. Obstet Gynecol 1990;75(1):33–7.
66. Goodwin H, Holmes JF, Wisner DH. Abdominal ultrasound examination in pregnant blunt trauma patients. J Trauma Inj Infect Crit Care 2001;50(4):689–94.
67. Richards JR, Ormsby EL, Romo MV, et al. Blunt abdominal injury in the pregnant patient: detection with US. Radiology 2004;233(2):463–70.
68. Smith KA, Bryce S. Trauma in the pregnant patient: an evidence-based approach to management. Emerg Med Pract 2013;15(4):1–19.
69. Hahn SA, Lavonas EJ, Mace SE, et al. Clinical policy: critical issues in the initial evaluation and management of patients presenting to the emergency department in early pregnancy. Ann Emerg Med 2012;60(3):381–90.e28.
70. Farmer DL, Adzick NS, Crombleholme WR, et al. Fetal trauma: relation to maternal injury. J Pediatr Surg 1990;25(7):711–4.
71. Lapinsky SE, Kruczynski K, Slutsky AS. Critical care in the pregnant patient. Am J Respir Crit Care Med 1995;152:427–55.
72. Sebring ES, Polesky HF. Fetomaternal hemorrhage: incidence, risk factors, time of occurrence, and clinical effects. Transfusion 1990;30(4):344–57.

# Care of Special Populations in an Observation Unit

## Pediatrics and Geriatrics

Sharon E. Mace, MD

### KEYWORDS

- Pediatrics • Infants and children • Geriatrics • Elderly • Special populations
- Observation medicine • Observation units

### KEY POINTS

- Special populations, such as pediatrics and the elderly, are a large and growing segment of the observation population.
- Special populations are complex, high-risk, vulnerable patients who present unique challenges and can be difficult to assess during a brief emergency department (ED) visit.
- An observation unit stay allows time to arrive at a diagnosis, evaluate, and/or treat these complex patients.
- Patients of all ages from newborns to the elderly with a wide variety of diagnoses can be safely and effectively treated in an ED observation unit.
- Benefits of observation unit care include better or equivalent patient outcomes, decreased cost, decreased lengths of stay, improved ED efficiency, and avoidance of unnecessary inpatient admissions with potential for iatrogenic complications.

## OVERVIEW: PEDIATRIC AND GERIATRIC DEMOGRAPHIC TRENDS AND EMERGENCY DEPARTMENT USE

Children and infants comprise about one-fourth of the population of the United States; 23% are less than 15 year old.[1,2] The elderly ($\geq$65 year old) make up 12% and are the fastest growing segment of the population. By the year 2030, it is estimated that the proportion of the population that is elderly will increase to 20%. These 2 population groups, pediatrics and geriatrics, currently comprise over one-third (37%) of the population and by 2030 will account for almost half (45%).[3]

According to an Institute of Medicine report, over 40% of emergency department (ED) visits are for a pediatric (27%) or geriatric (15%) patients.[4] The rate

Emergency Services Institute, Cleveland Clinic, Department of Emergency Medicine, Cleveland Clinic Lerner College of Medicine, Case Western Reserve University, 9500 Euclid Avenue, E-19, Cleveland, OH 44195, USA
E-mail address: maces@ccf.org

Emerg Med Clin N Am 35 (2017) 685–699
http://dx.doi.org/10.1016/j.emc.2017.03.011
0733-8627/17/© 2017 Elsevier Inc. All rights reserved.

of increase in ED visits is greatest for the elderly population.[5] Within the next 2 decades, the proportion of ED visits by geriatric patients is anticipated to increase to 25%.[3]

---

**Pediatric Vignette**

Sydney White is a 4-year-old girl with a history of asthma brought to the ED by her mother with increased respiratory distress and audible wheezing that started overnight. In the ED, she is febrile to 101.7°F; her pulse oximetry is 94% on room air. Respiratory rate is 45 breaths per minute, and heart rate is 140. She has a clear chest radiograph and tests positive for influenza A. Despite oseltamivir, ibuprofen, acetaminophen, nebulizer therapy, and oral corticosteroids, she shows only mild improvement and still has significant wheezing on pulmonary examination with low-grade fever. She is placed in the ED observation unit (EDOU), where she receives nebulized bronchodilator therapy every 3 hours, around-the-clock antipyretics, intravenous (IV) hydration, and serial examinations. Re-evaluation the next morning shows her work of breathing has significantly improved. She is discharged 17 hours after ED presentation with prescriptions for a short-term course of oral corticosteroids, a course of oseltamivir, and follow-up with her pediatrician the next day.

---

## INTRODUCTION: PEDIATRICS

Infants and children are a higher-risk, more vulnerable, and more complex patient population compared with adults. They can be challenging to assess, make a definitive diagnosis in, and institute appropriate treatment for.[6,7] Obtaining a history can be difficult, especially in preverbal infants/children because of limited ability to communicate symptoms and express experience of pain. Nonspecific complaints such as not eating, fever, vomiting, and caregiver concerns that "they are just not their usual self" are common. Physical examination may have subtle or limited findings. Children and adolescents may be reluctant to provide an accurate history for fear of punishment. Depending on their developmental stage and/or behavioral issues, the pediatric patient may not always be cooperative (**Box 1**). Physiologic and anatomic differences place the pediatric patient at greater risk. These patients have less physiologic reserve, greater susceptibility to infection, less developed organ systems (eg, liver, kidneys, and central nervous system), greater susceptibility to traumatic injury (eg, proportionally greater head size to rest of body, smaller size, weight, height, muscle mass, fat, subcutaneous tissue), greater reliance on heart rate rather than stroke volume to maintain cardiac output, and higher baseline respiratory rate, heart rate, oxygen consumption, and metabolic rate (see **Box 1**).

Most children and infants seen in the ED will have only a mild illness or injury. Differentiating serious limb- or life-threatening illness/injury from a benign condition can be difficult and sometimes impossible in a brief ED encounter.[8] Fever can be due to a viral upper respiratory infection (URI), bacteremia, meningitis, or sepsis. Abdominal pain can be present in gastroenteritis or appendicitis. Vomiting may be the only symptom of gastroenteritis, but, it may also be seen in diabetic ketoacidosis (DKA), central nervous system disease, and in surgical conditions of the abdomen (eg, intussusception, malrotation). There are nearly 15 million children with special health care needs (CSHCN) in the United States. This comprises nearly one-fifth (19.8%) of all children nationally from birth to 17 years of age.[9] Caring for CSHCN who have multiple medical problems adds another layer of complexity that requires significant time and/or resources to assess, diagnose, and initiate treatment in. Nonaccidental trauma should be considered in any pediatric complaint. Malpractice claims attest to the complexity of evaluating pediatric patients in the ED. Meningitis, followed by appendicitis, is the most frequent diagnosis in pediatric malpractice claims.[10]

**Box 1**
**Factors contributing to the difficulty in assessment and the increased vulnerability of the pediatric patient**

*History and social factors*

- Frequently present with nonspecific complaints
- Inability or limited ability to communicate (preverbal children and infants: inability to rely symptoms or pain, or give any history)
- Limited mobility
- Limited cognition
- Caregiver dependence
- Developmental stages: affects motor and verbal skills, psychological development and behavior
- Concern for radiation exposure (increased lifetime risk of malignancy)
- Behavioral or mental health issues: autistic, attention deficit hyperactivity syndrome, drug use
- Special health care needs or those with disabilities

*Physiology and anatomy*

- Subtle physical examination findings
- Increased susceptibility to infection
- Limited physiologic reserve
- Smaller total blood volume, same amount of blood loss may cause shock in a child or infant but not in an adult
- Airway: smaller diameter, larynx more anterior and cephalad; cricoid cartilage is narrowest part of airway, smaller lung volumes
- Immature kidneys: lesser ability to concentrate urine and purify toxins
- Immature liver: lesser ability to handle toxins
- Immature central nervous system: for example, not fully myelinated until 2 years of age
- Increased body surface area relative to weight, leads to a predisposition to dehydration and hypothermia
- Lesser total muscle mass
- Lesser total amount of body fat
- Thinner skin: affects absorption of drugs and toxins via the dermal route
- Smaller size including smaller stature or height
- Lesser weight
- Proportionately larger head to body ratio, leads to increased susceptibility to head trauma
- Increased susceptibility to general trauma compared with an adult: less protective fat, subcutaneous tissue, muscle to cushion internal organs from trauma and more likely to be thrown further since smaller size and weight, different types of traumatic injuries
- Increased heart rate in infants and young children compared with adults
- Greater reliance on increase in heart rate rather than stroke volume to maintain cardiac output
- Increased respiratory rate in infants and young children compared with adults
- Increased metabolic rate
- Increased oxygen consumption

The use of EDOUs allows time for more extended evaluation beyond the initial ED visit alone to determine which illnesses/injuries are more serious and may require inpatient admission. Another benefit of observation is the ability to perform serial examinations and avoid use of computed tomography (CT) scanning for conditions such as minor head trauma and abdominal pain.

---

**Geriatric Vignette**

Walter Jenkins is an 84-year-old man with a history of diabetes, chronic obstructive pulmonary disease (COPD) and mild dementia who lives with his wife and presents via ambulance to the ED after a fall from standing. Further history from the patient and his wife reveal several weeks of generalized weakness and 2 other falls during the period. In the ED, his trauma evaluation is reassuring, and laboratory analysis reveals serum glucose of 288 mg/dL, serum sodium level of 128 mEq/L, and pyuria. He also appears unsteady on his feet and mildly dehydrated on examination, but vital signs are normal. He is placed in the EDOU, where he receives an initial dose of intravenous antibiotics and hydration as well as endocrine, case management, and physical therapy consultations. The next day, he is transitioned to an oral antibiotic regimen with an improving sodium level and is safely ambulating with the assistance of a new walker. The endocrine team recommends a new diabetes regimen, and case management arranges for a visiting nurse to visit his home the next day. He is discharged home with a follow-up appointment scheduled with his primary care physician within 1 week.

---

## INTRODUCTION: GERIATRICS

Many factors make the elderly a high-risk, complex, and more vulnerable population.[11] These variables may be related to impairment of the senses, physical limitations, impaired cognition, psychosocial issues, and medical conditions (**Box 2**).

Many of the elderly have contagious conditions, are chronically ill, or may be in palliative or hospice care. They often need devices for assistance with mobility (eg, canes, walkers, or wheelchairs). Because of impaired mobility, they are at risk for falls, which often necessitate an ED visit. They may need assistance with the activities of daily living (ADLs): bathing, dressing, eating, toileting, transferring, and mobility. Should there be a problem or interference with the ADLs, such as poor oral intake causing dehydration, it often leads to an ED visit and admission. Elderly ED patients are more complex, use more resources, and have longer ED lengths of stay (LOS).[12]

Hospitalization of the geriatric patient frequently leads to iatrogenic complications related to the hospitalization itself: medication errors, acute psychosis, nosocomial infections, venous thromboembolic events, falls, and deconditioning. Thus, avoiding unnecessary hospital admission is a desired outcome. EDOUs serve to provide additional care while preventing these potentially avoidable admissions.[11]

Many of the common conditions evaluated and treated in EDOUs are seen more frequently in the elderly:

Cardiac—chest pain, mild congestive heart failure (CHF), atrial fibrillation
Respiratory—COPD, pneumonia, acute bronchitis
Neurologic—transient ischemic attack (TIA)
Metabolic—diabetes complications, hyperglycemia, hypoglycemia, diabetic ketoacidosis
Infections—cellulitis
Syncope[11–15]

It has been suggested that many of the common presenting symptoms of the elderly in the ED are well suited to EDOU evaluation and treatment, including falls and injuries, altered mental status, and acute abdominal pain.[11]

---

**Box 2**
**Factors contributing to the difficulty in assessment and the increased vulnerability of the geriatric patient**

*History and social factors*

- Impaired communication: aphasia (such as s/p stroke), incoherent or and/or disoriented (delirium, dementia)
- More complex psycho-social needs
- Fall risk: predisposition to falls because of impaired balance, poor vision, decreased muscle strength, limited exercise tolerance, deconditioning
- Inability to ambulate or difficulty in walking: need for assistive devices (eg, canes, walkers, wheelchairs), bedridden
- Limited cognition: Alzheimer disease, Parkinson disease, dementia, stroke patients
- Difficulties with the activities of daily living: bathing, dressing, eating, toileting, transferring, mobility

*Physiology and anatomy*

- Chronic health conditions
- Sensory impairment: decreased hearing or deaf, vision impairment or blindness
- Medication dependent
- Oxygen dependent: COPD, heart failure
- Technology dependent: cardiac – pacemaker, AICD, LVAD; respiratory: BiPAP. CPAP, ventilators, suctioning, tracheostomy: renal: dialysis: hemodialysis or peritoneal dialysis
- Wound/stoma care
- Urologic devices: Foley catheters, suprapubic catheters, nephrostomy tubes
- Feeding tubes/Special diets
- Monitoring: diabetics – blood sugar, hypertension – check of blood pressure

---

## THE EVIDENCE FOR EMERGENCY DEPARTMENT OBSERVATION UNIT CARE OF GERIATRIC PATIENTS

In a US study comparing EDOU nongeriatric with geriatric patients, chest pain was the leading diagnosis for both age groups, although the other diagnoses most frequently seen differed between the groups.[16] Admission rates were significantly higher for geriatric versus nongeriatric patients (26.1% vs 18.5%). Thirty-day return visit rate was higher for geriatric versus nongeriatric patients (9.4% vs 7.6%). LOS was significantly longer for geriatric (15.8 hours, 95% confidence interval [CI] 15.7–16) versus nongeriatric patients (14.5 hours, 95% CI 14.3–14.5), although the geriatric patients' LOS was similar to those previously reported; EDOU mean LOS was 15.3 hours,[17] and median LOS 19.5 hours.[13]

Another US study evaluated EDOU patients with coronary artery disease (CAD), defined as previous myocardial infarction, presence of coronary stent, or coronary bypass graft. There was a significant difference in the admission rate from the EDOU between geriatric and nongeriatric cohorts (31.3% vs 20.8%, $P = .013$). Geriatric patients had a significantly higher proportion of chronic conditions that increased risk for acute coronary syndrome: hypertension, diabetes, renal dysfunction and pre-existing heart disease. A history of CAD and renal dysfunction were independent predictors of inpatient admission.[14]

A study conducted in Wales by Harrop and Morgan[18] evaluated 100 geriatric (>70 years) patients in a short-stay unit (SSU) when no geriatric inpatient hospital beds were available. The overall SSU discharge rate of 72% is consistent with typical US EDOU discharge rates of 80%.[17] The discharge rate in the Wales study was likely lower than would be expected, because although some patients met inpatient criteria, they were placed in an EDOU and were not separated out from the other patients for data analysis.[18]

The most common diagnoses of geriatric patients in an EDOU study from the United Kingdom were: falls/injury 45%, infections 11%, constipation 5%, collapse 4%, stroke/TIA 3%, social 2%, and others 30%.[15] By diagnosis, admission rates were: falls/injuries 35%, infections 15%, collapse 6%, constipation 5%, stroke/transient ischemic attack (TIA) 3%, social 2% and others 34%. Overall, 71% of patients were discharged home and were usually discharged within 24 hours.

### Advanced Age as a Predictor of Inpatient Admission from the Emergency Department Observation Unit

Increasing age was a predictor of requiring inpatient hospital admission from the EDOU in some studies[19,20] but not in others.[21,22] A study of EDOU patients found that frailty and sociodemographic factors and not geriatric age are predictors of inpatient hospital admission. Frailty (measured by the Katz index of independence in daily living), disability insurance, and lower education were predictors of inpatient hospital admission from an EDOU. Age, race, gender, obesity as indicated by weight (body mass index), diagnosis category (surgical or medical), marital status, insurance, medical history (comorbidities [eg, number of, Charleston index], number of medications, anticoagulant use, antiplatelet use), smoking, and alcohol use were not predictors. Illicit drug use within 30 days was a predictor of Inpatient admission. Laboratory values that were not predictive of admission were hemoglobin, sodium, and creatinine; leukocytosis and hypercalcemia (although none of the patients included were cancer patients) were predictive.[22]

### Pediatric Observation Medicine: Historical Perspective

Pediatric EDs in the 1970s and 1980s often designated a room(s) in the ED, and they were used to treat children/infants of all ages, even very young infants, with all types of diagnoses for a short time period. These forerunners of today's pediatric EDOUs were termed ED holding room (HR), holding unit (HU) or SSU. They reported the same benefits of pediatric observation that are found today: significantly shorter LOS, lower costs, decreased inpatient admissions, fewer returns to the ED (reoccurrence rates), and high parent satisfaction. The most common diagnoses were similar to types of pediatric patients treated in our EDOUs today: respiratory, gastroenteritis/dehydration, neurologic, trauma, ingestion, and infections.[23–27]

### EVIDENCE FOR EMERGENCY DEPARTMENT OBSERVATION UNIT CARE OF PEDIATRIC PATIENTS

### Diagnoses/types of Pediatric Patients Placed in an Emergency Department Observation Unit

In studies of pediatric EDOU patients, respiratory illnesses (most commonly asthma) are the most frequent diagnosis, followed by gastroenteritis/dehydration, whether in a pediatric hospital,[28,29] academic general hospital,[8] or a community hospital.[30] In 1 study, these 2 categories accounted for about 80% of all EDOU patients: respiratory infections (asthma, pneumonia, bronchiolitis, croup) at 41.4% and gastrointestinal illnesses (gastroenteritis/dehydration, abdominal pain) 38%.[29] The most frequent diagnoses in a community hospital for EDOU patients were asthma (27%), gastroenteritis/dehydration (16%), infectious diseases (12%), and bronchiolitis (9%).[30] Other common diagnoses, whether in pediatric hospitals, academic tertiary general, or community hospitals are pneumonia, croup, neurologic (eg, seizures), infections, fever, trauma, and ingestions.[8,28–31]

### Ages of Children and Infants Placed in the Emergency Department Observation Unit

All ages of pediatric patients, even neonates, have been successfully treated in the EDOU. Reports indicate most pediatric EDOU patients are infants/toddlers rather than adolescents. The mean age in years reported in 3 separate studies from EDOUs at children's hospitals was 1.8,[32] 4.4,[29] and 4.7.[33] In another study, the mean age was 6 years, but 31% of the EDOU patients were less than 2 year old.[34] A community hospital reported placing patients from 0 to 18 years of age in observation status,[30] and a tertiary academic hybrid EDOU accepted all ages of pediatric patients except for neonates (<30 days).[8]

Studies performed at children's hospitals in the United States have provided statistics regarding age based on specific diagnoses. The average age of treatment for intussusception was 19 months in a study by Bajaj and colleagues[35] and 1.3 years in another study by Adekunle-Ojo and colleagues.[36] The mean age reported for the treatment of asthmatics in the observation unit was 3.9 years (Marks).[37] The median age reported for treatment of neonatal hyperbilirubinemia was only 5 days.[38]

In a report by Mallory and colleagues,[32] the median age for the treatment of dehydration and gastroenteritis was 1.2 years (mean 1.8 years). Other diagnoses where the mean age has been reported include croup (1.5 years),[39] poison exposures (2.3 years),[40] and closed head injuries (5.2 years).[41] These results indicate that infants, even neonates several days old, can be successfully treated in an EDOU. The fact that the studies were performed in various settings demonstrates that the care can be provided in EDOUs located in community hospitals and academic hospitals, as well as children's hospitals.

### Emergency Department Observation Unit Length of Stay for Pediatric Patients

Reported EDOU LOS (all diagnoses included) for pediatric patients is similar to or less than for adults, with a reported national mean LOS of 15.3 hours and a median LOS of 19.5 hours.[13,17] Furthermore, reported mean EDOU LOS of all diagnoses based on type of center where care was provided was 11.2 hours for academic tertiary general hybrid EDOU,[42] 13 hours for community hospital,[30] and 13 to 16.6 hours for children's hospitals.[28,33,34,41,43] Reported median LOS was 12 hours for community hospitals and 8.8 to 15.5 hours for children's hospitals.[31,44]

LOS varies based on diagnosis. Reported LOS for specific diagnoses was intussusception 7.2 hours (mean)[35] and 16 hours (median),[36] poison exposures 15.0 hours (mean),[40] asthma 16.5 hours (median),[43] neonatal hyperbilirubinemia 17.8 hours (median),[38] and closed head injury 15.5 hours (median).[41]

### Pediatric Patients Placed in Emergency Department Observation Unit from the Emergency Department

In studies of pediatric EDOUs, the percent of pediatric ED patients placed in an EDOU ranged from 2.9% to 4.8%.[28,32–34] The percent of ED patients that were direct inpatient admissions is reported as 6.3% to 7.4%.[28,34] Thus, about 88% to 91% of ED patients are discharged; 6% to 7% are admitted, and 3% to 5% are placed in the EDOU. This compares with about 10% of adult ED patients who are placed in EDOUs.[45]

A spike in pediatric EDOU visits during the winter months of January through March, coinciding with an increase in respiratory infections (eg, pneumonia, croup, bronchiolitis, influenza), has previously been noted.[8,31]

### Inpatient Admission Rates from the Emergency Department Observation Unit

Inpatient admission rates for EDOU pediatric patients (all diagnoses) range from 12% to 20.3%,[28,31,33] similar to adult inpatient admission rates from the EDOU of 15% to 20%.[4] Admission rates of EDOU patients by diagnosis at a children's hospital were hematochezia 60%, viral pneumonia 46%, bronchiolitis 43%, ventriculoperitoneal shunt issues 40%, bacterial pneumonia 30%, abdominal pain 27%, fever 26%, cyclic vomiting 25%, rule out sepsis 22%, and asthma 22%.[31] This compares to reported admission rates by diagnosis at a community hospital: pneumonia 50%, bronchiolitis 46%, infection 33%, asthma 23% and gastroenteritis 21% with an overall admission rate of 25%.[30]

### Factors Associated with Inpatient Admission

Studies show mixed results regarding age (eg, very young infants) and gender as predictors of inpatient admission from the EDOU. Increased resource utilization is a predictor of inpatient admission from the EDOU. In 1 study, predictors of inpatient admission from the EDOU were resource use: intravenous fluids or medications, cardiorespiratory monitoring, respiratory therapy, supplemental oxygen, subspecialty consultations, and esophageal foreign bodies. Age, gender, ethnicity, and insurance status were not associated with hospital admission.[33] Factors associated with inpatient admission in a study of patients placed in an EDOU for asthma were female gender ($P = .03$), fever (T $>38.5°C$) ($P<.01$), and oxygen requirement at the end of ED treatment ($P<.01$).[43] Another study of asthma patients placed in an EDOU found no difference in hospital admission rates for age groups (ie, very young infants did not have higher admission rates, and the highest admission rates were for respiratory diseases).[24] A French study reported age less than 1 year, need for intravenous fluids or medications, CT scan or MRI, and need for cardiorespiratory monitoring were associated with increased risk of admission.[46]

## THE INTERNATIONAL EXPERIENCE: ALL DIAGNOSES

The international experience is similar to the US findings. An Australian study performed after opening EDOUs at a children's hospital and at a general teaching hospital found annual cost savings of more than $1 million and approximately $300,000, respectively. Additionally, there were decreased inpatient admissions (14.7% and 10.3%, respectively) and high parental satisfaction.[47] A French study of pediatric short stay observation unit (SSOU) patients (all diagnoses), including those waiting for an inpatient bed and observation patients, reported a drop in the previously seen annual 5% increase in hospital admission rate from the ED in spite of a continuing rise in the ED census.[48]

A survey of clinicians placing patients in an SSOU in France demonstrated how the use of the observation unit helped to decrease inpatient hospitalizations. The researchers queried the likely disposition of pediatric patients if the option for placement in the SSOU was not available. The disposition decision would have been: inpatient hospitalization (77%), transfer to another hospital if inpatient beds were unavailable (7%), discharge home (10%), prolonged ED stay (4%), and unknown (2%).[49] Pediatric patients are frequently included in EDOUs in international settings. A survey of accident & emergency departments in the United Kingdom found that one-fourth of short-stay wards included children (ie, hybrid units with children and adults in the same EDOU).[50]

## BENEFITS OF OBSERVATION MEDICINE

The benefits of observation medicine noted for adults have been documented for - infants and children: decreased LOS, earlier time to initiation of treatment (with the presumption that earlier time to treatment improves outcomes), decreased costs, decreased inpatient admissions, shortened ED LOS, and high family satisfaction.[23,25–28,35,37,38,39,47,48]

Multiple studies demonstrate these findings. Compared with inpatients, patients who have undergone uncomplicated barium enema for intussusception at a children's hospital had a significantly decreased mean LOS with placement in the EDOU compared with inpatient admission (7.1 hours vs 22.7 hours, $P<.001$).[35] Inpatient versus EDOU treatment of neonates (median age 5 days) with hyperbilirubinemia treated with phototherapy has also been compared. Median time (hours) to phototherapy was shorter in the EDOU group (1.6 hours vs 6.7 hours, $P<.001$), and LOS was significantly shorter for EDOU patients (17.8 hours vs 41.8 hours, $P<.001$).[38] These 2 studies demonstrate that even young infants and neonates can be effectively and safely managed in an EDOU.

Significant cost savings were documented in 2 older randomized controlled trials (RCTs). In the RCT comparing inpatient versus holding room (HR) treatment of asthma patients, the mean LOS was less for those cared for in the HR compared with on an inpatient service (45.6 hours vs 11.8 hours). Additionally, this care was given in the HR at 44% lower cost than that given as an inpatient.[25] In an RCT comparing care provided to infants with dehydration, the mean LOS was ten-fold longer for inpatients than for in the EDOU (9.9 hours vs 103.2 hours). The mean cost was six-fold greater for inpatients than for HR patients ($P<.00001$).[27] More recent studies also noted significant cost savings with the use of an EDOU compared with inpatient units.[28,37,39]

A decrease in inpatient admissions frequently accompanies the opening of an EDOU.[37,48,51] In an Australian study, in the year following the opening of an SSU, inpatient admissions decreased by 10.3% at the general teaching hospital and 14.7% at the children's hospital.[37] At a US children's hospital, inpatient admissions for asthma from the ED decreased from 9.5% to 7.7% during the year following the opening of an SSU. It further decreased to 7.0% during the second year after opening. The overall decrease was 2.5% after 2 years, although other variables may have influenced the decrease.[37]

Cator and colleagues[44] sought to determine if the option to provide ED observational care within the ED itself, a so-called virtual EDOU, resulted in reduced admission rates and length of stay. Prior to initiation of the virtual EDOU, care protocols including inclusion/exclusion criteria and order sets were written for 9 common pediatric conditions: respiratory (asthma, bronchiolitis, pneumonia), dehydration, cellulitis/abscess, head injury, ingestion, allergic reaction, seizures, DKA, and headache. No additional ED bed capacity or staffing was added with implementation of the virtual EDOU. After opening the EDOU, a reduction in the rate of observation-eligible patients was not found, but other benefits were noted. The LOS was significantly shorter for patients discharged from the ED (5.6 hours vs 5.1 hours, $P<.001$) with a nonsignificant decrease in ED LOS for patients admitted to an inpatient unit (6.0 hours vs 5.8 hours, $P = .41$). It is possible that the failure to significantly decrease LOS for ED admitted patients is due to lack of ability to influence inpatient bed availability.

Rentz and colleagues performed a satisfaction survey among clinicians (pediatricians, family practitioners, pediatric subspecialists) who had patients cared for in a pediatric EDOU located within a children's hospital. The provider's satisfaction was measured using a 4-point Likert scale. They found high satisfaction rates in clinicians of all types surveyed. The median Likert score was 4 in each of the categories assessed (mean ± standard deviation [SD]): clinician's overall satisfaction (3.63 ± 0.79), notification (3.33 ± 0.88), quality of care (3.70 ± 0.78), and parental satisfaction (mean 3.49 ± 0.79).[52]

### Mixed Adult–Pediatric Observation Unit

Most EDOUs provide care for pediatric or adult patients but not both. In some instances, however, care may be provided to a mixed population of children and adults. There is no evidence comparing the care provided in these mixed units with age-restricted units. An academic tertiary care hospital hybrid EDOU, which accepted both adult and pediatric patients, cared for 5714 patients during the period reported from 1996 to 2000. Most patients placed in observation were adults, with only 6.7% under the age of 17. The average LOS for pediatric patients (age <17 years) was 11.2 hours. For adult patients 17 to 65 years of age, the average LOS was 15.1 hours, and for geriatric patients the average LOS was 15.4 hours.[42]

## SIMILARITIES BETWEEN PEDIATRIC AND ADULT OBSERVATION MEDICINE

The principles of observation medicine apply to any population. EDOU patients belong to one (or any combination) of 3 categories: they have an undifferentiated chief complaint that needs further evaluation to determine if they have a condition warranting inpatient admission; they have a known condition needing further treatment, or they need monitoring due to risk of development of some dangerous condition.[8] Examples of those with an unknown diagnosis requiring further testing to determine if they have a serious condition warranting inpatient admission are an adult with chest pain undergoing stress testing to determine if he or she an ischemic heart disease or a pediatric patient undergoing serial abdominal examinations to determine if he or she has appendicitis. Patients with asthma requiring further treatment with nebulized bronchodilators fall into the group of patients in whom the diagnosis is known but further treatment is required before discharge can be considered. Cardiac monitoring with pulse oximetry is frequently done for higher risk patients with syncope or in a pediatric patient with accidental ingestion.

Although specific protocols can be written for any diagnosis, the same tenets are applicable to any age group or diagnosis. Inclusion criteria include stable patients of low to moderate acuity or low to moderate severity (those who do not belong in an intensive care unit) and who do not need intensive nursing care or intensive physician care and have at least an 80% likelihood of being discharged within 24 to 48 hours.[8]

Protocols and order sets are an essential part of any EDOU and should focus on common complaints. There should be clear inclusion and exclusion criteria to ensure appropriate patient selection for the EDOU.[7] Adult patients tend to have more specialized testing such as stress tests, echocardiograms, CT scans and MRIs, while such use of ancillary services including radiology and cardiology is much less in the pediatric patients.[8]

The potential advantages of observation medicine, including improved patient outcomes, shorter LOS, lower cost, fewer missed diagnoses with better risk management and decreased liability, decreased ED crowding, improved ED throughput with decreased ED LOS, increased patient/family satisfaction, and decreased hospital admissions are the same no matter the age of the patient.[6–8]

## DIFFERENCES BETWEEN PEDIATRIC AND ADULT OBSERVATION MEDICINE

Obviously, the most common diagnoses cared for in EDOUs differ between adult and pediatric patients. In a combined adult and pediatric observation unit at an academic tertiary care referral hospital, the most common pediatric diagnoses were asthma, dehydration, gastroenteritis, pneumonia, abdominal pain, seizures, bronchiolitis, croup, poisonings, and trauma. The most common adult diagnoses were chest pain, abdominal pain, asthma, heart failure, COPD, syncope, TIA, ureterolithiasis, pyelonephritis, and skin and soft tissue infections such as cellulitis.[8]

Pediatric EDOU census has a seasonal variation. In the northern hemisphere, there is an upsurge in the EDOU census in the late fall/early winter during the cold and influenza season and a lesser upsurge in late winter/early spring when gastrointestinal pathogens, such as rotavirus, are in the community. In the summer, there is an increase in the traumatic injuries cared for in the EDOU, coinciding with the summer school recess. In adults, there is much less monthly and seasonal variation. Chest pain and other common adult diagnoses (eg, atrial fibrillation, syncope, and TIA) are much more consistent, with the exception of kidney stones, which are more frequent during the hot summer months.[8]

Equipment, supplies, and medications differ for pediatric and adult EDOU patients. The adult EDOU is primarily a cardiac monitoring unit, with the most common diagnoses being chest pain, syncope, atrial fibrillation, and heart failure. Patients with respiratory complaints including pneumonia and exacerbations of asthma or COPD are also frequently placed in EDOUs. Conversely, the pediatric EDOU is primarily a respiratory unit followed by an isolation unit, with the most frequent diagnoses being asthma, bronchiolitis and croup, followed by infectious processes such as gastroenteritis with vomiting and diarrhea resulting in dehydration, respiratory infections, and cellulitis. This has implications for equipment; adults need cardiac monitoring, repeat electrocardiograms (ECGs) and repeat blood draws for cardiac enzymes versus pediatric patients who mainly need respiratory care and intravenous fluids. For the pharmacy, cardiac medications from diuretics to antihypertensive and antiplatelet/antithrombotic medications tend to be ordered; aerosols, steroids, intravenous fluids, antiemetics, and to a lesser degree antibiotics are more frequently ordered in the pediatric EDOU.[6,8]

## UNDER-UTILIZATION OF OBSERVATION IN THE US AND CANADIAN HEALTH CARE SYSTEMS

Several studies indicate observation medicine is underutilized in the United States and internationally. A US study suggested that 70% of pediatric asthmatics could be treated in an alternative setting such as a pediatric observation unit, rather than as inpatients.[53] Similarly, "nearly all pediatric patients with simple acute gastroenteritis" could also be treated in an observation unit instead of as an inpatient.[54] Similar estimates have been published in an editorial in a US pediatric health care journal that estimated two-thirds to three-fourths of pediatric asthmatics could receive treatment in an EDOU instead of being admitted to an inpatient ward.[54] According to national data regarding hospitalized children, one-third of pediatric admissions in the United States are short stays with patients spending 1 night or fewer in an inpatient bed.[55] According to 1 study, only 18% of pediatric patients eligible for observation care were placed in a virtual EDOU with protocolized care plans.[44]

The American Academy of Pediatrics report on observation units, published in 2012 and reaffirmed in 2015, stated that "(ED)OUs may have an especially important effect on pediatric inpatient admissions, in part, because a significant number of inpatient admissions among children are of relatively short duration."[56] A Canadian health policy report in 1996 concluded one-fourth (25%) of adults and 39% of pediatric patients could be treated in an EDOU instead of being hospitalized as inpatients.[57]

## EMERGENCY DEPARTMENT OBSERVATION UNIT CARE OF GERIATRIC PATIENTS

Although the number of studies of geriatric patients cared for in an EDOU is far less than for pediatric patients, there were over 9000 geriatric patients included in only 4 studies. Elderly patients, just like pediatric patients, can be successfully evaluated and treated in EDOUs with the same benefits: equivalent or better outcomes than if an inpatient, inpatient admission rates comparable to national averages, LOS less than 24 hours, and similar LOS to national norms. Chest pain is the most frequent diagnosis for geriatric and nongeriatric adults, although the relative frequency of other diagnoses differed. The elderly may have somewhat different reasons for placement in the EDOU; they still have overall good results.

A short EDOU stay versus a longer inpatient admission may avoid some of the complications, especially in the elderly, experienced by hospital inpatients ranging from medication error, falls, deconditioning, psychosis, and venous thromboembolic events.

## SUMMARY

Infants and children and the elderly comprise a large and growing (especially the elderly) segment of the US population. Currently, these groups comprise over a third (37%) of the US population and are projected to be nearly half (45%) of the population by 2030. Similarly both of these groups account for 42% of ED visits, with estimates to be 52% of ED visits within the next 20 years. Although both pediatric and geriatric patients tend to be more complex, higher risk, more vulnerable, and more difficult to evaluate, they have both been successfully managed in an EDOU. Within the United States and internationally, the benefits of observation medicine have been documented in these 2 age groups: equivalent or better patient outcomes, decreasing missed diagnoses, better risk management, shorter LOS, decreased costs, earlier initiation of treatment, increased patient/family satisfaction, increased ED turnaround time with shorter ED LOS and decreased crowding, and avoidance of inpatient admissions with the many associated complications. Based on the success of observation medicine, and recognizing the growth of these special populations, it is likely that observation medicine will be expanding in the future, especially within the pediatric and geriatric populations. Future studies should be able to provide further evidence regarding the value of observation medicine in these 2 diverse population age groups.

## REFERENCES

1. National Commission on Children and Disasters 2010 Report to the President and Congress. Available at: http://archive.ahrq.gov/prep/nccdreport/index.html. Accessed October 1, 2016.
2. Kailes JI, Enders A. Moving beyond "special needs." A function-based framework for emergency management and planning. J Disabil Policy Stud 2007; 17(4):231–7.
3. Fernandez LS, Byard D, Lin C-C, et al. Frail elderly as disaster victims: emergency management strategies. Prehosp Disaster Med 2002;17(2):67–74.
4. Institute of Medicine. IOM report: the future of emergency care in the United States Health System. Acad Emerg Med 2006;13(10):1081–5.

5. Wilber ST, Gerson LW, Terrell KM, et al. Geriatric Emergency Medicine and the 2006 Institute of Medicine reports from the Committee on the Future of Emergency Care in the U.S. Health System. Acad Emerg Med 2006;13(12):1345–51.
6. Mace SE. Pediatric observation medicine. In: Mace SE, editor. Observation medicine principles and protocols. Cambridge (United Kingdom): Cambridge Medical Publishers; 2016. p. 291–9.
7. Ojo A. Pediatric observation medicine at a Children's Hospital. In: Mace SE, editor. Observation medicine principles and protocols. Cambridge (United Kingdom): Cambridge Medical Publishers; 2016. p. 300–3.
8. Mace SE. Pediatric observation medicine. Emerg Med Clin North Am 2001;19(1): 239–54.
9. 2011/2012 National survey of children with special health care needs. Data Resource Center for Child & Adolescent Health. A project of the Child and Adolescent Health Measurement Initiative. Available at: www.childhealthdata. org. Accessed September 30, 2016.
10. Selbst SM, Friedman MJ, Singh SB. Epidemiology nd etiology of malpractice lawsuits involving children in US emergency departments and urgent care centers. Pediatr Emereg Care 2005;21(3):165–9.
11. Hustey FM. Geriatric observation medicine. In: Mace SE, editor. Observation medicine principles and protocols. Cambridge (United Kingdom): Cambridge Medical Publishers; 2016. p. 304–8.
12. Strange GR, Chen EH. Use of emergency departments by elder patients: a five-year follow-up study. Acad Emerg Med 1998;5(12):1157–63.
13. Osborne A, Weston J, Wheatley M, et al. Characteristics of hospital observation services: a society of cardiovascular patient care survey. Crit Pathw Cardiol 2013; 12(2):45–8.
14. Madsen TE, Bledsoe J, Bossart P. Appropriately screened geriatric chest pain patients in an observation unit are not admitted at a higher rate than nongeriatric patients. Crit Pathw Cardiol 2008;7(4):245–7.
15. Khan SA, Millington H, Miskelly FG. Benefits of an accident and emergency short stay ward in the staged hospital care of elderly patients. J Accid Emerg Med 1997;14(3):151–2.
16. Ross MA, Compton S, Richardson D, et al. The use and effectiveness of an emergency department observation unit for elderly patients. Ann Emerg Med 2003; 41(5):668–77.
17. Mace SE, Graff L, Mikhail M, et al. A national survey of observation units in the United States. Am J Emerg Med 2003;21(7):529–33.
18. Harrop SN, Morgan WJ. Emergency care of the elderly in the short-stay ward of the accident and emergency department. Arch Emerg Med 1985;2:141–7.
19. Napoli AM, Mullins PM, Pines JM. Predictors of hospital admission after ED observation unit care. Am J Emerg Med 2014;32:1405–7.
20. Casalino E, Wargon M, Peroziello A, et al. Predictive factors for longer length of stay in an emergency department: a prospective multicentre study evaluating the impact of age, patient's clinical acuity and complexity, and care pathways. Emerg Med J 2014;31(5):361–8.
21. Caterino JM, Hoover EM, Moseley MG. Effect of advanced age and vital signs on admission from an ED observation unit. Am J Emerg Med 2013;31(1):1–7.
22. Zdradzinski MJ, Phelan MP, Mace SE. Impact of frailty and sociodemographic factors on hospital admission from an emergency department observation unit. Am J Med Qual 2016;21. 106286061664477.

23. Gururaj VJ, Allen JE, Russo RM. Short stay in an outpatient department: an alternative to hospitalization. Am J Dis Child 1972;123(2):128–32.
24. Ellerstein NS, Sullivan TD. Observation unit in children's hospital; adjunct to delivery and teaching of ambulatory pediatric care. N Y State J Med 1980;80(11): 1684–6.
25. Willert C, David AT, Herman JJ, et al. Short-term holding room treatment of asthmatics. J Pediatr 1985;106:707–11.
26. O'Brien SR, Hein EW, Sly RM. Treatment of acute asthmatic attacks in a holding unit of a pediatric emergency room. Ann Allergy 1980;45(3):159–1162.
27. Listernick R, Zieserl E, Davis AT. Outpatient oral rehydration in the United States. Am J Dis Child 1986;140(3):211–5.
28. Wiley JF, Friday JH, Nowakowski T, et al. Observation units: the role of an outpatient extended treatment site in pediatric care. Pediatr Emerg Care 1998;14(6):444–7.
29. LeDuc K, Haley-Andrews S, Rannie M. An observation unit in a pediatric emergency department: One children's hospital's experience. J Emerg Nurs 2002; 28(5):407–13.
30. Crocetti MT, Barone MA, Amin DD, et al. Pediatric observation status beds on an inpatient unit: an integrated care model. Pediatr Emerg Care 2004;20(1):17–21.
31. Zebrack M, Kadish H, Nelson D. The Pediatric Hybrid Observation Unit: An Analysis of 6477 Consecutive Patient Encounters. Pediatrics 2005;115(5):e535–42.
32. Mallory MD, Kadish H, Zebrack M, et al. Use of a pediatric observation unit for treatment of children with dehydration caused by gastroenteritis. Pediatr Emerg Care 2006;22(1):1–6.
33. Alpern ER, Calello DP, Windreich R, et al. Utilization and unexpected hospitalization rates of a pediatric emergency department 23-hour observation unit. Pediatr Emerg Care 2008;24(9):589–94.
34. Scribano PV, Wiley JF, Platt K. Use of an observation unit by a pediatric emergency department for common pediatric illnesses. Pediatr Emerg Care 2001; 17(5):321–3.
35. Bajaj L, Roback MG. Postreduction management of intussusception in a children's hospital emergency department. Pediatrics 2003;112(6):1302–7.
36. Adekunle-Ojo AO, Craig AM, Ma L, et al. Intussusception: postreduction fasting is not necessary to prevent complications and recurrences in the emergency department observation unit. Pediatr Emerg Care 2011;27(10):897–9.
37. Marks MK, Lovejoy FH, Rutherford PA, et al. Impact of a short stay unit on asthma patients admitted to a tertiary pediatric hospital. Qual Management Health Care 1997;6(1):14–22.
38. Adekunle-Ojo AO, Smitherman HF, Parker R, et al. Managing well-appearing neonates with hyperbilirubinemia in the emergency department observation unit. Pediatr Emerg Care 2010;26(5):343–8.
39. Greenberg RA, Dudley NC, Rittichier KK. A reduction in hospitalization, length of stay, and hospital charges for croup with the institution of a pediatric observation unit. Am J Emerg Med 2006;24(7):818–21.
40. Calello DP, Alpern ER, McDaniel-Yakscoe M, et al. Observation unit experience for pediatric poison exposures. J Med Toxicol 2009;5(1):15–9.
41. Holsti M, Kadish HA, Sill BL, et al. Pediatric closed head injuries treated in an observation unit. Pediatr Emerg Care 2005;21(10):639–44.
42. Hostetler B, Leikin JB, Timmons JA, et al. Patterns of use of an emergency department-based observation unit. Am J Ther 2002;9(6):499–502.
43. Miescier MJ, Nelson DS, Firth SD, et al. Children with asthma admitted to a pediatric observation unit. Pediatr Emerg Care 2005;21(10):645–9.

44. Cator AD, Weber JS, Lozon MM, et al. Effect of using pediatric emergency department virtual observation on inpatient admissions and lengths of stay. Acad Pediatr 2014;14(5):510–6.
45. Mace SE. Observation medicine: key concepts - how to start and maintain an observation unit: what you need to know. Clinical Issues. In: Mace SE, editor. Observation medicine: principles and protocols. Cambridge (United Kingdom): Cambridge University Press;; 2017. p. 2–10.
46. Najaf Zadeh A, Hue V, Bonnel Mortuaire C, et al. Effectiveness of multifunction paediatric short-stay units: a French multicentre study. Acta Paediatr 2011;100(11): e227–33.
47. Browne GJ. A short stay or 23-hour ward in a general and academic children's hospital: Are they effective? Pediatr Emerg Care 2000;16(4):223.
48. Lamireau T, Llanas B, Fayon M. A short stay observation unit improves care in the paediatric emergency care setting. Arch Dis Child 2000;83(4):369.
49. Martineau O, Martinot A, Hue V, et al. Effectiveness of a short-stay observation unit in a pediatric emergency department. Arch Pediatr 2003;10(5):410–6 [in French].
50. Beattie TF, Ferguson J, Moir PA. Short-stay facilities in accident and emergency departments for children. Emerg Med J 1993;10(3):177–80.
51. Gouin S, Macarthur C, Parkin PC, et al. Effect of a pediatric observation unit on the rate of hospitalization for asthma. Ann Emerg Med 1997;29(2):218–22.
52. Rentz AC, Kadish HA, Nelson DS. Physician satisfaction with a pediatric observation unit administered by pediatric emergency medicine physicians. Pediatr Emerg Care 2004;20(7):430–2.
53. McConnochie KM, Russo MJ, McBride JT, et al. How commonly are children hospitalized for asthma eligible for care in alternative settings? Arch Pediatr Adolesc Med 1999;153(1):49–55.
54. McConnochie KM, Conners GP, Lu E, et al. How commonly are children hospitalized for dehydration eligible for care in alternative settings? Arch Pediatr Adolesc Med 1999;153(12):1233–41.
55. Macy ML, Stanley RM, Lozon MM, et al. Trends in high-turnover stays among children hospitalized in the United States, 1993-2003. Pediatrics 2009;123(3): 996–1002.
56. Conners GP, Melzer SM, Betts JM, et al. Pediatric observation units. Pediatrics 2012;130(1):172–9.
57. DeCoster C, Peterson S, Karian P. Manitoba Centre for Health Policy and Evaluation: report summary alternatives to acute care. Winnipeg (Manitoba): University of Manitoba-Manitoba Centre for Health Policy and Evaluation; 1996.

# Additional Conditions Amenable to Observation Care

Matthew A. Wheatley, MD

## KEYWORDS

- Abnormal uterine bleeding • Emergency department observation unit
- Allergic reaction • Alcohol intoxication • Acetaminophen overdose
- Sickle cell vaso-occlusive crisis

## KEY POINTS

- There are many conditions that can be cared for in the EDOU that don't fit into larger protocols.
- This list isn't meant to be exhaustive.
- Any condition that complies with the definition of medical observation where the patient is 70–80% likely to be discharged in 15–18 hours is appropriate.

---

**Case study**

Victoria Woods is a 32-year-old woman who presents with complaints of heavy vaginal bleeding for 3 days. She is using four to five pads per day and is passing clots. This has been happening every month during her menses and she will occasionally have bleeding between her menses. She also endorses dizziness with standing and increased fatigue doing her daily tasks. Her physical examination is remarkable only for conjunctival pallor. Pelvic examination reveals no cervical lesions and a small amount of blood from the cervical os. Her uterus is slightly enlarged but nontender. Her urine pregnancy test is negative and hemoglobin (Hgb) concentration is 5.5 g/dL. She is placed in the emergency department observation unit (EDOU) for blood transfusion. While in the observation unit, the patient undergoes a transvaginal ultrasound that is unremarkable. She receives two units of packed red blood cells (PRBC) and her repeat Hgb is 7.5 g/dL. On reassessment, she states she is feeling better. In discussion with the on-call gynecologist, the decision is made to start her on progesterone hormone therapy. The patient is discharged with a diagnosis of abnormal uterine bleeding. She is started on iron supplementation in addition to her hormone therapy and instructions to follow-up with a gynecologist for further management of her condition.

---

## ABNORMAL UTERINE BLEEDING

Abnormal uterine bleeding (AUB), formerly known as dysfunctional uterine bleeding, is a common reason for presentation to the emergency department (ED). It is estimated

---

Disclosure: None.
Department of Emergency Medicine, Emory University School of Medicine, 49 Jesse Hill Jr. Drive Southeast, Atlanta, GA 30303, USA
E-mail address: mwheatl@emory.edu

Emerg Med Clin N Am 35 (2017) 701–712
http://dx.doi.org/10.1016/j.emc.2017.03.012     emed.theclinics.com

to affect 53 per 1000 women in the United States.[1] AUB is defined as abnormal quantity, duration, or timing of menstrual bleeding in nonpregnant females. Patients can seek medical care for the bleeding itself or for sequelae of blood loss, such as anemia. Etiologies for AUB are beyond the scope of this article, but have been classified by the International Federation of Gynecology and Obstetrics (**Box 1**).[2]

### Emergency Department Evaluation

The primary priorities of ED evaluation should be to rule out pregnancy, confirm the source of bleeding, and resuscitate patients who are hemodynamically unstable. The history taken in the ED should attempt to quantify the bleeding (ie, number of pads/hour, presence of clots) and evidence of symptomatic anemia (ie, fatigue, dyspnea, or chest pain with exertion). In addition, there should be an attempt to screen for causes of the bleeding, such as a menstrual history (ie, age of menarche, usual frequency, and duration of menses), presence of bleeding/clotting disorders, and the use of any anticoagulant or antiplatelet medications.

The physical examination should be used to identify signs of anemia or hemorrhagic shock with special note taken of resting tachycardia or hypotension. The clinician can also assess for conjunctival pallor or the presence of a flow murmur. A pelvic examination should be performed in the ED to confirm the uterus as source of bleeding, and rule out vulvar/vaginal trauma or cervical lesions. This can be deferred if the patient is not currently bleeding and has a history of AUB with an established diagnosis.

Laboratory tests should include a pregnancy test, complete blood count (CBC) with differential. A coagulation profile can be considered in patients with new presentations of AUB to screen for bleeding disorders. A qualitative urine human chorionic gonadotropin test is sufficient for low to moderate suspicion of pregnancy, whereas a quantitative serum test should be sent in cases where pregnancy is highly suspected. The CBC should be examined for Hgb and hematocrit levels and to rule out thrombocytopenia as a cause for bleeding. A type and screen should be sent during the initial evaluation and if the level of anemia requires blood product administration a crossmatch should be ordered.

---

**Box 1**
**Palm-COEIN classification system for abnormal uterine bleeding in nongravid reproductive-age women**

Polyp

Adenomyosis

Leiomyoma

Malignancy and hyperplasia

Coagulopathy

Ovulatory dysfunction

Endometrial

Iatrogenic

Not yet classified

*Data from* Munro MG, Critchley HO, Broder MS, et al. FIGO classification system (PALM-COEIN) for causes of abnormal uterine bleeding in nongravid women of reproductive age. Int J Gynaecol Obstet 2011;113:3.

Imaging in the ED is left to the discretion of the provider. A pelvic ultrasound is helpful in establishing a diagnosis in patients with a new complaint of AUB but probably does not add much to the treatment of patients with established diagnosis and recurrent bleeding.

## Observation Unit Care

### Red cell transfusion

The inclusion and exclusions for EDOU placement are listed in **Box 2**. In general, patients who are hemodynamically unstable, coagulopathic, have bleeding caused by a malignancy, or have heavy active bleeding are better served on an inpatient service because of suspected duration and intensity of treatment. The focus should be transfusion of patients who are hemodynamically stable and not having brisk active bleeding.

The primary EDOU intervention is blood transfusion. Recommendations on transfusion thresholds vary among specialty societies. The decision to transfuse should be made using clinical judgment taking into account not only the absolute Hgb or

---

**Box 2**
**EDOU abnormal uterine bleeding protocol**

*Inclusion*

- CBC, type, and crossmatch sent
- Transfusion consent signed and in chart

*Exclusion*

- Pregnancy
- Malignancy found or suspected on pelvic examination or imaging
- Coagulopathy, including use of warfarin or direct oral anticoagulants
- Known presence of circulating antibodies making blood match difficult
- Contraindication or refusal of transfusion
- Anemia with symptoms or signs of cardiac ischemia
- Anticipated need for greater than two units PRBCs (Hgb <5 mg/dL)

*Potential interventions*

- Red cell transfusion
- Pain control
- Gynecology evaluation
- Initiation of hormone therapy
- Pelvic ultrasound/imaging to investigate cause of bleeding

*Disposition*

- Home
  - Stable vital signs
  - Posttransfusion Hgb in acceptable range (7–8 mg/dL)
  - No symptoms with exertion
- Hospital
  - Prolonged heavy bleeding
  - Unstable vital signs
  - Inpatient procedure required

hematocrit levels, but also the presence of active bleeding, symptomatic anemia, and patient wishes. The American Association of Blood Banks recommends that transfusion is rarely indicated for Hgb greater than 10 g/dL.[3] Transfusion should be considered for patients with Hgb less than 10 g/dL if they have symptomatic anemia, ongoing bleeding, or evidence of myocardial ischemia. Transfusion is generally indicated with an Hgb of less than 7 g/dL in all populations. Hemodynamically stable patients should only be transfused to an Hgb of 7 to 8 g/dL, although symptomatic patients may require transfusion to a higher level.[3]

Each unit of PRBCs is expected to take 4 hours to complete and raises the Hgb approximately 1 mg/dL. Therefore, patients who might require more than three or four units of PRBCs should be considered for admission. Repeat Hgb can be sent 15 minutes after completion of the transfusion.[4]

### Other treatments

Some patients may be candidates to start medical hormone therapy to decrease the frequency and severity of bleeding. This should be discussed with the gynecology consultants. Nonsteroidal anti-inflammatory medications are the first line of therapy for pain control in patients with pain related to menstrual cramping. Nonsteroidal anti-inflammatory medications have the additional benefit of reducing the amount of menstrual blood loss by up to 50% through alterations in the cyclooxygenase pathway.[5] Low-dose opioids are used as needed for breakthrough pain.

### Disposition

The indications for hospital admission or discharge are summarized in **Box 2**. If a patient's Hgb responds to transfusion and they are no longer symptomatic with walking or performing normal activities, they may be discharged home with gynecology follow-up. Patients with continued heavy bleeding, who are symptomatic because of blood loss, or who continue to be orthostatic should be admitted.

## ALLERGIC REACTION

"Allergic reaction" is a general term for a type I (IgE-mediated histamine release) hypersensitivity reaction to various agents. Treatment algorithms in the ED and EDOU are the same for allergies and angioedema. The latter is histamine-mediated or bradykinin-mediated, as in hereditary angioedema and angiotensin converting enzyme inhibitor–induced angioedema. Patients may present to the ED with complaints ranging from hives or other rashes, difficulty breathing, tongue or throat swelling, gastrointestinal upset, to anaphylaxis involving respiratory distress and cardiovascular collapse. Offending agents are most commonly medications, insect exposure, or food, but may be unknown.

### Emergency Department Evaluation

Initial ED evaluation of patients with allergic symptoms involves rapid assessment for the presence of anaphylaxis. If anaphylaxis is present, the first-line treatment is with epinephrine. This may have been self-administered by the patient or paramedics before arrival. Patients may also receive treatment of symptoms, such as rash, wheezing, and lip and tongue swelling. These adjunctive medications, such as bronchodilators, antihistamines, and corticosteroids, are second line and should not delay or supplant the administration of epinephrine. Although these agents may help with symptoms of rash or itching, they have failed to show benefit in relieving airway obstruction or treating anaphylaxis.[6,7] Glucocorticoids, given to reduce the risk of biphasic reaction, take several hours to work and therefore are not effective for initial signs and symptoms of anaphylaxis.[8]

For patients with oral or laryngeal symptoms, emergent nasopharyngoscopy is indicated to assess airway involvement. This is performed by the emergency practitioner, or an otorhinolaryngologist or anesthesia consultant, depending on availability and provider comfort. Routine ordering of other imaging and laboratory studies do not generally change management.

Patients who did not require epinephrine and never had subjective or objective airway involvement can likely be discharged after ED treatment if their symptoms are resolving, or at least not progressing. Patients with rapidly progressing symptoms, worsening subjective or objective airway involvement, requiring multiple doses of epinephrine, or who have signs of cardiovascular collapse should be admitted to an inpatient service. Patients who received epinephrine either prehospital or in the ED and patients with severe symptoms should be watched carefully in the ED to make sure they do not develop airway or cardiovascular involvement. Although there is no consensus as to the optimal duration of observation in this patient population, an EDOU is an ideal disposition for these patients.

## Observation Unit Care

EDOU care for patients with allergic reaction is mainly supportive (**Box 3**). Intravenous (IV) fluids and repeated doses of antihistamines are given as needed. Patients need periodic reassessment for evolution of rash, involvement of airway, wheezing, or hemodynamic compromise. Patients whose symptoms improve or resolve can be

---

**Box 3**
**EDOU allergic reaction protocol**

*Inclusion Criteria*

- Response to therapy in the ED
- Erythroderma, urticaria, or angioedema not involving the airway
- Minimum 2 hours of stability or improvement in ED after treatment

*Exclusion Criteria*

- Hypotension (systolic blood pressure <100 mm Hg); tachycardia >110 bpm
- $SaO_2$ <94% on room air
- Suspicion of acute coronary syndrome
- Stridor, respiratory distress, hoarseness
- Intravenous vasopressors required

*Potential Interventions*

- Symptomatic management: antihistamines, corticosteroids

*Disposition*

- Home
  - Improvement or resolution of symptoms
  - Stable vital signs
- Hospital
  - Progression of symptoms
  - Involvement of airway or new hypotension
  - Need for epinephrine

discharged. Patients who received epinephrine prehospital or in the ED should be discharged with prescription for an epinephrine autoinjector. All patients should have followed up with an allergist. Patients with persistent, recurring, or evolving symptoms after 15 to 18 hours of observation should be admitted to an inpatient service.

## ALCOHOL INTOXICATION

Alcohol intoxication is a common reason for presentation to the ED. Patients can present via law enforcement, emergency medical services, or with friends or family and present for a variety of reasons including intoxication, trauma, or undifferentiated altered mental status.

### Emergency Department Evaluation

The primary ED priority for patients with known or suspected alcohol intoxication is to assess for and treat threats to airway, breathing, and circulation. Following this, secondary priorities are to rule out concomitant medical or traumatic conditions, such as sepsis, head injury, or ingestion of other substances; keep the patient safe while they metabolize the alcohol; achieve sobriety; and to monitor for signs of withdrawal. ED work-up is based on the clinician's gestalt as to the pretest probability that other conditions exist. Chronic alcoholics who admit to drinking may not need any work-up, whereas a patient with head trauma or polysubstance use that arrives obtunded requires laboratory studies and imaging. There is debate as to the utility of serum ethanol measurements. It is definitely recommended for the patient with unspecified alterations in consciousness, or other situations where the diagnosis is in question. In cases where the patient admits to alcohol consumption and the remainder of the history and examination are suggestive of this, serum alcohol measurement is probably of limited utility.

### Observation Unit Care

Decisions to use the EDOU for intoxicated patients are complicated by duration and level of service. Patients who are expected to achieve sobriety within 8 hours may not meet billing criteria for observation care. This is hard to predict, but is one argument for getting a serum ethanol level at presentation. The rate of ethanol clearance varies among patients. The classic understanding was that chronic alcoholics clear ethanol at a rate of 25 to 35 mg/dL per hour, whereas novice drinkers metabolize at a rate of 15 to 20 mg/dL per hour.[9,10] A more recent study of ED patients found a mean clearance rate of 20.43 mg/dL per hour with a standard deviation of 6.86 mg/dL per hour.[11] Despite these estimates, each patient reaches clinical sobriety at different ethanol levels; however, a serum ethanol level allows for a rough estimate of when the patient should be sober enough for discharge. In addition, intoxicated patients require close monitoring to prevent falls and to look for signs of alcohol withdrawal. For this reason, some sites perform "observation in place," where there is an order for observation services, but the patient remains in the acute care area of the ED. EDOUs with adequate nursing staff (at least 1:5 nurse to patient ratio) or the ability to have a one-on-one sitter at the patient's bedside may elect to move the patient to the EDOU for the observation period.

One important EDOU intervention (**Box 4**) is alcohol/substance abuse counseling and community resources. Providers should get an understanding from the patient as to their substance use patterns and their readiness to decrease or cease usage. Patients exhibiting for alcohol/substance abuse behavior should be counseled to quit and referred to the appropriate community resources. For patients expressing a desire to quit alcohol, the provider can consider discharging them with a prescription for a

---

**Box 4**
**EDOU alcohol intoxication protocol**

*Inclusion*

- Alcohol intoxication believed to take 8 hours or greater to resolve
- Traumatic brain injury, metabolic derangements, polyingestion ruled out in the ED (history alone is sufficient)
- No history of alcohol withdrawal

*Exclusion*

- Signs/symptoms of alcohol withdrawal
- Combative/delirious patients
- Patients requiring chemical sedation/restraints
- Patients with traumatic brain injury or other injuries identified on examination or imaging
- Alcoholic ketoacidosis
- Active comorbid condition

*Potential Interventions*

- IV or oral hydration as needed
- Alcohol cessation education
- Monitor for signs and symptoms of withdrawal

*Disposition*

- Home
  ○ Clinically sober: alert and oriented, able to ambulate unassisted and without difficulty
  ○ Stable vital signs
- Hospital
  ○ Failure to achieve sobriety in 15 to 18 hours
  ○ Development of signs and symptoms of withdrawal

---

chlordiazepoxide taper and information on local resources for outpatient detoxification follow-up.

Other EDOU interventions are at the discretion of the treating provider. IV crystalloid is used to treat dehydration but has not been shown to affect blood ethanol clearance.[12,13] Furthermore, there is little utility for routine use of IV multivitamins, thiamine, or folate.[14]

**Disposition**

Patients may be discharged as soon as they reach clinical sobriety. This is the point where they are deemed safe enough to leave the hospital from the standpoint of a mental status or fall risk. Patients are discharged sooner if they are in the care of a responsible, nonintoxicated adult. There is no need to follow serum alcohol levels or hold patients until they are below the legal limit of intoxication to operate a motor vehicle because some chronic alcoholics may exhibit withdrawal symptoms at lower serum ethanol levels.

## ACETAMINOPHEN OVERDOSE

Acetaminophen (APAP) is one of the most commonly used analgesics in the United States. It has also become the most common cause of overdose-related liver failure in the United States and other countries.[15,16] APAP overdose can be acute, in which the patient takes a single large supratherapeutic dose, or chronic, where the patient takes multiple smaller supratherapeutic doses at regular intervals. Toxicity is likely to occur with single ingestions greater than 250 mg/kg or greater than 12 g over a 24-hour period.[17,18]

### Emergency Department Evaluation

Patients with APAP poisoning may present to the ED as a suicidal patient who took an overdose or a patient may present with a painful condition and later be found to have taken multiple large doses. The emergency provider should have APAP toxicity in their differential for patients presenting with known or suspected overdose, altered mental status, jaundice, or with signs and symptoms of hepatitis or liver failure. An attempt should be made to quantify the amount and time the APAP was consumed and if it was an immediate or sustained-release preparation. Be sure to screen for all APAP-containing compounds, including over-the-counter cold and flu medications and prescription opioids.

ED management is similar as for all overdose patients. Priority should be to support the airway, breathing, and circulation issues. Gastrointestinal decontaminating agents, such as activated charcoal, are used based on the time of ingestion, cooperativity of the patient, and risk of aspiration. Laboratory studies should be sent including CBC, and comprehensive metabolic panel that includes a liver panel, coagulation profile, specifically prothrombin time, and international normalized ratio (INR). In addition a serum APAP level should be sent. For acute ingestions, this should be sent at 4 hours postingestion. For chronic ingestions or acute ingestions of unknown time, the level is sent at the time of presentation. Patients expressing suicidal ideation or who took the overdose intentionally should be placed on involuntary psychiatric hold and have a one-on-one sitter at their bedside to watch for attempts at self-harm or elopement. Psychiatry should be consulted for these patients. The local poison control center should be alerted regarding these patients and toxicology consulted for any overdose in the toxic range or evidence of hepatotoxicity on laboratory studies.

N-Acetylcysteine (NAC) is the treatment of APAP-induced liver toxicity and is most effective when started within 8 hours of acute ingestion. NAC is indicated in patients with a known ingestion time whose serum APAP concentration drawn 4 to 24 hours after ingestion is above the study line on the Rumack-Matthew nomogram (**Box 5**). Patients with an unknown ingestion time or chronic ingestions cannot be risk stratified using the nomogram. As a result of this, recommendations to start NAC may vary among poison centers. Most recommend NAC in an acute overdose of unknown time where there is a measurable serum APAP concentration, even in the absence of hepatic toxicity.[19] For chronic ingestions, there are recommendations to begin NAC if there is a supratherapeutic serum APAP concentration (>20 g/mL) or if there is any elevation in serum transaminases in the setting of ingestion of greater than 4 g per day.[19]

### Observation Unit Care

Patients must be carefully chosen for this protocol because there are numerous pitfalls and potential for critically ill patients to end up in the EDOU. As with intoxicated

---

**Box 5**
**Indications for N-acetylcysteine**

- Serum APAP concentration drawn between 4 and 24 hours following acute ingestion of immediate-release preparation above the study line on Rumack-Matthew normogram
- Unknown time of ingestion and measurable serum APAP concentration
- Chronic supratherapeutic ingestion with evidence of liver toxicity or serum APAP level >20 g/mL
- Recommendation from Poison Control Center or toxicology consultant

patients, the decision to take suicidal patients is EDOU specific. Necessary resources include a favorable nurse to patient ratio (1:4 or 1:5) and the ability to provide a one-on-one patient sitter. There also needs to be the ability to provide psychiatric consultation and disposition for patients once they are cleared from a medical standpoint. Patients sent to the EDOU must be started on NAC within 8 hours of ingestion and before elevation of transaminases or prolongation of INR.

The primary treatment modality in the EDOU is continuation of NAC protocol (**Box 6**). IV protocol is preferred for the EDOU because it is complete in 20 hours. The complete PO protocol lasts 72 hours. If the IV preparation is unavailable, or otherwise contraindicated, patients thought to require the entire protocol should be admitted. Patients require serial liver function tests, serum APAP levels, and INR monitored routinely while on the protocol. The treatment is discontinued when the serum APAP is undetectable, serum transaminases are decreasing or in normal range, and INR is less than two. These patients are suitable for discharge if otherwise stable. Patients with detectable APAP levels or persistently elevated transaminase levels at 15 to 18 hours require admission for continuation of their NAC protocol.

## SICKLE CELL VASO-OCCLUSIVE CRISIS

Acute painful episodes are the most common cause for individuals with sickle cell disease (SCD) to seek medical care. Nationally, vaso-occlusive crises accounts for more

---

**Box 6**
**EDOU acetaminophen overdose protocol**

*Inclusion*

- Known or suspected acute or chronic acetaminophen toxicity
- IV NAC started in ED within 8 hours of acute ingestion with no evidence of hypersensitivity
- Normal liver function tests and INR
- Hemodynamically stable

*Exclusion*

- Toxic ingestions in which NAC started after 8 hours from time of ingestion
- Patient is actively suicidal, at risk of further self-harm or elopement
- Signs/symptoms of acute liver injury (elevated transaminases, prolonged INR)
- Patient is obtunded or unable to comply with treatment

*Potential Interventions*

- IV or oral NAC treatment
- Routine liver function tests, INR, acetaminophen levels

*Disposition*

- Home
  - Acetaminophen level undetectable
  - No evidence of hepatic dysfunction
- Hospital
  - Acetaminophen level still detectable after 20-hours IV NAC protocol or 15 to 18 hours of oral NAC protocol
  - Elevation of alanine aminotransferase/prolongation of INR

than 230,000 ED visits every year and approximately $1.5 billion in annual health care expenditures.

### Emergency Department Evaluation

The goals of ED care of patients with SCD who present with acute painful episodes are to aggressively treat the pain and rule out other sickle cell crises, such as acute chest syndrome or infection. A careful history should be taken as to the location, duration, and severity of the pain in the current episode and how it compares with previous episodes. It is also helpful to assess for potential triggers to the episode, such as changes in medications, dehydration, overexertion, cold temperature, and hormonal changes. Patients presenting with pain outside their usual pattern should be carefully evaluated for an underlying condition.

Laboratory studies, such as a CBC, reticulocyte count, and comprehensive chemistry panel, should be sent to rule out infection and assess levels of anemia, but are not helpful in ruling out vaso-occlusive crises. Patients with chest pain, fever, shortness of breath, or cough should get a chest radiograph to assess for pneumonia or pulmonary infarct.

Aggressive treatment of acute painful episodes, similar to cancer pain, has been shown to decrease ED visits and hospital admissions.[20] IV opioids are the preferred treatment. If the previous opioid dose is unknown, morphine, 0.1 to 0.15 mg/kg, or hydromorphone, 0.02 to 0.05 mg/kg, is given initially with reassessment 15 to 30 minutes after the initial dose.[21] Fentanyl is recommended in cases of renal or hepatic dysfunction. Repeated dosing is often required.[22] This is given as intermittent doses of 0.02 to 0.05 mg/kg morphine every 20 to 30 minutes or via patient-controlled analgesia device. Use of patient-controlled analgesia has been shown to reduce hospital length of stay and improve patient satisfaction.[23,24]

### Observation Unit Care

Use of the EDOU for patients presenting with acute painful episodes caused by SCD is controversial. To date, there are no studies demonstrating this is an effective strategy. Specialty SCD clinics, however, have been shown to reduce length of stay, lower admission rate, and increased patient satisfaction when compared with ED care.[25–27] This is likely caused by the use of providers who are familiar with SCD care. Vaso-occlusive crises requiring care beyond the initial ED visit are likely to require greater than 15 to 18 hours recommended for EDOU cases. In addition, painful conditions most frequently require hospital admission from the EDOU or lead to ED recidivism.[28]

Meeting with stakeholders from internal medicine and hematology is essential before undertaking an EDOU protocol. This allows for agreement on patient selection and admission for those that require treatment past the EDOU period.

The goals of EDOU care are to continue the care established in the ED (**Box 7**). Patients should continue to receive IV fluids and IV opioids with frequent reassessment of the patient's pain level. Patients that are euvolemic are recommended to receive IV hydration with a hypotonic solution. Bolus dosing of IV fluids may increase the risk of developing acute chest syndrome. The use of incentive spirometers has been shown to decrease this risk. The routine use of oxygen in all patients with SCD is without evidence and there is a theoretic potential for harm with oxygen-induced vasoconstriction and formation of free radicals. Patients may be discharged home when they reach their goal pain level, provided their vital signs are stable and there are no comorbid conditions. Patients who are not at goal pain level at 15 to 18 hours should be admitted for continuation of therapy.

---

**Box 7**
**EDOU protocol for sickle cell disease vaso-occlusive crisis**

*Inclusion*

- Known sickle cell disease (HbSS, SC, or S/beta thalassemia)
- Not at pain goal after adequate dose of IV morphine or hydromorphone in ED

*Exclusion*

- Fever, hypotension
- Concern for acute chest syndrome, splenic sequestration
- History of prolonged hospitalizations for similar crises
- Active comorbid condition

*Potential Interventions*

- IV fluids
- IV opioids via intermittent dosing or patient-controlled analgesia

*Disposition*

- Home
  - Patient reaches goal pain level
  - Stable vital signs
- Hospital
  - Failure to reach goal pain level by 15 to 18 hours
  - Development of fever or other comorbid condition

---

## REFERENCES

1. Kjerulff KH, Erickson BA, Langenberg PW. Chronic gynecological conditions reported by US women: findings from the National Health Interview Survey, 1984 to 1992. Am J Public Health 1996;86(2):195–9.

2. Munro MG, Critchley HO, Broder MS, et al. FIGO classification system (PALM-COEIN) for causes of abnormal uterine bleeding in nongravid women of reproductive age. Int J Gynaecol Obstet 2011;113:3.

3. Carson JL, Grossman BJ, Kleinman S, et al. Red blood cell transfusion: a clinical practice guideline from the AABB. Ann Intern Med 2012;157(1):49.

4. Elizalde JI, Clemente J, Marin JL, et al. Early changes in hemoglobin and hematocrit levels after packed red cell transfusion in patients with acute anemia. Transfusion 1997;37(6):573–6.

5. Hartmann KE, Jerome RN, Lindegren ML, et al. Primary Care Management of Abnormal Uterine Bleeding. Comparative Effectiveness Review No. 96. (Prepared by the Vanderbilt Evidence-based Practice Center under Contract No. 290-2007-10065 I.) AHRQ Publication No. 13-EHC025-EF. Rockville (MD): Agency for Healthcare Research and Quality; 2013. Available at: www.effectivehealthcare. ahrq.gov/reports/final.cfm.

6. Sheikh A, Ten Broek V, Brown SG, et al. H1-antihistamines for the treatment of anaphylaxis: Cochrane systematic review. Allergy 2007;62(8):830.

7. Nurmatov UB, Rhatigan E, Simons FE, et al. H2-antihistamines for the treatment of anaphylaxis with and without shock: a systematic review. Ann Allergy Asthma Immunol 2014;112(2):126–31.

8. Choo KJ, Simons FE, Sheikh A. Glucocorticoids for the treatment of anaphylaxis. Cochrane Database Syst Rev 2012;(4):CD007596.
9. Bogusz M, Pach J, Stasko W. Comparative studies on the rate of ethanol elimination in acute poisoning and in controlled conditions. J Forensic Sci 1977;22:446.
10. Jones AW. Disappearance rate of ethanol from the blood of human subjects: implications in forensic toxicology. J Forensic Sci 1993;38:104.
11. Gershman H, Steeper J. Rate of Clearance of ethanol from the blood of intoxicated patients in the emergency department. J Emerg Med 1991;9(5):307–11.
12. Li J, Mills T, Erato R. Intravenous saline has no effect on blood ethanol clearance. J Emerg Med 1999;17(1):1–5.
13. Perez RS, Keijzers G, Steele M, et al. Intravenous 0.9% sodium chloride therapy does not reduce length of stay of alcohol-intoxicated patients in the emergency department: a randomised controlled trial. Emerg Med Australas 2013;25(6):527–34.
14. Li SF, Jacob J, Feng J, et al. Vitamin deficiencies in acutely intoxicated patients in the ED. Am J Emerg Med 2008;26(7):792–5.
15. Watson WA, Litovitz TL, Klein-Schwartz W, et al. 2003 annual report of the American Association of Poison Control Centers Toxic Exposure Surveillance System. Am J Emerg Med 2004;22(5):335.
16. Chun LJ, Tong MJ, Busuttil RW, et al. Acetaminophen hepatotoxicity and acute liver failure. J Clin Gastroenterol 2009;43(4):342–9.
17. Prescott LF. Paracetamol overdosage: pharmacological considerations and clinical management. Drugs 1983;25(3):290.
18. Makin AJ, Wendon J, Williams R. A 7-year experience of severe acetaminophen-induced hepatotoxicity (1987-1993). Gastroenterology 1995;109(6):1907.
19. Heard KJ. Acetylcysteine for acetaminophen poisoning. N Engl J Med 2008;359(3):285–92.
20. Brookoff D, Polomano R. Treating sickle cell pain like cancer pain. Ann Intern Med 1992;116(5):364.
21. Benjamin LJ, Dampier CD, Jacox AK, et al. Guideline for the management of acute and chronic Pain in sickle cell disease. Glenview (IL): APS Clinical Practice Guidelines Series No 1; 1999.
22. Bijur PE, Kenny MK, Gallagher EJ. Intravenous morphine at 0.1 mg/kg is not effective for controlling severe acute pain in the majority of patients. Ann Emerg Med 2005;46(4):362.
23. Gonzalez ER, Bahal N, Hansen LA, et al. Intermittent injection vs patient-controlled analgesia for sickle cell crisis pain. Comparison in patients in the emergency department. Arch Intern Med 1991;151(7):1372.
24. Melzer-Lange MD, Walsh-Kelly CM, Lea G, et al. Patient-controlled analgesia for sickle cell pain crisis in a pediatric emergency department. Pediatr Emerg Care 2004;20(1):2.
25. Benjamin LJ, Swinson GI, Nagel RL. Sickle cell anemia day hospital: an approach for the management of uncomplicated painful crises. Blood 2000;95(4):1130.
26. Wright J, Bareford D, Wright C, et al. Day case management of sickle cell pain: 3 years experience in a UK sickle cell unit. Br J Haematol 2004;126(6):878.
27. Aisiku IP, Penberthy LT, Smith WR, et al. Patient satisfaction in specialized versus nonspecialized adult sickle cell care centers: the PiSCES study. J Natl Med Assoc 2007;99(8):886–90.
28. Ross MA, Hemphill RR, Abramson J, et al. The recidivism characteristics of an emergency department observation unit. Ann Emerg Med 2010;56(1):34–41.

# Moving?

## Make sure your subscription moves with you!

To notify us of your new address, find your **Clinics Account Number** (located on your mailing label above your name), and contact customer service at:

**Email: journalscustomerservice-usa@elsevier.com**

**800-654-2452** (subscribers in the U.S. & Canada)
**314-447-8871** (subscribers outside of the U.S. & Canada)

**Fax number: 314-447-8029**

**Elsevier Health Sciences Division**
**Subscription Customer Service**
**3251 Riverport Lane**
**Maryland Heights, MO 63043**

*To ensure uninterrupted delivery of your subscription, please notify us at least 4 weeks in advance of move.

Printed and bound by CPI Group (UK) Ltd, Croydon, CR0 4YY

08/05/2025

01864701-0001